HEALTH INSURANCE *and* MANAGED CARE

What They Are and How They Work

FOURTH EDITION

PETER R. KONGSTVEDT, MD, FACP

Senior Health Policy Faculty

Department of Health Administration and Policy
George Mason University
Fairfax, VA

Principal, P. R. Kongstvedt Company, LLC
McLean, VA

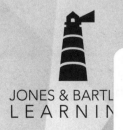

JONES & BARTL
LEARNIN

D0202269

World Headquarters
Jones & Bartlett Learning
5 Wall Street
Burlington, MA 01803
978-443-5000
info@jblearning.com
www.jblearning.com

Jones & Bartlett Learning books and products are available through most bookstores and online booksellers. To contact Jones & Bartlett Learning directly, call 800-832-0034, fax 978-443-8000, or visit our website, www.jblearning.com.

Substantial discounts on bulk quantities of Jones & Bartlett Learning publications are available to corporations, professional associations, and other qualified organizations. For details and specific discount information, contact the special sales department at Jones & Bartlett Learning via the above contact information or send an email to specialsales@jblearning.com.

Copyright © 2016 by Jones & Bartlett Learning, LLC, an Ascend Learning Company

All rights reserved. No part of the material protected by this copyright may be reproduced or utilized in any form, electronic or mechanical, including photocopying, recording, or by any information storage and retrieval system, without written permission from the copyright owner.

The content, statements, views, and opinions herein are the sole expression of the respective authors and not that of Jones & Bartlett Learning, LLC. Reference herein to any specific commercial product, process, or service by trade name, trademark, manufacturer, or otherwise does not constitute or imply its endorsement or recommendation by Jones & Bartlett Learning, LLC, and such reference shall not be used for advertising or product endorsement purposes. All trademarks displayed are the trademarks of the parties noted herein. *Health Insurance and Managed Care: What They Are and How They Work, Fourth Edition*, is an independent publication and has not been authorized, sponsored, or otherwise approved by the owners of the trademarks or service marks referenced in this product.

There may be images in this book that feature models; these models do not necessarily endorse, represent, or participate in the activities represented in the images. Any screenshots in this product are for educational and instructive purposes only. Any individuals and scenarios featured in the case studies throughout this product may be real or fictitious, but are used for instructional purposes only.

This publication is designed to provide accurate and authoritative information in regard to the subject matter covered. It is sold with the understanding that the publisher is not engaged in rendering legal, accounting, or other professional service. If legal advice or other expert assistance is required, the service of a competent professional person should be sought.

Production Credits

VP, Executive Publisher: David D. Cella
Publisher: Michael Brown
Associate Editor: Nicholas Alakel
Associate Production Editor: Rebekah Linga
Senior Marketing Manager: Sophie Fleck Teague
Manufacturing and Inventory Control Supervisor: Amy Bacus
Composition: Cenveo Publisher Services

Cover Design: Scott Moden
Rights and Media Manager: Joanna Lundeen
Rights and Media Research Coordinator: Mary Flatley
Media Development Assistant: Shannon Sheehan
Cover Image: © Unscrew/ShutterStock, Inc.
Printing and Binding: Edwards Brothers Malloy
Cover Printing: Edwards Brothers Malloy

To order this product, use ISBN: 978-1-284-04325-9

Library of Congress Cataloging-in-Publication Data
Kongstvedt, Peter R. (Peter Reid), author, editor.
  [Managed care]
  Health insurance and managed care : what they are and how they work / Peter R. Kongstvedt. -- Fourth edition.
      p. ; cm.
  Preceded by Managed care : what it is and how it works / Peter R. Kongstvedt. 2009.
  Some of the chapters are adapted from previously published works by the same author.
  Includes bibliographical references and index.
  ISBN 978-1-284-08711-6 (paper)
  I. Title.
  [DNLM: 1. Managed Care Programs—organization & administration—United States. 2. W 130 AA1]
  RA413.5.U5
  362.1'0425—dc23
                                                        2014047770

6048
Printed in the United States of America
19 18 17 16 15   10 9 8 7 6 5 4 3 2 1

Contents

Preface

This fourth edition of *Health Insurance and Managed Care: What They Are and How They Work* is significantly changed and updated from the third edition, beginning with the title.* The reason for the changed title is not because health insurance was not addressed in prior editions—it always has been part of the text's content—but rather because the terms "health insurance" and "managed care" are now commonly used to refer to the same thing, to the point that many people simply call any type of health benefits plan "health insurance."

High-level descriptions of what is new in this edition and what has changed are found in the New to This Edition section that follows this Preface. First, however, it is necessary to point out the biggest change affecting every single chapter: the Patient Protection and Affordable Care Act (ACA), which was passed by the U.S. Congress and signed into law by President Barack Obama on March 23, 2010. The ACA is addressed specifically in the *Laws and Regulations in Managed Care* chapter, but it is also covered throughout the entire text wherever it applies, which is pretty much everywhere.

Like this industry overall, the history of the ACA, including its current state, has been subject to many political forces and regulatory changes, meaning certain elements of the ACA described in this text may, in fact, change or no longer apply after the text's publication. Changes continue to take place outside the ACA as well, which is why I have provided some sources from which to obtain updated information (see the Keeping Current section that follows).

As we continue to add new laws, new regulations, new plan designs, new payment methodologies, and new means of managing utilization and quality, it becomes increasingly challenging to keep the overall size of this text down. The

---

* All of the prior editions were titled *Managed Care: What It Is and How It Works.*

only way I have found to address this issue is to focus only on the most important aspects, and to keep most descriptions at about the same level. As a result, readers who have no knowledge of how health insurance and managed care actually work will at times feel overwhelmed with detail. In some cases it may make sense to complete a chapter and then go back and reread any confusing sections, which will have become more understandable in the context of the rest of the material. In contrast, readers who are veterans of the industry will be struck by how much has been left out. If that second group of readers wants more detail, they can find it in this text's big sister, *The Essentials of Managed Health Care, Sixth Edition*, also published by Jones & Bartlett Learning.

Change is a constant, and whenever you hear someone complain about how the healthcare system in the United States is undergoing turbulent times, you should recognize that it has actually been in a state of flux for close to a century. As one acquaintance of mine remarked, "Health care is in permanent white water." Wishing we could return to the calm and placid times in the past is the same as wishing we could return to the world of *Leave It to Beaver*; both are fiction and never actually existed.*

The *causes* of this ongoing turbulence *also* continue to change, and not just as the result of new laws and regulations. Health costs keep rising, but where once that trend was due primarily to overutilization, it now reflects a great many factors, including pricing, advances in technology, and changing demographics and consumer demands. The industry's dynamic nature is the reason that health insurance and managed care are now so difficult to distinguish from each other. It is also the reason for this text, and the reason you are reading it.

While health insurance and managed care might change, the main goal of this text has not. Its purpose is very simple—to provide its readers with a broad understanding of how health insurance and managed care actually work. If it succeeds in doing that, then some who are reading these words right now will be in a position to better contribute to the future evolution of this dynamic industry, thereby benefiting us all.

Peter Reid Kongstvedt
McLean, VA

---

* The second fantasy—that of living in the world of a 1950s sitcom—does, however, make for a wonderful movie titled *Pleasantville* (1998, New Line Cinema), starring Tobey McGuire, Reese Witherspoon, William H. Macy, Jeff Daniels, Joan Allen, and among many others, the terrific Don Knotts.

New to This Edition

So what new information makes this edition different from previous editions? Too much to describe fully here. To do so would essentially rewrite the book, so what follows is a very high-level description of some of the more important changes.

CHAPTER 1: A HISTORY OF MANAGED HEALTH CARE AND HEALTH INSURANCE IN THE UNITED STATES

This chapter, cowritten with another author, is probably the least changed chapter in the book. Obviously, events that occurred after the prior edition was published are included, but some other historical events have been added and/or clarified. For example, a rather important new law affecting health insurance and managed health care—the Patient Protection and Affordable Care Act (ACA)—was passed in 2010.

CHAPTER 2: HEALTH BENEFITS COVERAGE AND TYPES OF HEALTH PLANS

Much of this chapter is entirely new. Previously, the focus was on the different types of insurers and managed care organizations, as well as integrated delivery systems (IDSs). IDSs have been relocated to the chapter on the provider network, and updated descriptions of plan types remain in this chapter.

Before getting to those descriptions, however, the chapter now includes entirely new descriptions and discussions of the following topics:

- Health benefits plans, and defined benefits plans in particular, and the elements that apply to all of them

- Essential health benefits under the ACA
- Cost-sharing in general, and the related topic of the "metallic level" benefits tiers under the ACA
- Coverage requirements in the individual market, the small group market, large groups, and "grandfathered" health benefits plans
- Coverage mandates for individuals and employers
- Guaranteed issue requirements for insurers
- Sources of coverage and ways that coverage is obtained
- Who bears the risk for coverage costs and how it is paid for
- Reinsurance and how it differs from health insurance

This new material provides an added foundation for understanding how and why the rest of the hugely complex system works.

CHAPTER 3: THE PROVIDER NETWORK

In prior editions, all of the material in Chapters 3 and 4 in this book were addressed in a single chapter. In this edition, an updated discussion of what a network is and how it is managed is now separated from the discussion of how providers are paid. This reflects better how the world actually works, and it keeps the issue of money where it belongs—as a distinct issue requiring the focused descriptions and discussion it deserves.

The concepts of service areas and access standards have been clarified and updated, as has the discussion on credentialing. The description of IDSs is both updated and compressed. New types of provider organizations and relationships have also emerged in the last five years, though one has mercifully disappeared—the provider-sponsored organization, though even that structure is making a type of comeback under different labels. We have also seen new types of provider organizations come into being, such as the accountable care organizations (ACOs) that are part of the ACA, and some new dynamics develop around some older approaches such as hospital employment of physicians. All of these changes affect the larger U.S. healthcare system.

The content of this chapter also provides more detail than is found in other chapters because this content is so critical to (here it comes again) understanding the how and why of the hugely complex system's workings.

CHAPTER 4: PROVIDER PAYMENT

The chapter on provider payment is the expanded and updated other half of what was formerly in a single chapter. Like Chapter 3, it contains more detail than what is found in other chapters. Unlike all other nations on earth, the U.S. healthcare system uses about eleventy-eight zillion different payment strategies and methodologies, and an equal number of variations of each. We have even created more new approaches by law such as the shared savings program in Medicare, a new value-based purchasing mechanism, and other new approaches to payment that were spawned by the ACA.

In the case of payment (and as discussed in this text, the proper term is "payment," not "reimbursement"), there is one more reason to describe at least some of the ways we pay for health care, which is summed up by the singer/songwriter Randy Newman: "It's money that matters, in the USA."*

CHAPTER 5: UTILIZATION MANAGEMENT, QUALITY MANAGEMENT, AND ACCREDITATION

Besides moving and updating the section on accreditation from a different chapter, the most significant updates to this chapter deal with the approaches to managing utilization in special populations, such as people with multiple chronic conditions. The discussion about medical necessity and its impact on benefits coverage has been expanded, as has the description of the use of evidence-based clinical guidelines for coverage determinations. Management of the prescription drug benefit is also evolving as specialty pharmaceuticals grow in importance and cost.

CHAPTER 6: SALES, GOVERNANCE, AND ADMINISTRATION

As with the other chapters, this chapter is affected by the ACA. In particular, the means by which health plans underwrite, create and manage premium rates and rebates, and access the market through sales and distribution channels; the appearance of new health insurance exchanges for individuals and small groups; and management of appeals of coverage denials warrant new and updated descriptions due to the ACA. The discussion of enrollment and billing has also been expanded, and aspects of financial management have been clarified. The now-standardized eligibility, special eligibility based on life events, and coverage extensions are addressed here as well.

CHAPTER 7: MEDICARE AND MEDICAID

Implementation of the ACA has required major updates to this chapter as well, and the chapter has been essentially rewritten. For example, the ACA changed

---

* Randy Newman, "It's Money That Matters" from *Land of Dreams*, Reprise/Warner Bros. 1988.

how the Part D drug benefit is constructed and managed, and it changed (or modified) how Medicare Advantage plans are paid, including the Quality Bonus Program. A section on eligibility and enrollment has been added. Marketing and sales in these markets are also fundamentally different than the corresponding functions found in the commercial market, so the chapter now includes a discussion of what is allowed and what is prohibited. Finally, Medicaid expansion under the ACA—something that not all states have undertaken—is addressed, as is the increasing reliance of states on managed Medicaid plans.

CHAPTER 8: LAWS AND REGULATIONS IN MANAGED CARE

Chapter 8 is the only chapter that I did not write or coauthor. It was entirely rewritten by contributor Tom Wilder and provides descriptions of the major state and federal laws and regulations affecting health plans. It also provides an excellent summary of the key elements of the ACA that have an impact on health benefits plans.

GLOSSARY

The Glossary has nearly doubled in size in terms of pages, and more than doubled in the number of entries compared to the previous edition's glossary. Along with adding new terms (and even removing a few), changes include updates and clarifications of some of the definitions, spelling out many of the acronyms that prior versions included only through their initials, expansion of some definitions to include new meanings or uses of terms, and modification of terms due to their redefinitions under the ACA.

IS THAT ALL?

Of course not. This breakdown provides only a glimpse of the overall revisions, updates, and new material in this edition. The health insurance and managed care industry is always undergoing change, but the combination of the ACA and the political, social, and economic forces have yet again accelerated the pace of change since the previous edition's publication. Said another way, changes and updates to this text are equal to the changes in the industry, which have been massive. But if I have done my job right, the new content should all fit together once again. At least until the next edition comes out.

Acknowledgments

Although I cannot name them all, because to do so would double the size of this text, I thank the many colleagues, clients, and friends in the health insurance, managed care, and consulting industries with whom I have had the pleasure to work beside over the years. Likewise, I thank my students and acknowledge their contributions to keeping me on my game. I also want to give sincere thanks to the many readers of previous editions of this text for their support, kind words, observations, and suggestions that have contributed to improvements over the years. Acknowledging the contributions of others does not, however, mean that any of them contributed to any errors or misstatements; those are solely mine.

About the Author

Dr. Peter Kongstvedt is a highly regarded national authority on the healthcare industry with particular expertise in health insurance and managed health care. He is principal of the P. R. Kongstvedt Company, LLC, and advises healthcare executives on strategy, operations, and effective decision making. Dr. Kongstvedt is also a Senior Health Policy Faculty member in the Department of Health Administration and Policy at George Mason University. In March 2014, he was appointed by Virginia Governor Terry McAuliffe to serve on the board of Virginia's Board of Medical Assistance Services (Virginia Medicaid).

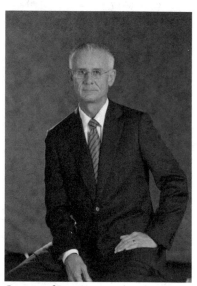

Courtesy of Peter Kongstvedt

Dr. Kongstvedt's unique business expertise comes from the varied roles he has performed over his long career. Prior to his most recent positions as partner and senior executive in global consulting firms, Dr. Kongstvedt held the most senior-level executive positions at a number of health plans and insurers. His roots as a practicing physician also give him firsthand understanding of the totality of the healthcare profession.

Renowned as the primary author and editor of "the bibles of managed care," Dr. Kongstvedt's books are used by more than 256 graduate and undergraduate health administration and policy programs. These books include *The Essen-*

tials of Managed Health Care, Sixth Edition (Jones & Bartlett Learning, 2013), and *Managed Care: What It Is and How It Works, Third Edition* (Jones and Bartlett Publishers, 2008), now updated as *Health Insurance and Managed Care: What They Are and How They Work, Fourth Edition* (Jones & Bartlett, Learning, 2015).

As a healthcare industry thought leader, Dr. Kongstvedt has been quoted in dozens of trade publications and presents frequently at industry conferences and corporate events. He has consulted to and made several appearances on *The CBS Evening News*, and has appeared on NBC's *Today Show*, CNN, and National Public Radio's *All Things Considered*. He has also been quoted in the *Wall Street Journal*, the *Washington Post*, and the *Los Angeles Times*, as well as in numerous trade publications.

A licensed physician, a board-certified internist, and a Fellow in the American College of Physicians, Dr. Kongstvedt received his BS and MD degrees at the University of Wisconsin, where he also completed his internal medicine training and residency. He resides in McLean, Virginia. Further information may be found on his website: www.kongstvedt.com.

Contributors

Peter D. Fox, PhD

Independent Consultant
Denver, Colorado

Tom Wilder, JD

Senior Counsel
America's Health Insurance Plans
Washington, DC

Keeping Current

Keeping current on trends and data presents a significant challenge, particularly in regard to trends and data presented in a book. Fortunately, there are several useful resources accessible via the web that periodically provide updated data and trend information, and discussion of important health policy issues relevant to health insurance and managed health care. Some examples of such sources are provided here; web addresses were current at the time of publication, but are always subject to change.

Examples of Federal Sources of Information	
HealthCare.gov, the federal exchange portal	https://www.healthcare.gov
Centers for Medicare & Medicaid Services (CMS)	http://www.cms.gov
CMS main page for Regulations and Guidance	http://www.cms.gov/home/regsguidance.asp
CMS's Center for Consumer Information and Insurance Oversight (CCIIO)	http://www.cms.gov/cciio/index.html
Department of Labor's (DOL) Employee Benefits Administration	http://www.dol.gov/ebsa
Agency for Healthcare Research and Quality (AHRQ)	http://www.ahrq.gov
Medicare Payment Advisory Commission (MedPAC)	http://www.medpac.gov
Medicaid and CHIP Payment and Access Commission (MACPAC)	http://www.macpac.gov

Policy and Research Organizations That Provide (Relatively) Unbiased Data and Information	
Henry J. Kaiser Family Foundation	http://www.kff.org
Commonwealth Fund	http://www.commonwealthfund.org
Robert Wood Johnson Foundation	http://www.rwjf.org

Publications (may require a subscription)	
Health Affairs	http://www.healthaffairs.org
American Journal of Managed Care and *American Journal of Accountable Care*	http://www.ajmc.com
Sanofi-Aventis's Yearly *Managed Care Digest* Series	http://www.managedcaredigest.com
Managed Care Online	http://www.mcol.com

These and many, many more useful links are also available through my website. Either navigate to http://www.kongstvedt.com and click on the "Useful Links" tab, or go directly to http://www.kongstvedt.com/useful_urls.html (also current at the time of publication but subject to change).

Attribution Note

Portions of the material in this text are adapted in part from their more detailed counterparts in *The Essentials of Managed Health Care, Sixth Edition* (Jones & Bartlett Learning, 2013). Interested readers wanting additional information about health insurance and managed care are advised to consult this reference. In addition, certain portions and exhibits were created and copyrighted by the P. R. Kongstvedt Company, LLC. All such material is used with permission, but not always identified or attributed any further.

CHAPTER 1

A History of Managed Health Care and Health Insurance in the United States*

Peter D. Fox, PhD and Peter R. Kongstvedt, MD, FACP

LEARNING OBJECTIVES

- Understand how health insurance and managed care came into being
- Understand the forces that have shaped health insurance and managed care in the past
- Understand the major obstacles to managed care historically
- Understand the major forces shaping health insurance and managed care today

---

* This chapter is adapted from Fox PD, Kongstvedt PR. A history of managed health care and health insurance in the United States. In: Fox PD, Kongstvedt PR, eds. *The Essentials of Managed Health Care*. 6th ed. Burlington, MA: Jones & Bartlett Learning; 2013.

INTRODUCTION

Health insurance and managed health care are inventions of the 20th century. For a long time, they were not considered to be "insurance" but rather "prepaid health care"—i.e., a way of accessing and paying for healthcare services rather than protecting against financial losses. From its inception, this set of arrangements has been in a never-ending state of change and turbulence. This chapter explores the historical roots and evolutionary forces that have resulted in today's system. The dates mentioned in this chapter are specific for such events as the passage of laws and the establishment of an organization but only approximate for trends.

1910 TO THE MID-1940s: THE EARLY YEARS

The years before World War II saw the development of two models of providing and paying for health care besides the patient simply paying for the service. The first were early forms of what is now called a health maintenance organization (HMO), though this term was not actually coined until the early 1970s. Such a model relied on an organization that was capitated (i.e., that charged a preset amount per member, or per enrollee, per month) and that provided services directly through its facilities and personnel, thereby combining the functions of financing and delivery. The second was the early Blue Cross and Blue Shield plans, which paid for services provided by contracted community doctors and hospitals, which also regularly served patients not covered by these plans.

Prepaid Medical Group Practices

The Western Clinic in Tacoma, Washington, is often cited as the first example of prepaid medical group practice. Started in 1910, the Western Clinic offered, exclusively through its own providers, a broad range of medical services in return for a premium (capitation) payment of $0.50 per member per month.[1] The program, which was offered to lumber mill owners and employees, served to assure the clinic a flow of patients and revenues.

1929 was a remarkable year in the history of health plans. In that year, Michael Shadid, MD, established a rural farmers' cooperative health plan in Elk City, Oklahoma, by forming a lay organization of leading farmers in the community. Participating farmers purchased shares for $50 each to raise capital for a new hospital in return for receiving medical care at a discount.[2] For his troubles,

Dr. Shadid lost his membership in the county medical society and was threatened with suspension of his license to practice. Some 20 years later, however, he was vindicated by a favorable out-of-court settlement resulting from an antitrust suit against the county and state medical societies.

Also in 1929, Doctors Donald Ross and H. Clifford Loos established a comprehensive prepaid medical plan for workers at the Los Angeles Department of Water and Power. It covered physician and hospital services. From the outset, it focused on prevention and health maintenance.[3] For that reason, some consider it to be the first real HMO. Doctors Ross and Loos were also expelled from their local medical society for their actions.

Despite opposition from the American Medical Association (AMA), prepaid group practice formation continued for many reasons, including employers' need to attract and retain employees, providers' efforts to secure steady incomes, consumers' quest for improved and affordable health care, and even efforts by the housing lending agency to reduce the number of foreclosures caused by health-related personal bankruptcies. Two prominent examples from this time period are the Kaiser Foundation Health Plan in California and the Group Health Association of Washington, D.C., which subsequently became part of the Kaiser system. They, too, were opposed by local medical societies.

The organization that evolved into the Kaiser Foundation Health Plan was started in 1937 by Dr. Sidney Garfield at the behest of the Kaiser Construction Company. It sought to finance medical care, initially for workers and families who were building an aqueduct in the southern California desert to transport water from the Colorado River to Los Angeles and, subsequently, for workers who were constructing the Grand Coulee Dam in Washington State. A similar program was established in 1942 at Kaiser ship-building plants in the San Francisco Bay area.

In 1937 the Group Health Association (GHA) was started in Washington, D.C., at the behest of the Home Owners' Loan Corporation to reduce the number of mortgage defaults that resulted from large medical expenses. It was created as a nonprofit consumer cooperative with a board that was elected by the enrollees.* The District of Columbia Medical Society vehemently opposed the formation of GHA. It sought to restrict hospital admitting privileges for GHA physicians and threatened expulsion from the medical society. A bitter antitrust battle ensued, culminating in the U.S. Supreme Court's ruling in favor of GHA.

---

* Its governance structure was quite similar to that required for the new consumer-owned and -operated plans (CO-OPs) enabled under the Patient Protection and Affordable Care Act (ACA) of 2010.

In 1994, faced with insolvency despite an enrollment of some 128,000, GHA was acquired by Humana Health Plans, a for-profit, publicly traded corporation. It was subsequently divested by Humana and incorporated into Kaiser Foundation Health Plan of the Mid-Atlantic.

The Blues

1929 also saw the origins of Blue Cross (BC), when Baylor Hospital in Texas agreed to provide some 1500 teachers with prepaid inpatient care at its hospital. The program was later expanded to include participation by other employers and hospitals. State hospital associations elsewhere created similar plans. Each was independent of the others, as they are today. In 1939 the American Hospital Association (AHA) adopted the Blue Cross emblem and created common standards. The symbol and was subsequently transferred to the Blue Cross Association (BCA) in the early 1960s, and the AHA ended its involvement with the BCA a decade after that.

The first type of organization that would become the basis for Blue Shield (BS) plans elsewhere, though it was not itself a BS plan, originated in the Pacific Northwest in 1939, when lumber and mining companies sought to provide medical care for their injured workers. Those companies entered into agreements with physicians, who were paid a monthly fee through a service bureau—a type of organization that would evolve into the service plans found at the core of most BC and BS plans today (see the *Health Benefits Coverage and Types of Health Plans* chapter).[4]

Beyond establishing the first appearance of the organizational type that would be adopted by BS plans, the appearance of the first *actual* BS plan is somewhat difficult to establish due to differences among sources. One source states that the BS logo first appeared in Buffalo, New York, as early as 1930.[5] Most sources state that the first official BS plan was the California Physicians' Service plan created by the California Medical Association in 1939.[6-8] In all events, other state medical societies soon emulated this model. Like the BC plans, the new BS plans were independent of both each other and the BC plans in their respective states, but were nevertheless associated with them.

The earliest BC and BS plans were also considered to offer prepayment for health care. However, unlike the prepaid group practices and cooperatives, BC and BS plans relied on providers in independent private practices rather than employing physicians or contracting with a dedicated medical group. To define the payment terms between a BC plan and a hospital, hospitals created cost-based charge lists, the forerunners of today's hospital chargemaster, and BS plans developed payment rates for defined procedures based on profiles (i.e., statistical distributions of what physicians charged).*

Initially, BC plans provided coverage only for hospital-associated care (including skilled nursing home care), while BS plans provided coverage for physician and related professional services (such as physical and speech therapy). Over time, many BC plans merged with their local BS counterparts to become joint BCBS plans, although some remain separate even now. Most of these BC and BS plans were statewide and did not compete with each other, albeit with some exceptions; for example, Pennsylvania and New York both have several BC and/or BS plans. From the beginning, the BC and BS plans, collectively referred to as the "Blues," operated independently from each other. In the past few decades, however, a significant number of BC and BS plans have merged.

Historically, in only a few cases did the Blues plans compete with each other; rather, they mostly respected each other's geographic boundaries and cooperated in selling to multistate accounts. More recently, they have begun to enter each other's territory and now do compete, although only one may use the BC and/or BS logo in a defined territory.

Hospitals and physicians retained control of the various Blues plans until the 1970s. In that decade, these plans changed to either a community governance model with a self-perpetuating nonprofit board not controlled by the providers or a structure under which the board was elected by the insureds (i.e., a mutual insurer). In recent decades, many Blues have converted to publicly owned for-profit corporations.

Importantly, the formation of the various BC and BS plans in the midst of the Great Depression, as well as the emergence of many prepaid group practices, was not driven by consumers' demands for coverage or entrepreneurs' seeking to establish a business but rather by providers' desire to protect their incomes.

THE MID-1940s TO MID-1960s: THE EXPANSION OF HEALTH BENEFITS

In the United States, World War II produced both inflation and a tight labor supply, leading to the 1942 Stabilization Act. That act imposed wage and price controls on businesses, including limiting their ability to pay higher wages to

---

* The chargemaster is the price list a hospital creates for all services for which it charges. The Current Procedural Terminology (CPT) charge codes, which define the procedures for which doctors and other providers bill, were created by the AMA in 1966; the AMA has maintained this list ever since. The chargemaster, CPT codes, and fee schedules are addressed in the *Provider Payment* chapter.

attract scarce workers. However, the act did allow workers to avoid taxation on employer contributions to certain employee benefits, including health benefits. Also, health benefits were not constrained by wage controls. The twin effects of favorable tax treatment and the exemption from wage controls fueled the growth of commercial health insurance as well as greater enrollment in the Blues. Before World War II, only 10% of employed individuals had health benefits from any source, but by 1955 nearly 70% did, although many of these plans covered only inpatient care.

HMO formation and enrollment growth also continued, albeit at a slower pace. Newly formed plans included (1) the Health Insurance Plan (HIP) of Greater New York, created in 1944 at the behest of New York City, which wanted coverage for its employees,* and (2) Group Health Cooperative of Puget Sound (GHC), organized by 400 Seattle families, each of whom contributed $100. GHC remains a consumer cooperative to this day.

The McCarran-Ferguson Act, passed in 1945, exempted insurance companies from federal regulation. As a result, regulation of health insurance devolved to the states. The McCarran-Ferguson Act also provided limited antitrust immunity for certain activities such as pooling of claims data for pricing purposes. In the absence of federal authority, the regulation of insurance companies and premium levels became the responsibility of the states, which varied widely in their level of oversight.

In the 1950s, as a competitive reaction to group practice–based HMOs, HMOs evolved that resemble today's independent practice association (IPA) model. In an IPA, an HMO contracts either directly with physicians in independent practice or indirectly with an organization that in turn contracts with these physicians. In contrast, early HMOs had their own dedicated medical staffs. The basic IPA structure was created in 1954 to compete with Kaiser when the San Joaquin County Medical Society in California formed the San Joaquin Medical Foundation. The Foundation paid physicians using a relative value fee schedule, which it established; heard consumer grievances against physicians; and monitored quality of care. This organization became licensed by the state to accept enrollee premiums and, like other HMOs, performed the insurance function, but under a different regulatory structure than standard insurance. In most states, HMOs—then and now—have faced different regulatory requirements than insurance companies.

---

* HIP subsequently merged with New York–based Group Health Incorporated (GHI) to form EmblemHealth.

THE MID-1960S TO MID-1970S: THE ONSET OF HEALTHCARE COST INFLATION

In the early 1960s, President John F. Kennedy proposed what eventually became Part A of Medicare. This program, which was financed through taxes on earned income (i.e., not investment income) similar to Social Security, was intended to cover mostly hospital services. The Republicans in Congress then proposed to cover physician and related professional services as well, in what became Part B of Medicare. This program was financed through a combination of general revenues and enrollee premiums. Following Kennedy's assassination, President Lyndon B. Johnson worked aggressively to achieve some of the late president's domestic goals, including covering persons age 65 and older. In 1965, Congress established two landmark entitlement programs: Medicare for the elderly (Title XVIII of the Social Security Act) and Medicaid (Title XIX of the Social Security Act) for selected low-income populations. In 1972, the Medicare Act was amended to cover selected disabled workers (but not their dependents), mostly those who had permanent disabilities starting 29 months after the onset of the disability. The benefits and provider payment structures of Medicare of the time were similar to those of BC and BS plans, with separate benefits for hospitalization paid through Medicare Part A and physician services paid through Medicare Part B. This system remains in place for traditional (i.e., for beneficiaries not enrolled in capitated health plans, as described below) Medicare today.

The combination of Medicare, Medicaid, private insurance, and medical care (other federal programs, for example) resulted in the majority of health care being paid for by third-party payers. The third-party payment system severs the financial link between the provider of the service and the patient—a disconnect that fostered increases in both the price of services and their utilization.

These developments marked the beginning of a long history of healthcare cost inflation, attributable to the combination of the third-party payment system, advances in medical science, and increased demand by consumers. To illustrate, in 1960, 55.9% of all healthcare costs nationally were paid by the patient, but that percentage has declined steadily, leveling out at 11–12% by 2012.[9] At the same time, national health expenditures as a percentage of the gross domestic product (GDP) rose from 5.2% in 1960 to 5.8% in 1965, the year before Medicare was implemented; it reached 7.4% in 1970 and 17.2% in 2012.[10]

Nevertheless, isolated examples of early attempts to control costs beyond seeking provider discounts can be cited:

- In 1959, Blue Cross of Western Pennsylvania, the Allegheny County Medical Society Foundation, and the Hospital Council of Western

Pennsylvania performed retrospective analyses of hospital claims to identify utilization that was significantly above average.[11]

- Around 1970, California's Medicaid program initiated hospital precertification and concurrent review in conjunction with medical care foundations in that state, typically county-based associations of physicians who volunteered to participate, starting with the Sacramento Foundation for Medical Care.*

- The 1972 Social Security Amendments authorized professional standards review organizations (PSROs) to review the appropriateness of care provided to Medicare and Medicaid beneficiaries. In time, PSROs became known as peer review organizations (PROs), and then as quality review organizations (QIOs). QIOs continue to oversee clinical services on behalf of the federal and many state Medicaid agencies today.

- In the 1970s, a handful of large corporations initiated precertification and concurrent review for inpatient care, to the dismay of the provider community. Some companies took other measures such as promoting employee wellness, sitting on hospital boards with the intent of constraining their costs, and negotiating payment levels directly with providers.[12]

Although unrelated to costs, and initially only peripherally related to health benefits plans or health insurance, another significant event occurred at the end of this period: the passage in 1974 of the Employee Retirement Income Security Act (ERISA). Although the focus of ERISA was on retirement benefits, it also addressed employers' pretax employee health benefits. Among other things, ERISA established appeal rights for denial of benefits, requirements for handling benefits claims, and various other new regulations for employers that self-funded their benefits plans, topics that are addressed further in the chapters titled *Health Benefits Coverage and Types of Health Plans* and *Sales, Governance, and Administration*.

The problem of healthcare costs rising faster than costs in the economy as a whole, thereby consuming an ever larger share of the GDP, increasingly became a subject of public discussion in the 1970s. Throughout the 1960s and into the early 1970s, HMOs played only a modest role in the financing and delivery of health care, although they were a significant presence in a few communities such

---

* Precertification, also known as prior authorization, requires that health plan approval be obtained for a service to be covered; concurrent review entails requiring approval to continue the service, such as determining whether the hospitalized patient still needs to be in the hospital.

as in the Seattle area and parts of California. In 1970, the total number of HMOs ranged between 30 and 40, with the exact number depending on one's definition. That would soon change.

THE MID-1970s TO MID-1980s: THE RISE OF MANAGED CARE

Between 1970 and 1977, national health expenditures as a percentage of GDP rose from 7.4% to 8.6%. The acceleration in healthcare cost increases, driven in large measure by a high percentage of the medical dollar being paid for by insurance, private or public (notably Medicare and Medicaid), rather than by the patient became widely discussed and led to the next major development: managed health care as we know it today. In particular, this period saw the growth of HMOs; the appearance of a new model, the preferred provider organization; and widespread adoption of utilization management by health insurers.

HMOs

In 1973, the U.S. Congress passed the HMO Act.[13] This legislation evolved from discussions that Paul Ellwood, MD, had in 1970 with the leadership of the U.S. Department of Health, Education, and Welfare (which later became the Department of Health and Human Services)[14] as the Richard M. Nixon administration sought ways to address the rising costs of the Medicare program.

These discussions resulted in a proposal to allow Medicare beneficiaries the option of enrolling in HMOs, which were to be capitated by the Medicare program—a change that was not actually adopted until 1982. However, the legislative debate resulted in the enactment of the HMO Act of 1973. The desire to foster prepaid HMOs reflected the view that third-party (insurance) payments on a fee-for-service basis gave providers incentives to increase utilization and fees. Ellwood is also widely credited with coining the term "health maintenance organization" at that time as a substitute for "prepaid group practice" because it had greater cachet.

The HMO Act included three important features:

- It made federal grants and loan guarantees available for planning, starting, and/or expanding HMOs.
- The federal legislation superseded state laws that restricted the development of HMOs.
- The "dual choice" provision required employers with 25 or more employees that offered indemnity coverage to also offer at least one group or

staff model and one IPA-model federally qualified HMO, but only if the HMOs formally requested to be offered. (Types of HMOs are described in detail in the *Health Benefits Coverage and Types of Health Plans* chapter.)

The dual choice mandate was used by HMOs of the time to get in the door of employer groups to become established. Because the federal mandate applied to only one HMO of each type, opportunities to exercise the mandate were limited, although employers were free to offer as many HMOs as they liked. The dual choice requirement expired in 1995. Nevertheless, even more than the other provisions, the dual choice mandate is widely regarded as providing a major boost to the HMO industry at a time when it was in its infancy.

To be federally qualified, HMOs had to satisfy a series of requirements such as meeting minimum benefit package standards, demonstrating that their provider networks were adequate, having a quality assurance system, meeting standards of financial stability, and having an enrollee grievance process. Many states ultimately adopted these requirements for all state-licensed HMOs.

Unlike a state license to operate, federal qualification as an HMO was voluntary. However, many HMOs became federally qualified to avail themselves of the HMO Act's features and because such qualification represented a type of "Good House-keeping Seal of Approval" that employers and consumers would trust. Although federal qualification no longer exists, it was an important step when managed care was in its infancy and HMOs were struggling for inclusion in employment-based health benefits programs. The expiration of federal qualification inspired the creation of health plan accreditation as a replacement "seal of approval."

The HMO Act imposed requirements on HMOs that were not levied on indemnity health insurers. Examples of requirements that applied to HMOs but not to standard insurance included the following:

- A level of comprehensiveness of benefits, including little cost sharing* and the coverage of preventive services, that exceeded what insurers at the time typically offered
- The holding of an annual open enrollment period during which HMOs had to enroll individuals and groups without regard to health status
- Prohibiting the use of an individual's health status in setting premiums

---

* Cost sharing is the amount of a covered benefit that is paid by the enrollee and has three major forms: (1) deductibles, an amount paid before any benefits are paid; (2) coinsurance, the percentage of the bill above any deductible for which the patient is responsible; and (3) copayments, a fixed dollar amount for which the patient is liable for a particular service or product (e.g., prescription drugs). Cost sharing and other benefits design issues are discussed in the *Health Benefits Coverage and Types of Health Plans* chapter.

These provisions applied only to federally qualified HMOs, making them potentially uncompetitive compared to traditional health insurance plans. The HMO Act was amended in the late 1970s to lessen this problem.

The HMO Act was largely successful. During the 1970s and 1980s, HMOs grew and began displacing traditional health insurance plans. What was not anticipated when the original HMO Act was passed was the rapid growth in IPA-model HMOs. By the late 1980s, enrollment in IPAs exceeded enrollment in group and staff model HMOs, a difference that has increased over time. This dynamic accelerated as commercial insurers and BCBS plans acquired or created their own HMOs, most of which followed the IPA model.

The original concept of using federally qualified HMOs in the Medicare program finally came into being in 1982 with the enactment of the Tax Equity and Fiscal Responsibility Act (TEFRA). The intent, which was largely achieved, was that the ability of HMOs to control healthcare costs would encourage these plans to offer more comprehensive benefits than traditional Medicare. For example, the new Medicare HMOs typically required less cost sharing than did traditional Medicare and offered coverage of prescription drugs and selected preventive. However, considerable debate arose as to whether HMOs were able to offer the additional benefits within the Medicare capitation amount because they were more efficient or because of favorable selection (they attracted a disproportionate share of healthy patients).

Also in 1982, the federal government granted a waiver to the state of Arizona that allowed it to rely solely on capitation, and not offer a fee-for-service alternative, in the state's Medicaid program.[15] A number of states had previously made major efforts, in some cases under federal demonstration waivers, to foster managed care in their Medicaid programs but had not done so statewide. That practice is now widespread. (Medicare managed care is discussed in the *Medicare and Medicaid* chapter.)

HMOs were increasingly accepted by consumers, due not only to their lower premiums and reduced cost sharing but also because of their more extensive benefits, such as coverage of preventive services, children's and women's preventive health visits, and prescription drugs, most of which were not covered by the typical traditional insurance or BCBS plans of the time. In contrast, HMOs were not required to offer coverage of prescription drugs but most did so to attract enrollees. In response to the competition from HMOs, many traditional insurance carriers and BCBS plans began to add coverage of prescription drugs and preventive services to their non-HMO products.

Preferred Provider Organizations and Utilization Management

The growth of HMOs led to the development of another type of managed care plan: preferred provider organizations (PPOs). PPOs are generally regarded as having originated in Denver, Colorado. In that city in the early 1970s, Samuel Jenkins, a vice president of Martin E. Segal Company, a benefits consulting firm, negotiated discounts with hospitals on behalf of its self-insured clients.[16] Hospitals granted discounts in return for enrollees having lower cost sharing if they used the contracting hospitals, thereby attracting patients away from competitor hospitals.

The concept soon expanded to include physicians and other types of providers. The term PPO arose because hospitals and doctors who agreed to discounted fees were considered to be "preferred" by the health insurance plan. People covered under the PPO faced lower cost sharing if they saw a PPO provider rather than a noncontracted, or "out of network," provider.

Unlike most HMO coverage at the time, PPO benefits did not require authorization from the patient's primary care physician (PCP) to access care from specialists or other providers. PPO providers also agreed to certain cost-control measures. For example, they agreed to comply with precertification requirements for elective hospitalizations, meaning that for the service to be covered, the doctor had to obtain approval before ordering any elective hospital admission or selected high-cost outpatient service. Precertification programs remain common today. Second-opinion programs were also instituted, whereby patients were required to obtain a second opinion from a different surgeon for selected elective procedures to be covered. Second-opinion programs are rarely mandated today.

Another development in indemnity insurance, which occurred mostly during the 1980s, was the widespread adoption of large case management—that is, the coordination of services for patients with expensive conditions requiring treatment by multiple providers, but did not coordinate with each other. Examples include patients who had experienced accidents, cancer cases, patients with multiple chronic illnesses causing functional limitations, and very low-birth-weight infants.* Utilization review, the encouragement of second opinions, and large case management all entailed at times questioning physicians' medical judgments, something that had been rare outside of the HMO setting. These activities were crude by today's standards of medical management but represented a radically new role for insurance companies in managing the cost of health care. They sometimes met with ferocious opposition in the medical community, with physicians' complaining that the programs constituted "cookbook medicine" or interfered with the "right" of the doctor to make unfettered medical decisions.

---

* The lack of coordination of medical services remains a persistent problem in the healthcare system—one that managed care was supposed to alleviate, which it has done to a limited extent.

Utilization management by HMOs contributed to practice pattern changes, including shifting care from the inpatient setting to the outpatient setting and shortening the length of hospital stays. Shortening length of stay was also strongly encouraged by legislation enacted in 1982 under which the Medicare payment system no longer paid a hospital's actual cost (albeit with upper limits on payments that affected particularly expensive hospitals) but instead paid a fixed amount per admission within a given class or grouping of diagnoses—an approach that some private health plans also adopted.

THE MID-1980s TO THE LATE 1990s: GROWTH AND CONSOLIDATION

From the mid-1980s through the mid-1990s, managed care grew rapidly while traditional indemnity health insurance declined, creating new strains on the U.S. healthcare system. At the same time, new forms of managed care plans and provider organizations appeared, and the industry matured and consolidated. That growth was not trouble free, however.

Managed Care Expands Rapidly

HMOs grew rapidly, growing from 3 million in 1970 to over 80 million in 1999.[17] Initially, PPOs lagged behind, but by the early 1990s enrollment was roughly equal: By 1999, PPOs had a 39% market share, compared to HMOs at 28%. This growth came at the expense of traditional indemnity health insurance. In the mid-1980s, traditional indemnity insurance accounted for three-fourths of the commercial market; by the mid-1990s, it represented less than one-third of the market and that share would decline to single digits by 2000.[18]

A new product was also introduced during this period—the point-of-service (POS) plan. In a POS plan, members had HMO-like coverage with little cost sharing if they both used the HMO network and accessed care through their PCP; unlike in a "pure" HMO, however, they still had coverage if they chose to get non-emergency care from out-of-network providers but were subject to higher cost sharing if they did. Members typically had to designate a PCP, who approved any referral to specialists and other providers (e.g., physical therapists) except in emergency situations. Though they were initially very popular, POS plans would stall out due to their high costs. These and other hybrid products make statistical compilations related to managed care trends difficult. As new types of plans appeared, the taxonomy of health plan types expanded and lines were blurred, with the term managed care organization (MCO) eventually coming to represent HMOs, POS plans, PPOs, and a myriad of hybrid arrangements. Medicare and Medicaid also witnessed significant managed care growth. Medicare enrollment in capitated plans—that is, plans such as HMOs that set premiums and assumed the risk for the delivery of services—grew from 1.3 million to 6.8 million between 1990 and 2000.[19] During that same time period, Medicaid managed care grew from 2.3 million (10% of Medicaid beneficiaries) to 18.8 million (56%).[20]

As is the case with dandelions, rapid growth is not always good. Some MCOs outstripped their ability to run their businesses, as evidenced by overburdened management and poorly functioning information systems, resulting at times in poor service and mistakes. In their quest to continually drive down utilization, some HMOs became increasingly aggressive. More ominously, the industry began to see health plan failures or near-failures.

Consolidation Begins

Beginning in the early 1990s, the pace of consolidation quickened among both MCOs and health systems. Entrepreneurs, sensing financial opportunities, acquired or started HMOs with the goal of profiting by later selling the HMO to a larger company. In other cases, they acquired smaller plans to build a regional or national company, enhancing their ability to issue stock. However, not all plans could be sold at a profit, and in some cases troubled MCOs made good acquisition targets, allowing larger plans to acquire market share at minimal expense. Although uncommon, MCOs that were getting close to failure might be seized by a state insurance commissioner, who would then either sell the MCO to another company or liquidate it and divide the membership among the remaining MCOs.

As the market consolidated, smaller plans were at a disadvantage. Large employers with employees who are spread out geographically favored national companies at the expense of local health plans. For smaller plans, the financial strain of having to upgrade computer systems continually and adopt various new technologies mounted. In addition, unless they had a high concentration in a small market, smaller plans found themselves unable to negotiate the same discounts as larger competitors. At some point, many simply gave up and sought to be acquired.

Not all mergers and acquisitions were large companies acquiring small ones. This trend also affected large companies. By 1999, multistate firms, including Kaiser Permanente and the combined Blue Cross and Blue Shield plans, accounted for three-fourths of U.S. enrollment in managed care plans.

Another trend saw health plans convert from not-for-profit to for-profit status. For example, the largest publicly traded managed care company in the

United States is currently United Health Group, the corporate parent of United Health Care, which started as a nonprofit health plan in Minnesota. Likewise, US Health Care, a Pennsylvania HMO company, converted from nonprofit to for-profit status and was eventually acquired by Aetna.

Many years earlier, the actual Blue Cross and Blue Shield trademarks had become the property of the Blue Cross Blue Shield Association (BCBSA) representing member plans. The BCBSA created standards that member plans had to meet to license the Blues trademarks, including a prohibition on being a for-profit company.

Breaking with that tradition, in 1994 the BCBSA voted to allow member plans to convert to for-profit status.[21] The reasons leading to this shift were financial. Since their beginnings, Blues plans had been tax-exempt as "social welfare plans," but the Tax Reform Act of 1986 revoked that exemption because Congress determined that Blues plans were selling insurance in an open market.* At the same time, BCBS plans were losing market share and were not able to keep up with changing operational demands because of a lack of capital—something that publicly traded companies were able to obtain through the sale of stock. Converting to for-profit status would therefore have little impact on the Blues' tax status, but would allow them to access capital to improve their competitive position.

Blue Cross of California was the first to convert to for-profit status under its corporate name WellPoint. The Indiana Blues soon followed under the corporate name Anthem. Other Blues plans also converted and were subsequently acquired by WellPoint or Anthem, and in 2004 Anthem merged with WellPoint to create what is now the second largest commercial health plan company in the United States. These conversions required the creation and funding of foundations, commonly known as "conversion foundations," holding the assets of the nonprofit plan. Many of these entities are among the largest grant-giving foundations in their respective states.

Consolidation also took place among health plans that were not publicly traded, albeit at a slower rate. By the end of 2013, among the top 10 largest health plans, four were non-investor owned:[22]

- Kaiser Foundation Group, with group model HMOs in nine regions, is the third largest.
- Health Care Services Corporation (Health Care Services Corporation), the largest mutual health insurer (i.e., owned by its enrollees), which has BCBS plans in five states, is the sixth largest.

---

* The Tax Reform Act did, however, allow for some special tax treatments for nonprofit BCBS plans acting as "insurers of last resort."

- Highmark Group, with BCBS plans in three states, is the eighth largest.
- EmblemHealth in New York, a company formed through a combination of Group Health, Inc. (GHI) and the Health Insurance Plan of Greater New York,[23] is the 10th largest.

Provider Consolidation and the Appearance of Integrated Delivery Systems

Among physicians, there was a slow but discernable movement away from solo practice and toward group practice in the 1990s. There was nothing slow, however, about the amount of hospital consolidation that began on a regional or local level in the 1990s. According to a study conducted by the Rand Corporation, more than 900 mergers and acquisitions occurred during the 1990s, and by 2003 90% of the metropolitan areas in the country were considered "highly concentrated" in terms of healthcare systems.[24] Hospital and health system mergers and consolidations continued after that study was published.

Hospital consolidation was commonly justified in terms of its potential to rationalize clinical and support systems. A clearer impact, however, has been the increased market power that enables such entities to negotiate favorable payment terms with commercial health plans (see the chapters titled *The Provider Network* and *Provider Payment*). Consolidation also meant that health plans could no longer selectively contract with individual hospitals. Systems with "must have" hospitals or even "must have" services, such as very specialized cardiac or oncology services, could refuse to enter into contracts that did not cover all of the services that the health system offered. As a result hospital prices to private payers rose by a total of 20% nationally between 1994 and 2001 and by 42% between 2001 and 2008.[25]

Consolidation, both among health plans and providers, diminished competition to the point of bringing into question the viability of the competitive model in the delivery of healthcare services. Instead of competition among multiple buyers and sellers, what evolved was closer to what economists call "bilateral monopolies," with health plans and providers in local markets having little choice but to reach agreements with each other.

Provider consolidation was not the only response to managed care. In many communities, hospitals and physicians collaborated to form integrated delivery systems (IDSs), principally as vehicles for contracting with payers and with HMOs in particular. Types of IDSs are discussed in the chapter titled *The Provider Network*.

Most IDSs were rather loose organizations consisting of individual hospitals and their respective medical staff, the most common of which was the physician–hospital organization (PHO). Most PHOs and IDSs required that health plans contract with all physicians with admitting privileges at the hospital that met the HMO's credentialing criteria, rather than with only the more efficient ones. Indeed, under the fee-for-service method of payment, physicians with high utilization benefited the hospital financially. Also, physicians were commonly required to use the hospital for outpatient services (e.g., for laboratory tests) that might be obtained at lower cost elsewhere.

Some hospitals chose to purchase PCP practices to increase their negotiating leverage with HMOs, although they did little to integrate those practices. Most IDSs of the time suffered, at least initially, from organizational fragmentation, payment systems to individual doctors that were misaligned with the goals of the IDS, inadequate information systems, inexperienced managers, and a lack of capital. In addition, hospitals that had purchased physician practices quickly discovered that physician productivity declined once those doctors were receiving a steady income, albeit with incentives to enhance volume, and no longer felt the financial pressures of independent practice. In most cases, those practices became a financial drag on the hospital and were eventually spun off at a net loss.

At the time, none of these factors stopped many of the systems from seeking to "cut out the middleman" and become risk-bearing organizations themselves—a decision they would soon regret. Provider organizations lobbied hard to be allowed to accept risk and contract directly with Medicare. The Balanced Budget Act of 1997 (BBA 97)* permitted them to do so as provider-sponsored organizations (PSOs) if they met certain criteria. With a few exceptions, these efforts failed and the PSOs lost millions of dollars in a few short years. The federal waiver program for PSOs expired, although not until most had failed, and only a handful exist today.†

Some IDSs and provider systems pursued another route to accepting full risk by forming a licensed commercial HMO. The existence of hospitals, physicians, and a licensed HMO and/or PPO under one corporate umbrella is called vertical integration. For a while, this model was touted as the future of health care. Like so many future scenarios confidently predicted by pundits, it mostly did not come to pass. Instead, provider-owned HMOs mostly failed for the same reasons PSOs failed—namely, the system was conflicted by, on one hand, the need to promote volume for patients under the fee-for-service system and, on the other

---

* The BBA 97 also reduced payments to Medicare HMOs, which many believe led to a decline in Medicare HMO enrollment in the early 1990s.

† The acronym "PSO" is now used by Medicare to mean "patient safety organization."

hand, the desire to be efficient in the delivery of services to capitated patients. Not all vertically integrated organizations failed, however. Those that did succeed typically managed their subsidiary HMOs as stand-alone entities. Many HMOs started by large, well-run medical groups also did well and continue to do so today. The rest were sold, given away, or ceased to operate.

Many large provider systems and physician practice management companies nevertheless accepted global capitation risk from HMOs, entailing their receiving a percentage of premium revenues (e.g., 80%) in return for being at risk for most covered medical services. Most of those also failed, with the exception of California, the number of provider systems contracting to accept full risk for medical costs dropped dramatically.

Utilization Management Shifts Focus

As hospital utilization became constrained, the focus of utilization management shifted to encompass the outpatient setting including prescription drugs, diagnostics (which have become increasingly expensive with the development of new technologies), and care by specialists. Perhaps even more important was the recognition of the large expense incurred by a small number of patients with chronic, and often multiple, conditions, resulting in significantly more attention being paid to these high-cost patients.

The role of the PCP also changed. In a traditional HMO, that role was to manage a patient's medical care, including access to specialty care. This "gate-keeper" function was a mixed blessing for PCPs, who at times felt caught between pressures to reduce costs and the need to satisfy the desires of consumers, who might question whether the physician had their best interests at heart in light of a perceived financial incentive to limit access to services. Likewise, patients might resent the administrative hassle entailed in having to get the PCP's referral. The growth of PPOs as compared to HMOs also led to a shift away from PCP-based "gatekeeper" types of plans. However, most plans (including PPOs) continued to set lower copayments for services delivered by a PCP rather than by a specialist, thereby retaining a primary care focus.

The focus of utilization management was also sharpened through the growth of carve-out companies—that is, organizations that have specialized provider networks and are paid on a capitation or other basis for a specific service. Among services that lend themselves to being "carved out" are prescription drug benefits as well as behavioral health, chiropractic, and dental services. The carve-out companies market principally to health plans and large self-insured employers since they are generally not licensed as insurers or HMOs and, therefore, are limited in their ability to assume risk. In recent years, some of the large health plans that contracted for such specialty services have reintegrated them, typically because the carved-out services made it difficult to coordinate services and/or because the plans had grown large enough to manage the services in question themselves.

Industry Oversight Spreads

Health insurance and managed care have always been subject to oversight by state insurance departments and (usually) health departments. The 1990s saw the spread of new external quality oversight activities. Starting in 1991, the National Committee for Quality Assurance (NCQA) began to accredit HMOs. This organization was launched by the HMOs' trade associations in 1979 but became independent in 1990. The majority of its board seats are now held by representatives of employers, unions, and consumers rather than health plans. Interestingly, this board structure was proposed by the Group Health Association of America, which represented closed-panel HMOs at the time. Many employers require or strongly encourage NCQA accreditation of the HMOs with which they contract to serve their employees, and accreditation came to replace federal qualification as the "seal of approval." NCQA, which initially accredited only HMOs, has evolved with the market to encompass a wide range of plan types and services and continues to broaden its programs. This is also the case with the two other bodies that accredit managed health care plans: URAC* and the Accreditation Association for Ambulatory Health Care, also known as the Accreditation Association (AAAHC). (For further discussion of these organizations, see the *Utilization Management, Quality Management, and Accreditation* chapter.)

Performance measurement systems (report cards) were also introduced, with the most prominent being the Healthcare Effectiveness Data and Information Set (HEDIS).† HEDIS was initially developed by the NCQA at the behest of several large employers and health plans. Medicare and many states now require HEDIS reporting by plans, and the federal government's involvement in this effort has grown. Other forms of report cards appeared as well and continue to evolve as a result of the market demanding increasing levels of sophistication and accountability.

---

* URAC is its only name and is no longer an acronym. At one time, it stood for Utilization Review Accreditation Commission.

† HEDIS now stands for Healthcare Effectiveness and Data Information Set.

At the federal level, the Health Insurance Portability and Accountability Act of 1996 (HIPAA) was enacted. Among other provisions, it limits the ability of health plans to (1) deny insurance based on health status to individuals who were previously insured for 18 months or more and (2) exclude coverage of preexisting conditions (i.e., medical conditions that exist at the time coverage is first obtained). A decade earlier, a provision in the Consolidated Omnibus Budget Reconciliation Act of 1985 (COBRA) allowed individuals who lost eligibility for employment-based group coverage to continue that coverage for up to 18 months, although they could be required to pay the full cost plus 2% themselves.*

HIPAA was designed in part to provide a means for individuals to have continued access to coverage once they exhausted their COBRA benefits. COBRA had only limited success because the coverage was usually expensive. In particular, a young person could often obtain coverage as an individual for less than the group rate, which was priced to include all individuals in the group, including older ones, who on average consume more services. Furthermore, the cost of COBRA coverage was often unaffordable because the loss of employer coverage often occurred as a result of someone becoming unemployed. However, until guaranteed issue requirements went into effect in 2014 under the 2010 Patient Protection and Affordable Care Act (ACA), continued coverage under HIPAA was the only way a person with serious medical problems could purchase insurance. Even fewer people took advantage of the HIPAA coverage provisions than was the case with COBRA. More important to the industry were the standards that HIPAA created for privacy, security, and electronic transactions.

THE LATE 1990s TO THE EARLY 2000s: THE MANAGED CARE BACKLASH[26]

Anti-managed care sentiment, commonly referred to as the "managed care backlash," became a defining force in the industry as the United States approached the new millennium. As a society, Americans expected managed care to reduce the escalation of healthcare costs but became enraged at how it did so. In retrospect, why that happened is obvious: Managed health care was the only part of the healthcare sector that ever said "no." The emotional overlay accompanying health care outstrips almost any other aspect of life. The health problems of a

---

* Coverage also had to be offered to select other groups, such as persons who lose coverage as a result of being newly widowed or divorced as well as children who lose dependent status. These individuals are eligible for coverage for as long as 36 months.

spouse or child causes feeling in ways that a house fire or losing one's employment does not.

The roots of the backlash date back to the early 1990s. At that time, most employers allowed their employees to choose between an HMO and a traditional health insurance plan, although their payroll deduction was typically higher if they chose the traditional health plan. Eventually, to control costs, many employers began putting employees into a single managed care plan without offering the choice of an indemnity plan.

One source of contention with some consumers—particularly those who had not chosen to be in an HMO—was the requirement that they obtain authorization from their PCP to access specialty care. Arguably, this provision both reduces costs and increases quality by assuring that PCPs are fully apprised of the care that their patients receive. Also, consumers under the care of a specialist who was not in the HMO's network were required to transition their care to an in-network doctor—another burden resented by individuals who had not voluntarily chosen to be in an HMO.

There was more to the backlash, however. As noted earlier, rapid managed care growth increased the risk of problems arising. Some of the problems were largely irritants, such as mistakes in paperwork or claims processing in health plans with information systems that were unable to handle the expanded load. Rapid growth also affected the ability to manage the delivery system. Where clinically oriented decisions on coverage were once made with active involvement of medical managers, some rapidly growing health plans became increasingly bureaucratic and distant from both their members and their providers, causing the plans to be seen as cold and heartless and the errors, and delays in payment as intentional.

Sometimes, rapid growth led to inconsistent coverage decisions. The public's perception that decisions regarding coverage of clinical care were made by "bean counters" or other faceless clerks may not have been fair or accurate in the opinion of managed care executives, but neither was it always without merit. Some HMOs, especially those whose growth outstripped their ability to manage, did delegate decision-making authority to individuals who lacked adequate training or experience and were not supported by the comprehensive algorithms that are common today. Furthermore, some plans were accused of routinely and intentionally denying or delaying payment of claims, caving in only when the member appealed—an accusation disputed by the plans. Regrettably, the managed care industry during this period did a poor job of self-policing and lost the confidence of large segments of the public.

Other problems were emotional and not a threat to health, such as denial of payment for care that was not medically necessary—for example, an unnecessary diagnostic test or an additional day in the hospital. For doctors and patients who are unaccustomed to *any* denial of coverage, it was easy to interpret these actions as overzealous utilization management, which, indeed, they were in some instances. How often such denials occurred is impossible to know, not only because of the turbulence of the era but also because standardized medical practices were only first coming into being, and there are no studies on which to rely.

Finally, while uncommon, some problems did represent potential threats to health such as difficulties in accessing care or denial of authorization for payment for truly necessary medical care, thereby causing subsequent health problems. Sometimes, the denial was due to the care not being a covered benefit, as in the case of certain experimental procedures. This occurred with indemnity health insurance as well but was not viewed the same way. The public expects low premiums but demands coverage for all medically related services, including ones that might be judged unnecessary or outside of the scope of the defined benefits; the public also expects access to any provider an individual chooses to consult.

Whether a service is medically necessary or simply a convenience can be a matter of interpretation or dispute. Is a prescription for a drug to help with erectile dysfunction medically necessary? What about growth hormone therapy for a child who is short because her or his parents are short, not as a result of a hormonal deficiency? Should fertility treatments be unlimited? Some interventions may be medically necessary for some patients but not others. For example, in a patient with droopy eye lids but no impairment of vision, surgery is primarily cosmetic, although it often progresses until it is medically necessary because vision is impaired. The most damning of all accusations was that health plans were *deliberately* refusing to pay for necessary care to enrich executives and shareholders—a perception enhanced by media stories of multimillion-dollar compensation packages of senior executives. Putting aside the fact that financial incentives drive almost all aspects of health care to varying degrees, this charge was particularly pernicious for health plans in light of the increasing number of for-profit plans.

Serious, even if isolated, problems make good fodder for news using the well-proven reporting technique of "identifiable victim" stories in which actual names and faces are associated with anecdotes of poor care or problems accessing coverage. Whether the problems portrayed were fair was irrelevant. When added to the disgruntlement caused by minor or upsetting (although not dangerous) irritants caused by health plan operations, the public was not liable to be sympathetic to managed care, particularly given the backdrop that few insurance companies are loved.

Politicians were quick to jump on the bandwagon, especially during the debate over the Health Security Act of 1993, legislation proposed by President

Bill Clinton but not enacted. Many states passed "patient protection" laws specifying prudent layperson standards for emergency care,* stronger appeal and grievance rights, and requirements for HMOs to contract with any provider willing to agree to the HMO's contractual terms and conditions. Whether the "any willing provider" provision protects consumers is debatable, and not all states passed laws to require it. Most states did pass laws requiring prudent layperson standards and appeal rights, which later were incorporated into the Affordable Care Act.

Another example of a "patient protection" law that arose out of the managed care backlash was the prohibition of "gag clauses" in HMO contracts with physicians in which an HMO's contract supposedly prevented a physician from informing patients of their best medical options. So prevalent was the belief that such constraints existed that it made the cover of the January 22, 1996, edition of *Time* magazine; that cover showed a surgeon being gagged with a surgical mask and a headline reading "What Your Doctor Can't Tell You. An In-Depth Look at Managed Care—And One Woman's Fight to Survive."† The Government Accountability Office (GAO), an agency of the U.S. Congress, investigated the practice at the request of then-Senators Lott, Nickles, and Craig and issued its report on August 29, 1997. The GAO reviewed 1150 physician contracts from 529 HMOs and could not find a single instance of a gag clause or any reported court cases providing guidance on what constitutes a gag clause.[27] This report had no impact on public perception, however. Laws prohibiting "gag clauses" became widespread, and years later this element was also incorporated into the Affordable Care Act.

The popular press continued to run regular "HMO horror stories." For example, the cover of the July 12, 1998, issue of *Time* magazine showed a photo of stethoscope

---

* Prudent layperson emergency standards require coverage when an enrollee who is not medically trained visits an emergency room in a situation that is not a true emergency, but the enrollee could reasonably have thought it might be (e.g., chest pains caused by a indigestion but that could have been symptomatic of a heart attack).

† The cover story was called "Medical Care: The Soul of an HMO" and dealt with a woman's dispute with a California HMO over coverage for a procedure for her disseminated breast cancer, known as autologous bone marrow transplantation. Authorization was denied because the treatment was considered experimental and investigational by a committee of the HMO's private oncologists. The story reported a considerable amount of communication, meetings, phone calls, medical visits and so forth, as well as the salaries and bonuses of HMO executives.

The woman sued and succeeded in getting the procedure covered, and an arbitration panel awarded her family punitive damages from the HMO. This case was only one of a number of lawsuits that finally forced HMOs and insurers to pay for this procedure. The woman died soon after the procedure was performed. Rigorous scientific study of autologous bone marrow transplantation eventually found that that the procedure was worse than conventional treatment alone, and it is no longer performed. The story highlights another dynamic in the U.S. health system: the practice of medicine by judge and jury.

tied in a knot and a headline that read "What Your Health Plan Won't Cover…" with the word "Won't" in bold red letters. In another example, the November 8, 1999, cover of *Newsweek* magazine featured a furious and anguished woman in a hospital gown with the words "HMO Hell" displayed across the image. HMOs were disparaged in movies, cartoons, jokes on late night TV, and even the comic sections of newspapers. The number of lawsuits against HMOs increased, with many alleging interference in doctors' decision making. Many also alleged that capitation incented physicians to withhold necessary care, although this charge lacked empirical support, as shown in a series of research studies discussed in the *Provider Payment* chapter.

In a futile attempt to counter the rising tide of antipathy, the managed care industry repeatedly tried to point out the good things it did for members such as coverage for preventive services and drugs, the absence of lifetime coverage limits, and coverage of highly expensive care—but there was nothing newsworthy about that. A reporter for a major newspaper, who did not himself contribute to the backlash, said at the time to one of this chapter's authors, "We also don't report safe airplane landings at La Guardia Airport."

In response to public complaints, HMOs expanded their networks and reduced how aggressively they undertook utilization management. Some eliminated the PCP "gatekeeper" requirement, thereby allowing members open access to any specialist, albeit at higher copayment levels than applied visits to the PCP. To borrow words used a decade earlier by President George H. W. Bush in his inaugural address, HMOs became "kinder and gentler," and healthcare costs began once again to rise faster than general inflation or growth in the GDP.

The managed care backlash eventually died down. The volume of HMO jokes and derogatory cartoons declined, news stories about coverage restrictions or withheld care became uncommon, and state and federal lawmakers moved on to other issues. However, the HMOs' legacy of richer benefits combined with the general loosening of medical management and broad access to providers collided with other forces by the end of the millennium, and the return of healthcare cost inflation resulted in the cost of health benefits rising as well, leading to an increase in the number of uninsured and greater cost sharing for those with coverage.

2000 TO 2010: HMOs AND POS PLANS SHRINK, COSTS GROW, AND COVERAGE ERODES

Economic growth was steady early in the first decade of the new millennium but slowed late in the decade, with GDP actually declining in 2008 and 2009 as the United States entered the "Great Recession." During that decade, healthcare costs rose seemingly inexorably, with national health expenditures increasing from 13.8% to 17.9% of GDP.[28] The increases reflected a variety of factors, including the decline in HMO market share, looser utilization management, the adoption of new and expensive (and often unproven) technologies, increased consumer expectations, direct-to-consumer marketing, the provider community's quest for new sources of income, and the practice of defensive medicine by providers who feared malpractice suits. During this decade, many employers responded to the tight economic situations by increasing deductibles and other forms of cost sharing and, in some cases, dropping employee coverage altogether rather than by promoting more tightly managed care. For some people in the individual market, health insurance became unaffordable, and healthcare costs strained many family budgets.

The Decline of HMO and POS Market Share

HMOs' share of the commercial enrollment market stood at 29% in 2000. It declined thereafter, reaching 25% in 2004, and then hovered around 20–21% from 2005 to 2009, before dropping further to 13% by 2014. POS plans, which had enjoyed a 24% market share in 1999, also steadily declined but then leveled out at around 10% by 2009. PPOs, in contrast, gained market share—growing from 39% in 1999 to 61% by 2005, before declining slightly after 2009.[29]

Medicare managed care enrollment also reversed itself, declining from 6.4 million in 1999 to 4.6 million by 2003.[30] This trend occurred not because of the managed care backlash but rather largely as a result of a provision in the Balanced Budget Act of 1997 that reduced what Medicare paid the health plans, resulting in those plans' reducing benefits, which in turn made them less attractive to Medicare beneficiaries. However, the situation changed with the enactment in 2003 of the Medicare Modernization Act (MMA), which increased payment to managed care plans from below the estimated cost of delivering services in the fee-for-service system to an amount that in years leading to the ACA exceeded 10% of what Medicare would have spent had enrollees remained in the fee-for-service system. The MMA also changed the name of the Medicare managed care program from Medicare+Choice to Medicare Advantage (MA) and promoted new forms of managed care that were more like traditional insurance policies than like HMOs. In turn, enrollment grew to 11 million in 2010 and to 15.5 million in 2014, representing 29% of all Medicare beneficiaries.[31] HMOs remain the largest form of MA plan, however, accounting for approximately 78% of all MA enrollees.

The MMA also created the first major benefit expansion in Medicare since the passage of the initial legislation in 1965: the Part D drug benefit. Interestingly, rather than paying for the benefit on a fee-for-service basis as in traditional

Medicare, the government capitated private companies, some of which specialized in processing drug claims (such as ExpressScripts and CVS Caremark) and were known as pharmacy benefits managers (PBMs); others were insurers or HMOs that had the same capability. This method of administering the Part D benefit was intended to provide beneficiaries with a choice among competing plans. Existing MA managed care plans were also required to offer at least one plan that incorporated the drug benefit. Providing the new drug coverage benefit entirely through private companies was highly controversial, in part because it had never been done before. It was also regarded by some at the time as unworkable. Nevertheless, Medicare Part D's benefit has survived, albeit with administrative problems at the beginning.

Growth in the Medicaid managed care program followed a smoother trajectory. Cash-strapped states increasingly turned to private managed care plans, whose Medicaid enrollment grew from 18.8 million in 2000 to 42.2 million in 2011, representing 74% of all Medicaid beneficiaries.[32] Expanded Medicaid eligibility under the ACA is also increasing the number of people covered under managed Medicaid plans.

The Toll of Rising Healthcare Costs[33]

The toll of rising healthcare costs on the economy in the first decade of the new millennium was considerable. In the commercial group market, employers continued to pay approximately 70% of the cost, with the remainder coming from payroll deductions.* However, with healthcare costs rising so rapidly, employees' absolute dollar contribution rose considerably. Rising costs, along with a weakened economy, resulted in the percentage of Americans without health insurance rising from 14% in 1999 to 17% in 2009.[34] One reason for this trend was that some businesses, particularly small ones, found coverage to be unaffordable. Another reason was greater number of employees declining employer-sponsored coverage so as to avoid the payroll deduction. Although statistics vary, bankruptcies resulting from medical debt during this period were also widely estimated to account for more than half of all personal bankruptcies; whether this will change under the ACA is unknown at this time.

Increasing payroll deductions were not the only way in which costs to consumers rose. In an effort to limit premium increases, employers also increased cost sharing, especially the size of deductibles (i.e., the amount an individual must pay

---

* Larger employers typically contribute more than do smaller employers.

out-of-pocket before benefits are paid). By 2013, more than 28% of large firms and 58% of all small firms had an annual deductible of $1000 or more, whereas $250 was typical in the prior decade. Cost sharing also increased for both routine visits and prescriptions. Whereas once the typical office copayment was $5, it now averaged $23 for visits to a PCP and $35 for visits to specialists. In addition, coverage of prescription drugs once required a single copayment no matter which drug was purchased; in the 2000s, this benefit typically became subject to complex tiered copayments, with lower copayments required for generic drugs (where available) and higher levels of copayments required for brand-name drugs. Cost sharing in benefits design is addressed in more detail in the *Health Benefits Coverage and Types of Health Plans* chapter, and management of the drug benefit is discussed in the *Utilization Management, Quality Management, and Accreditation* chapter.

The middle of this decade also saw the appearance of high-deductible health plans (HDHPs) and related consumer-directed health plans (CDHPs), both of which confer savings in federal income taxes. The main benefit to the enrollee in such a plan is savings in taxes and premiums. The amount of the minimum deductible required to qualify for favorable tax treatment has varied over the years but amounted to $3300 per year in 2014 for individuals and $6550 for a families. Embedded in CDHPs is the notion that consumer choice and accountability should be enhanced. The initial focus was to provide members with better information regarding quality and cost of care along with information to help them understand their health care. However, such plans are controversial because, whatever the resulting savings, people with high incomes disproportionately gain from tax savings because they are in higher tax brackets, whereas persons with high medical expenses—notably those individuals with chronic conditions—face higher out-of-pocket expenses, often year after year.

2010 TO PRESENT: THE ACA AND THE ONGOING EVOLUTION OF THE U.S. HEALTHCARE MARKET

The Patient Protection and Affordable Care Act (ACA, also known as "Obamacare"), signed into law on March 23, 2010, is the most sweeping healthcare legislation passed in the United States since 1965, when Medicare and Medicaid were enacted. It is also the most important legislative development in the health insurance and managed care industry to occur in this millennium. It is not, however, the only development of note.

The Patient Protection and Affordable Care Act

At nearly 1000 pages in length, the ACA affects the entire healthcare sector, but its two areas of greatest impact are on the health plan industry and on access to coverage. Because the ACA is so sweeping, it is not possible to cover it all within the confines of this text, much less in this chapter. The specific provisions of the ACA that are most important to understand are addressed throughout this text. The ACA affects health insurance and managed healthcare plans in several ways, with many of the provisions being phased in over time. Particularly important provisions include the following:

- Health benefits plans are required to cover dependents until age 26.
- Health insurance and HMO coverage is required to be "guaranteed issue," meaning health plans cannot deny coverage or vary premiums based on preexisting conditions or health status. Premiums can, however, reflect geographic location, age (within prescribed limitations), and tobacco use. Guaranteed issue is confined to an annual limited period of "open enroll-ment" when individuals and groups can apply for coverage.*
- Health insurance "exchanges" are established by states, and by the federal government if a state either fails or refuses to do so. Such exchanges are largely computer-based systems where individuals and small businesses can purchase insurance from private health plans.
- All Americans not otherwise covered are required to purchase an approved private insurance policy or pay a penalty, with some exceptions, the most important being individuals deemed to be subject to undue hardship as a result. Individuals and families with incomes less than 400% of the poverty level who are not eligible for Medicaid can qualify for premium subsidies. Ironically, the idea of requiring that Americans obtain health insurance—which was vehemently opposed by most Republicans as an infringement on personal liberties—is commonly attributed to the Heritage Foundation, a conservative think-tank; the Foundation proposed this concept in 1989, and it was supported by many Republicans at the time.
- The Medicaid program was expanded to cover all families and individu-als with incomes of less than 133% of the federally established poverty line, with the federal government paying states 100% of the cost of

---

* The ACA requires that open enrollment periods be no less than one month per year, which is typically a month in the fall for coverage beginning the following January 1. Nevertheless, states are free to require open enrollment on a more frequent basis. No state, however, requires continuous open enrollment—that is, enrollment throughout the year.

covering the expansion population in 2014–2016, declining gradually to 90% in 2020 and thereafter.

The ACA, which passed narrowly, was the subject of a hard-fought battle prior to its enactment and remains controversial. Lawsuits pertaining to its legitimacy reached the U.S. Supreme Court after being litigated in lower courts. The two main Supreme Court decisions, both reached on 5 to 4 votes, were that the mandate that individuals obtain health insurance was constitutional but not the requirement that states expand their Medicaid programs so dramatically as a condition for receiving *any* federal matching funding. According to the Kaiser Family Foundation, "As of June 2014, 27 states, including [the District of Columbia], were expanding Medicaid, three states were actively debating the issue, and 21 states were not moving forward." The nonparticipating states can elect to expand their Medicaid programs at any time.

In a later case heard by the U.S. Supreme Court, the court ruled that the ACA's provision that all benefits plans must cover contraception did not apply to certain types of closely held corporations that have religious objections to covering such care. At the time of publication, there were other outstanding legal cases.

Taken as a whole, the provisions of the ACA had the effect of expanding the number of individuals in both Medicaid and private healthcare plans—one reason why the health insurance industry was generally supportive of the legislation. Nevertheless, the ACA continues to face challenges, both political and legal, and the law may even be amended by the time this text reaches readers; for example, as of this writing, the U.S. Supreme Court has agreed to hear a case involving the federal government's ability to provide subsidies to eligible individuals who purchase coverage through an exchange operated by the federal government rather than a state, but it has not yet made a ruling.

The Healthcare Market Continues to Evolve

As significant as the ACA is, it is not the only change in the U.S. healthcare system in recent years. The four examples given here are in many ways reminiscent of events of 15 or more years ago.

Accountable Care Organizations and Provider–Payer Joint Initiatives

The ACA authorizes the creation of accountable care organizations (ACOs), which entails a provider entity assuming responsibility for the total costs of the Medicare

Part A and Part B benefits for a defined population of beneficiaries in the traditional Medicare fee-for-service program, with that entity sharing in any savings or losses relative to a target. The target is intended to approximate what would have been spent absent the ACO agreement. What is unique about this arrangement is that Medicare beneficiaries are attributed to the ACO based on past utilization patterns rather than their choosing to enroll. Those beneficiaries can use any Medicare participating provider, unlike in an HMO. In fact, the ACO is essentially invisible to the beneficiary. The ACO program was included in the ACA as a permanent (not a pilot) program, despite the fact that it was an untested model.

Some of the early ACOs have dropped out over what they perceive as long delays in the Government's provision of data that determine whether they met the expenditure targets. In addition, ACOs sometimes questioned the accuracy of the data. How successful the ACO program will be, and whether it is scalable nationally, remains to be seen.

Physician Employment by Hospitals

Group and staff model HMOs declined in prominence throughout the late 1980s and into the early 1990s as the market turned toward open-panel HMOs and PPOs. At the same time, many hospitals that felt threatened by managed care reacted by purchasing physician private practices, mostly those of PCPs but of some other specialties as well. The intent was to make it difficult for an HMO or PPO to exclude the facility in question from its network and to gain negotiating strength by employing the PCPs whom health plans most needed. For most hospitals, this expansion was a costly effort that was subsequently reversed.

This dynamic has returned in recent years as hospitals have consolidated to create major health systems. In many cases, the hospitals have once again purchased practices, increasingly attracting physicians who seek employment because they recently finished their training programs, require a steady income to repay student debts, or do not want the burden of practicing privately. One aspect of this burden is government efforts to induce providers to adopt electronic medical records, which are beneficial but costly and time consuming for the provider to learn to use when first installed.

As before, hospitals have purchased private practices, initially at least to further strengthen their already strong negotiating position with health plans and thereby obtain more favorable pricing agreements. However, while PCP practices continue to be acquired, there is now greater focus on specialties such as cardiology that rely heavily on ancillary services, particularly diagnostic tests that the hospital offers.

Employed physicians are expected to direct patients to use the health system's ancillary services instead of those with potentially lower cost. This expectation creates a significant problem for both private payers and Medicare. To illustrate this dilemma, the traditional Medicare program pays more for services and procedures rendered by physicians at a hospital facility than if the same services and procedures were delivered by non-hospital-affiliated physicians in their offices. Proposals have been advanced to change Medicare's "site of service" differential, which some view as an anomaly, but as yet this has not occurred.

In many markets, individual healthcare systems may employ more than 1000 physicians—numbers that were unheard of the last time this strategy was attempted. The consolidation that is occurring brings into question the viability of the competitive model when large provider systems dominate the market, leaving insurers little opportunity to select the providers with whom they contract.

While hospital employment of physicians is by far the more significant dynamic, some health plans have also purchased existing physician practices. They have done so in some cases to ensure that they would have network physicians who were not employed by a hospital and in other cases to create an alternative for medical groups that did not want to become part of a large hospital system.

"Cutting Out the Middleman" Is Back

Provider interest is growing in "cutting out the middleman" (i.e., the insurance carrier) by developing health plans that providers fully own and control. Unlike the last time this phenomenon occurred, the providers in question are health systems with large panels of employed physicians rather than smaller hospitals dependent on physicians in private practice.

Compared to 15 years ago, more managers with health plan experience are available, and computer support systems are better. Theoretically at least, employing the physicians provides greater ability to manage care and costs. Whether this is enough to offset the other problems that provider-owned plans face is still unknown, with the most notable unresolved issue being the tension between being efficient and the need to generate revenues from fee-for-service patients. Although the number of people seeking insurance has expanded under the ACA, there is less room in the market for new entrants than there was the last time this strategy became popular.

The Narrowing of Networks

During the heyday of early HMO growth in the 1970s and early to mid-1980s, the expectation among many pundits (including the authors) was that managed care plans would select providers based on their efficiency, resulting in relatively small provider networks in comparison to the total number of physicians in a geographic area. This by and large did not come to pass. Indeed, particularly after the managed care backlash, health plans broadened their networks by accepting any providers into their networks who met the health plan's terms and requirements.

Stimulated by the ACA, the strategy of having a broad network is now changing, at least for some health plans or for some of their products. Specifically, some health plans participating in the state and federal insurance exchanges are being selective in terms of who they accept as participating providers. In those cases, the networks for the products being offered in the exchanges are smaller than those offered to large employer groups. The goal of these health plans is to manage better the higher costs and utilization associated with providing coverage to individuals with significant medical problems who had not been able to obtain insurance before.

The limitations in network size have rankled many consumers and consumer activist organizations as well as some state regulators. Some states are considering requiring plans that participate in their exchanges to offer out-of-network benefits with higher cost sharing. So far, only a few states have required this type of expanded access for coverage sold through an exchange. As one of its provisions, the ACA reduced capitation payments to Medicare managed care plans from 10% or more above fee-for-service levels to amounts that are closer to parity. Instead of responding to this change in reimbursement by trimming benefits, many plans have sought to narrow the network by contracting with providers whom they view as efficient. This narrowing of networks has caused disgruntlement among enrollees accustomed to being able to go to almost any provider and has raised questions regarding whether some of the networks are too small, although Medicare closely regulates networks to assure reasonable access to providers. Consumers will likely increasingly have to decide whether to pay more for an inclusive network offering very broad provider choice, albeit not necessarily higher quality, or accept a more limited (albeit adequate) network.

CONCLUSION

Managed health care has affected the U.S. healthcare delivery system in significant ways—many positive, but some negative. HMOs, for example, demonstrated that many procedures that were once performed only on an inpatient basis could be performed equally well in an outpatient setting. HMOs also showed that inpatient length of stay could be reduced without ill effect. Over time, these changes have become the norm of practice, including in the fee-for-service system. Likewise, HMOs' early emphasis on prevention is now reflected in certain laws including those pertaining to the ACA and Medicare.

The early HMOs were also the source of considerable research on quality of care, far more so than the unmanaged fee-for-service system. This research contributed to policy makers' and large employers' becoming comfortable contracting with them. Furthermore, it helped accelerate the overall broadening of quality measurement and management beyond the hospital setting to which it had traditionally been confined.

The initial and ongoing public and regulatory mistrust of managed health care and health insurers in general led to the creation of standard measures to evaluate health plans. Most notable among these measures are the Healthcare Effectiveness Data and Information Set (HEDIS) and the Consumer Assessment of Health Care Providers and Systems (CAHPS) survey (see the *Utilization Management, Quality Management, and Accreditation* chapter).

Of note is the synergistic relationship between the public and private sectors. HMOs, which are private entities, have proved themselves to be viable mechanisms for delivering care to Medicare and Medicaid beneficiaries. Government at all levels has stimulated managed care growth in other ways as well. One of the earliest examples of a large employer contract with HMOs on a dual-choice basis was that between the U.S. Office of Personnel Management (OPM) and the Kaiser Foundation Health Plans, an approach that was subsequently adopted by many large employers. Today, federal, state, and local government employees constitute the largest accounts of many managed care plans. In addition, the HMO Act of 1973 spurred HMO development through grants, loans, and—most importantly—the dual choice mandate. Finally, many health plans have adopted Medicare's methodology for paying physicians and, less commonly, hospitals.

On a negative note, the managed care industry did not respond well to the managed care backlash of the late 1990s and the early 2000s. It did not at the time make sufficient efforts at self-regulation, although many health plans were supportive of the NCQA. At first, the industry handled the backlash as a public relations problem. In opposing legislation to address the backlash, MCOs opposed what most people viewed as sensible requirements, notably the layperson emergency rule and the right to appeal coverage denials to an independent body, giving the impression that the managed care industry was putting money ahead of patient care.

Rising costs meant rising numbers of uninsured individuals, which was the impetus behind the passage of the ACA in 2010. The lingering negative view of health insurers and managed care played a prominent role in the debate and the ACA's ultimate passage. Whether the ACA will accomplish its intended goals is unknown, but it is fair to say that its primary focus is on ensuring access to health insurance and not on restraining costs.

The issue of cost containment continues to be featured prominently in the media. Unfortunately, everyone has his or her "silver bullet" to solve the costs problems: if we could only solve the malpractice problem *or* if we could only institute higher cost sharing so that patients would seek out efficient providers *or* if provider payment could be changed to avoid the incentives in fee-for-service plans to deliver more, and more expensive, care *or* fill-in-your-favorite-solution-here. Each of these measures has a place as part of a comprehensive strategy, as do other approaches such as promoting wellness and addressing the problem of untested, questionable, expensive, and marginally effective technologies. In the past several years, attention has also been focused on pricing by providers and drug manufacturers, but such reports usually generate only a brief flurry of indignation before fading away.

An inherent problem in controlling healthcare costs is that one person's cost is another person's revenues—and providers seeking to protect their incomes are better organized than are patients or, for that matter, the citizenry as a whole. In addition, at the time of needing services, patients have little concern with costs. For their part, politicians commonly issue demagogic statements identifying any limitation as "rationing," hampering informed public discussion.

Health plans can do only so much. In the short run, they must respond to the desires of their customers—individuals, employers, or unions—who themselves may be neither willing to address the issues nor well informed. Health plans must also respond to state and federal regulators as well as new ACA requirements, and those regulators may likewise be unwilling or unable to address cost concerns. Managed health care has and will continue to make important contributions, but it is not the panacea some had hoped for.

NOTES

1. Mayer TR, Mayer GG. HMOs: origins and development. *N Engl J Med.* 1985;312(9):590–594.
2. MacLeod GK. An overview of managed care. In: Kongstvedt PR, ed. *The managed care handbook.* 2nd ed. Gaithersburg, MD: Aspen; 1993:3–11.
3. Starr P. *The social transformation of American medicine.* New York, NY: Basic Books; 1982:295–310.
4. Blue Cross and Blue Shield Association. Blue beginnings. Available at http://www .bcbs.com/about/history/blue-beginnings.html. Accessed April 23, 2011.

5. Lichtenstein M. Health insurance from invention to innovation: A history of the Blue Cross and Blue Shield companies. BlueCross BlueShield Blog. Available at: http://www.bcbs.com/blog/health-insurance.html. Accessed January 5, 2015.

6. Austin DA, Hungerford TL. The market structure of the health insurance industry. *Congressional Research Service*, April 8, 2010.

7. Consumers Union. Blue Cross and Blue Shield: A historical compilation. Available at: http://consumersunion.org/wp-content/uploads/2013/03/yourhealthdollar.org_blue-cross-history-compilation.pdf. Accessed January 5, 2015.

8. This is also stated on the websites of many BCBS plans; for example, see Wellmark Blue Cross Blue Shield at http://www.wellmark.com/AboutWellmark/CompanyInformation/History.aspx; accessed January 5, 2015.

9. http://www.cms.gov/Research-Statistics-Data-and-Systems/Statistics-Trends-and-Reports/NationalHealthExpendData/Downloads/PieChartSourcesExpenditures2012.pdf. Accessed July 22, 2014.

10. http://www.cms.gov/Research-Statistics-Data-and-Systems/Statistics-Trends-and-Reports/NationalHealthExpendData/Downloads/highlights.pdf. Accessed July 22, 2014.

11. Fielding JE. *Corporate cost management*. Reading, MA: Addison-Wesley; 1984.

12. Ibid.; Fox PD, Goldbeck WB, Spies JJ. *Health care cost management, private sector initiatives*. Ann Arbor, MI: Health Administration Press; 1984.

13. HMO Act of 1973, 42 U.S.C. § 300e.

14. Strumpf GB. Historical evolution and political process. In: Mackie DL, Decker DK, eds. *Group and IPA HMOs*. Gaithersburg, MD: Aspen; 1981:17–36.

15. Kaiser Family Foundation. Medicaid: A timeline of key developments. 2011. Available at http://www.kff.org/medicaid/timeline/pf_entire.htm. Accessed April 4, 2011.

16. Spies JJ, Friedland J, Fox PD. Alternative health care delivery systems: HMOs and PPOs. In: Fox PD, Goldbeck W, Spies, JJ, eds. *Health care cost management: private sector initiatives*. Ann Arbor, MI: Health Administration Press; 1984:43–68.

17. *InterStudy Extra*, Vol. 1, Issue 4, December 2000.

18. Kaiser/HRET survey of employer-sponsored health benefits, 1999–2013; KPMG survey of employer-sponsored health benefits, 1993, 1996; Health Insurance Association of America (HIAA), 1988.

19. Ibid.

20. Ibid.

21. http://www.hschange.org/CONTENT/644/. Accessed August 10, 2014.

22. http://health.usnews.com/health-news/health-insurance/articles/2013/12/16/top-health-insurance-companies. Accessed July 24, 2014.

23. http://www.emblemhealth.com/About-Us.aspx. Accessed August 10, 2014.

24. Vogt WB. *Hospital market consolidation: trends and consequences*. NIHCM Expert Voices; November 2010. Available at http://www.nihcm.org/pdf/EV-Vogt_FINAL.pdf. Accessed March 27, 2011.

25. Ibid.

26. The description of the managed care backlash is based on the author's own experiences as well as many academic papers, including the following: Blendon R, Brodie M, Benson J, et al. Understanding the managed care backlash. *Health Affairs*. 1998;17(4):80–94; Rodwin M. Backlash: as prelude to managing managed care. *J Health Politics Pol Law*. 1999;24(5):1115–1126; Draper D, Hurley R, Lesser CS, et al. The changing face of managed care. *Health Affairs*. 2002;21(1):11–23.

27. Government Accountability Office. AO HEHS-97-175 HMO Gag Clauses.

28. Martin AB, Lassman D, Washington B, et al. Growth in US health spending remained slow in 2010: health share of gross domestic product was unchanged from 2009. *Health Affairs.* 2012;31(1):208–219.

29. Kaiser/HRET survey of employer-sponsored health benefits, 1999–2013.

30. *MedPAC data book: health care spending and the Medicare program.* June 2014.

31. Ibid.

32. Centers for Medicare & Medicaid Services. *Medicaid managed care enrollment report: summary of statistics as of July 1, 2011.*

33. All citations for data and figures described in the section titled "Out-of-Pocket Spending Increases" are from the Kaiser/HRET survey of employer-sponsored health benefits, 1999–2013, 3.

34. U.S. Census Bureau. Health insurance coverage status and type of coverage all persons by age and sex: 1999 to 2009. Health insurance historical tables. Available at: http://www.census.gov/hhes/www/hlthins/data/historical/index.html. Accessed May 13, 2011.

Health Benefits Coverage and Types of Health Plans

> **LEARNING OBJECTIVES**
>
> - Understand the core components of health benefits coverage
> - Describe the sources of health benefits coverage
> - Explain the differences in risk bearing
> - Understand the basic health insurer and managed care organization models
> - Describe the differences between models

INTRODUCTION

At its simplest, the U.S. healthcare system is made up of five types of people or organizations:

1. *Patients*
2. *Providers*, which include not only doctors and hospitals, but all licensed professionals and medical facilities
3. *Manufacturers*, such as drug and medical device manufacturers as well as the vendors that sell those drugs and devices
4. *Payers*, referring to health insurers and managed care organizations
5. *Regulators*, referring to those who apply the various state and federal laws and regulations

The fundamental obligation of any payer is to manage benefits for healthcare goods and services, meaning which goods and services will be paid for and under which circumstances, how much will be paid by the benefits plan when something is covered, and how much will be paid by the patient who is covered under that plan. This simple description, however, quickly becomes complex in the real world when done by different types of payer organizations.

The generic terms "health plan," "payer," and "payer organization" apply to any type of organization that pays for healthcare benefits. A great many different types of payers exist, and defining these different types is an ever-evolving challenge. Thirty years ago, it was relatively easy to distinguish among different types of payers. Back then, health insurers, health maintenance organizations (HMOs), preferred provider organizations (PPOs), and point-of-service (POS) health plans were distinct types of organizations and were identified as such. Later, the broader term "managed care organization" (MCO) came into common use for many different types of plans; this term continues to be used today, albeit less frequently. Around 20 years ago, there was no such thing as a consumer-directed health plan (CDHP), but that entity has joined the fray. The Patient Protection and Affordable Care Act of 2010 (ACA) has directly affected the definitions of health benefits and health plans as well.

The clear distinctions between types of payers have become progressively blurred over time, and organizational elements and features that had appeared previously in only one type of payer have found their way into other types of payers. For all these reasons as well as in recognition of the widespread use of managed care techniques in all types of plans, we will refer to these organizations as "payers," "MCOs," "health plans," or simply "plans" when addressing them broadly, but will identify the specific types of payers when it is important to distinguish between them.

DEFINED BENEFITS, COST SHARING, AND COVERAGE LIMITATIONS

Before describing the different types of payers, it is important to understand the core components in place in any type of health benefits plan. While managing benefits is the fundamental obligation of any type of payer organization, it is important to bear in mind that a health plan does not actually provide health care (with the exception of group and staff model HMOs). It can only manage what services it will and will not pay for, and under which circumstances. In other words, health plans cannot prevent someone from receiving a medical service, but it can determine that this service will or will not be paid for by the plan. This is not to say that health plan benefits coverage policies and decisions have no impact: It is hard to argue that a plan's denial of coverage for a $50,000 elective procedure would have no impact on a person's decision to have that procedure done. Nevertheless, it is critical to keep in mind that health plans manage benefits, meaning payments for medical goods and services, but do not provide the care and cannot actually prevent a doctor from doing a procedure or a patient from getting a treatment, drug, or device.

There are three interrelated core components of healthcare benefits:

- Defined benefits
- Cost sharing
- Coverage limitations

Defined Benefits and Cost Sharing

"Benefits" means that a health plan provides some type of coverage for particular types of medical goods and services, and under particular circumstances. "Cost sharing" means that some amount of a covered benefit is not paid by the plan, but rather is paid out-of-pocket by someone covered under the benefit plan. Each term is a reflection of the other, so they are addressed together here.

Defined Benefits in General

Defined benefits refer to what is covered, and under which circumstances coverage applies. In other words, the actual benefit is defined, regardless of what it ultimately costs to provide coverage for that benefit, although coverage may depend on meeting various requirements. This mechanism differs from a defined contribution benefits plan, which defines a fixed amount of money that may be put toward a benefit. For example, a defined benefit would be coverage of an inpatient stay regardless of cost. A defined contribution, in contrast, would be coverage of only $250 of the cost of that stay, regardless of what it actually costs. All types of health plans discussed in this text, as well as in the ACA, are defined benefits plans.

Even in a defined benefits plan, the rules and requirements governing when coverage may apply also vary by type of health plan. For example, HMOs typically cover nonemergency services only when they are authorized or when authorization is not required per the HMO's policies; they will not cover the cost of nonemergency care provided by noncontracting providers or nonauthorized costly services. Other plan types may provide some level of coverage for nonemergency care provided by noncontracting providers that HMOs do not, although the amounts and conditions vary by plan type. Coverage may also depend on whether a treatment is considered reasonable based on a person's medical condition, particularly when there is more than one way to treat that condition.

To review a plan's defined benefits, existing members and individuals looking for coverage are required under the ACA to be provided with a standardized document called the summary of benefits and coverage (SBC), also called a summary of coverage (SOC). This document also summarizes how the plan defines "medical necessity," meaning how it determines whether coverage is appropriate based on a person's clinical condition and other factors, as discussed in the *Utilization Management, Quality Management, and Accreditation* chapter.

Defined Benefits Under the ACA

The ACA also defines essential health benefits (EHBs), meaning services or goods that must be covered. EHBs apply to all types of plans, but the amount of cost sharing or levels of coverage may differ for various plans (with one exception—no cost sharing is allowed for preventive and wellness services). Table 2-1 lists the EHBs as defined by the ACA. The ACA also limits plan participation in the insurance exchanges to qualified health plans (QHPs) covering the EHBs. The details of EHBs may differ slightly from state to state for reasons discussed shortly.

State-Mandated Benefits Coverage

In addition to the overall EHBs under the ACA, states have mandated benefits coverage requirements. In other words, state laws may require health plans to cover the costs of certain defined types of care and medical services as well as services provided by certain types of providers. States typically have multiple mandated benefits.

Table 2–1 Essential Health Benefits Under the ACA

Benefit	Cost Sharing Allowed
Ambulatory patient services	Yes
Emergency services	Yes
Hospitalization	Yes
Maternity and newborn care	Yes
Pediatric services	Yes
Preventive and wellness services	No; first-dollar coverage required
Prescription drugs	Yes, but type may differ from cost sharing for medical benefits
Laboratory services	Yes
Mental health and substance use disorder services	Yes, but may *not* differ from cost sharing for medical benefits
Chronic disease management	Yes
Rehabilitative and habilitative services and devices	Yes

Coverage mandates in the states apply only to insured plans; that is, they do not apply to self-funded plans (the difference between insured and self-funded plans will be described a bit later). Examples of typical state coverage mandates for clinical conditions include in vitro fertilization, cancer screening, and the treatment of autism. Examples of mandates involving types of provider include requirements to cover care provided by chiropractors or by nonphysician mental and behavioral healthcare providers.

Detailed definitions of EHBs are defined by each state, although they must comply with the broader definitions used in the ACA. States construct their unique definitions by looking at the largest commercial plans in the state and basing coverage definitions on their offerings. As a result, mandated benefits are incorporated into coverage sold through the exchanges.

Coverage Mandates for Individuals and Employers

The ACA also addresses defined benefits by requiring almost everyone to be covered under an individual plan, an employer-sponsored plan, Medicare, Medicaid, or some other equivalent benefits plan. This mandate is intended to balance out the guaranteed issue requirement under the ACA, which specifies that health insurers and HMOs must sell coverage to any individual or employer group that requests it, at least during the open enrollment period in each state. Without the mandate that all people obtain coverage, sicker people would seek coverage while healthier people might avoid it, thereby increasing the cost of coverage (money paid in by healthy people covers the costs for sicker people).

These mandates actually refer to potential financial penalties for individuals and for employers that fail to obtain health insurance. There is no enforcement provision in the ACA and failure to pay the penalty is not a crime. However, the Internal Revenue Service, which is charged with determining and enforcing these penalties, can withhold unpaid penalty amounts from any tax refunds.

For individuals, this penalty started out relatively low in 2014, but increases each year until it reaches the greater of $695 or 2.5% of taxable income in 2016. After 2016, the amount is increased every year by any increase in the overall cost of living. Many exemptions to the individual penalty exist, however, with most being related to low income.

For employers that have 50 or more full-time employees (FTEs) and that do not offer a health plan, if even one FTE receives a tax-credit subsidy for coverage purchased through a health insurance exchange, then the employer must pay a penalty of $2000 per employee, not counting the first 30 employees. The penalty is even higher for employers with 50 or more FTEs that *do* offer coverage, but where at least one FTE receives the premium tax credit through an exchange. Employers with fewer than 50 FTEs are exempt from any penalties, but the ACA provides tax incentives to encourage them to offer coverage.

Cost Sharing in General

Cost sharing refers to the amount of money a member must pay out-of-pocket for each type of covered benefit. It applies only to services that are covered by the plan, not to services or goods for which there is no coverage. The three basic types of cost sharing are as follows:

- **Copayment**, meaning a fixed amount of money per type of service—for example, $30 each time a member goes to the doctor
- **Coinsurance**, meaning a percentage of the total dollar amount that is covered—for example, 20% of what the plan will cover for a hospital stay
- **Deductible**, meaning the amount a member must pay out-of-pocket before coverage begins to apply—for example, a $1000 deductible for hospital stays, after which coinsurance applies

All three types of cost sharing may be found in a typical health benefits plan. Deductibles and coinsurance may apply to the same benefit, whereas copayments typically apply to services that are not usually subject to a deductible. For example, a visit to a primary care physician (PCP) who is in the network of a PPO may have a $20 copayment, while a visit to a physician who is not in the network may be subject to a $500 deductible before the PPO makes any payment, but even then the member must pay 20% of the covered amount as well as any amount over what the plan covers.

Cost sharing may also differ by type of service. For example, PCP visits may have a $20 copayment, whereas a hospital stay may be subject to a $1000 deductible and then 10% coinsurance after the deductible is met.

Cost Sharing Under the ACA

The ACA defines levels of allowable cost sharing for QHPs and insured coverage (self-funded plans may be somewhat different). For preventive services, the ACA does not allow any cost sharing at all for any type of plan. For other covered benefits listed in Table 2-1, the ACA defines four basic levels of cost-sharing percentages for EHBs in the individual, group, and insured markets:

- Platinum, defined as 10% or less total cost sharing
- Gold, defined as 20% total cost sharing

- Silver, defined as 30% total cost sharing
- Bronze, defined as 40% total cost sharing

The ACA also defines a special type of benefits plan that may be offered to individuals younger than the age of 30, which has a higher level of cost sharing but a very low premium.

Cost sharing is based on the average total amount of cost sharing for nonemergency services provided by network providers. In other words, it is the combination of copayments, coinsurance, and deductibles—not just one type of cost sharing. It is based on the average total amount of cost sharing for all members, rather than the amount of cost sharing by any particular member. The percentages also reflect how much a plan pays its network providers, such that members who receive nonemergency care from non-network providers are covered only up to the amount a plan would pay based on in-network services. These different tiers apply only to plans sold to individuals and small groups, but all plans must offer at least 60% coverage regardless of plan type.

The ACA also limits the maximum out-of-pocket cost for individuals and for families, after which no further cost sharing may be applied. The dollar amounts are set by the U.S. Treasury Department each year. For example, in 2014, the maximum out-of-pocket costs could be no more than $6350 for an individual and $12,700 for families.

Grandfathered Benefits Plans

Grandfathered health benefits plans refer to plans that were in effect on March 23, 2010, the date of enactment of the ACA. Such plans do not need to comply with all of the ACA's requirements as long as they maintain the grandfathered status. A grandfathered plan loses that status if it changes in any substantial way, such as by changing the benefits or amounts of cost sharing, changing the employee contribution to the cost, or changing insurers.

Grandfathered plans may be exempt from many of the ACA's requirements, but not all of them. Even they must comply with certain requirements, some of which went into effect upon passage of the ACA and others of which went into effect in 2014:

- Grandfathered plans cannot exclude individuals because of a preexisting condition or discriminate based on health status for children younger than age 19.
- They cannot have any lifetime limits on coverage.

- They cannot have any annual limits on coverage.
- They must extend coverage to an employee's dependents until age 26.

Coverage Limitations

Several different types of coverage limitations exist, including the following:

- A benefit may be covered only if it is provided through a contracted provider. For example, a plan that has different levels of coverage for nonemergency services provided by in-network versus out-of-network providers may cover long-term rehabilitative services only when they are provided by a contracted provider.
- The maximum dollar amount of coverage may be based on what the plan pays providers in its network, not what a provider charges.
- Limits may be placed on the number of services or devices covered in a time period. For example, coverage may be limited to one pair of foot orthotics every two years.
- Coverage may be based on medical necessity. For example, the plan may not provide any coverage for care that is experimental or investigational (unless part of an authorized study as defined in the ACA), care that is for the convenience of the patient or provider, and so forth.
- Some services may not be covered under any circumstances. For example, coverage is usually not provided for people who need custodial care because they cannot care for themselves.

In the past, many plans used to limit coverage to a total dollar amount paid in a year, in a person's lifetime, or both. The ACA, however, now prohibits this.

SOURCES OF BENEFITS COVERAGE AND RISK

The sources of benefits coverage refer to where an individual's health benefits come from, while risk refers to who or what is at risk for the cost of payment for those benefits. These two concepts are closely related, but are not identical and are not the same for each group or individual. At its most basic, there are three basic types of coverage sources and three basic types of risk bearing.

Three basic sources of benefits coverage include the following:

- Entitlement programs
- Individual coverage
- Group health benefits plans

Three broad forms of risk bearing include the following:

- Government bears the risk
- Health insurer bears the risk
- Employer bears the risk

These sources of coverage and risk are not mutually exclusive, and health insurance or health benefits coverage for any individual will be some combination of them. Table 2-2 summarizes the sources of coverage and risk.

Sources of Coverage

The sources of coverage refer to where that coverage comes from. This entity may be the company handling the claims, but is not always the same. It is also not always clear what that source is depending on which type of payer is providing the coverage. Nevertheless, the easiest way to consider this issue is to look at these three sources:

- Government entitlement programs
- Individual health insurance
- Employer group health benefits plans, also referred to as group health benefits plans (dropping the word "employer")

Entitlement Programs

In the United States, the federal and state governments actually pay for more than 40% of healthcare costs. Coverage is provided to anyone who is eligible to

Table 2–2   Sources of Coverage and Risk

		Sources of Benefits Coverage		
		Entitlement Programs	**Individual Coverage**	**Group Health Benefits Plans**
Bears Risk for Costs of Covered Health Benefits	**Government**	Traditional Medicare and Medicaid	N/A	Military health benefits plans
	Health Insurer	Medicare Advantage, managed Medicaid	Individual Health Insurance	Employment-based group health insurance
	Employer	Retiree health benefits coverage	N/A	Employment-based group health benefits coverage

get it, meaning that person is entitled to that coverage. Government entitlement programs, which may or may not include all or some managed care features, include the following:

- Medicare
- Medicaid
- Military programs (both direct care by military providers and the Tricare program under the Civilian Health and Medical Program of the Uniformed Services [CHAMPUS])
- Veterans Administration
- U.S. Public Health Service
- Indian Health Service

The largest entitlement programs are Medicare and Medicaid. The Centers for Medicare & Medicaid Services (CMS), a branch of the U.S. Department of Health and Human Services (DHHS), administers Medicare. Medicare provides healthcare benefits for the elderly, for many individuals with end-stage renal disease, and for individuals with some other conditions and disabilities. The states manage their own Medicaid programs, which rely on state and federal funds and provide healthcare benefits to the poor and many disabled or institutionalized individuals. Managed care techniques have been applied to all types of government programs, with specific types of health plans being developed for Medicare and Medicaid. The ACA included language to broaden eligibility for low-income individuals and families for Medicaid; the U.S. Supreme Court invalidated that part of the law, however, so some states have not expanded their Medicaid coverage.

In traditional Medicare and Medicaid programs, the federal or state government uses private payers, such as Blue Cross Blue Shield plans or commercial health insurers, to administer the program. Those private entities, which are called intermediaries, provide only administrative services, so the government (i.e., taxpayers) remains at risk. In contrast, in some private Medicare Advantage and managed Medicaid plans, the risk is transferred from the government to the private plan.

The Federal Employees Health Benefit Program (FEHBP) is an employee benefits program for federal employees. Likewise, state and local governments typically provide benefits to their full-time employees. These are not entitlement programs, however, but rather employer group health benefit plans.

Individual Health Insurance

Several different sources of coverage are available to individuals. For example, individuals may purchase health insurance policies directly from commercial insurance companies. In general, individual health insurance policies are more expensive for the same level of coverage than are group health benefits plans. Under the ACA, as of January 2014 individuals became able to purchase coverage either directly from a health insurer or through a health insurance exchange, as discussed in the *Sales, Governance, and Administration* chapter. Prior to 2014, individuals often needed to pass "medical underwriting," meaning their health status determined whether they could get coverage. That is no longer the case: Individuals cannot be refused coverage based on health status.

Except in the case of "life events," individuals can buy such coverage only during designated periods of the year, typically one month per year, although the ACA allows states to extend these open enrollment periods if they so choose. Individuals' benefits and premiums are affected by provisions of the ACA but managed by the states. The ACA also created an obligation for most people to have coverage, either through their employer or as individuals. Individuals with low incomes or other hardships may be excluded from that requirement, but others face a financial penalty for not purchasing coverage. Subsidies are also available for qualifying low-income individuals and families.

Individuals may also obtain coverage following certain "life events," also called "special eligibility events," such as marriage or divorce, losing a job, or child birth or adoption. They must apply for this coverage within 60 days of the life event or they will lose their eligibility. One option is to obtain coverage through the health insurance exchange.

Another option following a "life event" is to obtain coverage through the Consolidated Omnibus Budget Reconciliation Act of 1985 (COBRA). COBRA requires employers with 20 or more employees to offer certain former employees, retirees, spouses, former spouses, and dependent children the right to temporary continuation of health coverage at group rates. The individual must pay the full cost of that coverage, but it is usually less expensive than an individual policy unless the individual qualifies for subsidized coverage under the ACA. Coverage under COBRA is limited to 18 months in most cases, and the end of that period of coverage is considered a life event for purposes of obtaining coverage through the insurance exchange. (See the chapters titled *Sales, Governance, and Administration* and *Laws and Regulations in Managed Care* for further discussion of the ACA and COBRA.)

When COBRA coverage runs out, that is also a "life event," and in the past, individuals with medical problems could obtain coverage only under the terms of the Health Insurance Portability and Accountability Act of 1996 (HIPAA). This was an important right for individuals who had medical conditions that made it difficult or impossible for them to buy coverage because insurers would not sell to people with preexisting conditions. HIPAA coverage was (and still is) very costly and the benefits poor, however. When the ACA made coverage available to all individuals during an open enrollment or following a life event, that became a far better option than is coverage under HIPAA.

Group Health Benefits Plans

Employer-based group health benefits plans are the largest source of health benefits coverage in the United States, accounting for almost half of all coverage. While employers are not compelled to provide coverage, the ACA requires all employers with more than 50 full-time employees to offer qualified health benefits coverage plans or pay a penalty,* and it provides tax incentives to encourage small employers to offer coverage. Large employers must automatically enroll new employees into their plan, though the employee can opt out. Even when an employer does offer health insurance, not all employees may be considered eligible, however; in fact, temporary or part-time employees are seldom eligible to participate in an employer's health insurance benefits plan.

Group health benefits plans have several advantages:

- The cost of the coverage is paid on a pretax basis.
- Employers can either purchase group health insurance or self-fund the benefits plan.
- Employers, especially large employers, are usually able to obtain more favorable pricing than individuals can.
- Large employers often provide employees with different options for type of health plan or amount of cost sharing.
- Healthcare coverage benefits may be combined with other types of benefits (e.g., flexible spending accounts, health payment accounts, or life insurance).
- The employer—not the individual employee—manages administrative needs such as payroll deductions and payment of premiums.

If costs for a group health benefits plan increase, as they usually do each year, the employer generally absorbs much of that cost increase. Employees typically contribute part of their pretax earnings toward the cost of the coverage, usually around 25% of the total cost. As a consequence, as health plan costs rise, the dollar amount

---

* The penalty applies only if any employees receive subsidized coverage through an insurance exchange. This penalty also applies if the employer does offer a benefits plan, but it is not considered "affordable," and at least one employee obtains subsidized coverage through the exchange.

of the payroll deduction also rises even though it is the same on a percentage basis. An employer may set that payroll deduction (i.e., the amount that the employee must pay) to favor lower-cost choices; for example, there may be a lower payroll deduction if the employee chooses a lower-cost plan. Because healthcare costs usually rise faster than overall inflation, some of the money an employer might have used for pay raises ends up being used to pay for health benefits, so that higher employee payroll deductions affect the amount of total take-home pay.

In all cases, however, the cost of the benefits plan paid by the employer as well as the payroll deduction are pretax expenses, meaning they are not considered taxable income to employees. That is not the case for individual health insurance: Individuals must pay their premiums with after-tax dollars, meaning they cannot deduct it from their income taxes (with some exceptions).

Bearing Risk for Medical Costs

Bearing risk for medical costs refers being responsible for paying for covered healthcare benefits, not the cost of the insurance premium. Contrary to popular belief, a health insurance company does not always bear the financial risks associated with the medical costs of its customers or members. In fact, insurers bear the risk in fewer than half of all group benefits plans, and it is the employers who bear the risk. In other cases, the federal and/or state government bears the risk.

Because many day-to-day payer operations are not tied to who is bearing the risk for medical costs, distinctions about who bears the financial risk will be made throughout this text only when this issue is important, such as its impact on benefits design or on how a plan is regulated.

Government Entitlement Programs

The government is at risk for the traditional entitlement programs. However, commercial Medicare Advantage plans and commercial managed Medicaid plans may contract with the government to provide and administer those benefits, in which case they assume the risk for medical costs (though some managed Medicaid plans share the risk with the state), though most operate under different requirements than purely commercial plans do. Managed care plans in both of the entitlement programs are discussed further in the *Medicare and Medicaid* chapter.

Health Insurance

People purchase healthcare insurance to protect themselves from unexpected medical costs. The insurer provides coverage of medical costs and charges premium rates to groups or individuals that are calculated to cover those costs on average. This is often referred to as "private" or "commercial" health insurance. A private or commercial insurer can be a for-profit or nonprofit organization.

The central point of health insurance is that the risk for medical expenses belongs to the payer. In other words, in exchange for the payment of insurance premiums, the payer is responsible for paying some or most of the cost of medical care provided to individuals, subject to cost sharing and coverage limitations. Whether the actual costs for a group or an individual are higher or lower than average, the premium payment does not change during the period the insurance policy is in effect.

Federal laws and regulations under the ACA, HIPAA, and Employee Retirement Income Security Act of 1974 (ERISA) apply to health insurance, but generally speaking, regulation of insurance is the responsibility of the state governments. Because the regulatory system is highly complex, it is described throughout this text when applicable and addressed specifically in the *Laws and Regulations in Managed Care* chapter.

Self-Funded Employer Health Benefits Plans

Most large corporations do not actually purchase health insurance to cover their employees. Instead, it is the employer that bears the risk benefits plan, a practice called "self-funding." Said another way, in a self-funded plan, the employer is the insurer and the entity that is at risk. Self-funding is mostly used in large groups, although some medium-sized employer groups have also moved to this practice. It is found in large groups because a risk pool (i.e., a group of covered people) must be large enough to be able to predict costs In a small group, the impact of chance and luck—good and bad—is higher than in a large group, where chance and luck average out.

Assuming the risk of medical costs makes it possible for a large employer to avoid paying state premium taxes, offering state-mandated benefits, or being subject to state laws regarding health insurance. Costs in a self-funded group are based only on who is actually covered under the plan (i.e., the company's employees and their dependents, and in some cases the company's retirees) and are not affected by costs incurred by other groups or individuals. Self-funded plans also do not pay the charge that insurers build into their premiums for the cost of taking on risk and to ensure the insurer's profits or margin contributions. The cost of taking on risk is real, however, so self-funded employers also purchase reinsurance.

Self-funded benefits plans are not regulated by the states, but they are regulated by the U.S. Department of Labor and to some degree by the U.S. Department of the Treasury. Self-funded plans are also exempt from some, but not all, requirements under the ACA—although as a practical matter, they do comply with most of the important requirements. As long as an employer complies with the benefits plan requirements under ERISA and the ACA, there is very little regulation involved.

Self-funded plans may mimic any type of health plan. Employers with self-funded plans typically contract with third-party administrators (TPAs) to perform the plan's administrative activities, such as handling enrollment and eligibility, processing claims, and managing appeals. In many cases, the third-party administrator is actually a large health insurance company, a Blue Cross Blue Shield plan, or an HMO, which may cause confusion among both members and providers as to who the insurer actually is. Such commercial payers not only provide administrative services but also pass along to the employers any discounts from the providers. In other cases, a TPA that is not itself an insurer administers the plan but remains behind the scenes, and the self-funded plan contracts with different companies for different services such as accessing a discounted provider network, managing utilization, managing drug benefit claims and so forth.

Provider Risk

In some forms of provider payment, a contracted provider may assume some portion of risk. The most common arrangement is HMO capitation, in which the provider receives a fixed payment for each member each month regardless of which services those members actually obtain from the provider. This type of provider risk is usually limited and does not apply to all medical costs, although some large health systems may take on substantial risk in the form of fixed payments. This important topic is discussed in more detail in the Provider Payment chapter.

Reinsurance

Reinsurance is a high-level type of indemnity insurance that applies only to high-cost cases or higher than predicted overall costs. Large payers are often able to manage risk themselves, but other payers purchase reinsurance that usually is uniform across all of its insured policies. For example, a reinsurer will pay 80% of costs above $1,000,000 for a single case, up to a limit of $5,000,000; or 60% of total costs if they exceed 120% of projected costs, up to a limit of $20,000,000.

Almost all self-funded employer groups also purchase reinsurance. Most states have rules regarding how much reinsurance a self-funded health benefits plan can have before it is considered a commercial group health insurance plan and, therefore, becomes subject to state regulation. For example, if an employer purchases reinsurance to cover expenses that are less than 10% higher than what was budgeted for, the state may claim that the employer is insured and not self-funded, which means it must comply with all state laws and regulations for health insurance.

Reinsurance is not the same as health insurance. It comes in many different forms and is regulated differently from health insurance. A reinsurer can, however, apply different rules for defining when something is covered and when it is not. Benefits plans must treat all of their beneficiaries equally and cannot deny ongoing coverage to an individual based on that person having high medical costs—but a reinsurer can do just that, resulting in the self-funded plan having to continue to pay the benefits costs but having no financial protection from the expenses incurred by the individual.

Prior to 2014, self-funded plans facing reinsurance coverage exclusions or dramatic rate hikes had no options because other reinsurers would include the same coverage exclusions or high premium rates, and health insurers would refuse to underwrite the group as a whole. However, the ACA now requires insurers and HMOs to provide coverage to any individual or group that seeks it, at least during an open enrollment season, although large groups with high costs would still face high premiums.

TYPES OF PAYER ORGANIZATIONS

Serious challenges are associated with attempting to describe the types of payer organizations in a field as dynamic as health insurance and managed care. The healthcare system has been continually evolving in the United States, and change is the only constant. Nevertheless, distinctions remain between different types of payers.

Originally, HMOs, PPOs, and traditional forms of indemnity health insurance were distinct, mutually exclusive products with different approaches to providing healthcare coverage. Today, an observer might be hard pressed to uncover the differences among these and many newer products without reading the fine print. Further confusing this issue is the existence of provider-based integrated delivery systems (IDSs), described in the chapter titled *The Provider Network*.

As a result of these changes, the descriptions of the different types of payer organizations that follow provide only a guideline to the various types of payer organization models or structures. In many cases (or in most cases in some markets), a specific payer will be a hybrid of several specific types.

Nonprofit, For-Profit, and Member-Owned Payer Organizations

There are three different ways that most payer organizations are structured around ownership and governance. These arrangements are described only briefly here because the types of ownership and governance have little real impact on general operations or marketplace behavior.

In a **nonprofit** plan, the payer is not owned by investors or members and cannot therefore distribute profits to its owners. Any profits or margins that a nonprofit organization earns belong only to the nonprofit plan. If a nonprofit organization is sold to a for-profit company, or if it converts from nonprofit to for-profit status, that is considered a type of sale. The nonprofit's assets and marketplace value must benefit the community overall, not any private person or group.

In a **for-profit plan**, the company is owned by investors and has the ability to distribute profits to its investors. Many of these organizations are publicly traded, meaning their stock is listed on the stock market. Others are owned as a for-profit subsidiary of either a for-profit or a nonprofit company; nonprofit companies typically establish for-profit subsidiaries so that the subsidiary's profits can be paid to its corporate parent.

Member-owned means the plan's members own the plan on a collective basis, albeit not in the same way as the shareholders own a publicly traded company. Member-owned plans are technically neither nonprofit nor for-profit entities. Three types of member-owned plans exist:

- Mutual insurers in which policy holders own the company on a mutual (shared) basis.
- Cooperatives (co-ops), which are similar to co-ops found in agriculture or other industries, in which the members of the co-op receive the co-op's services.
- Consumer-owned and -operated plans (CO-OPs), a plan type that was created specifically under the ACA as a means of increasing competition in the health insurance exchanges. CO-OPs are similar to co-ops or mutual insurers but have specific requirements that co-ops and mutual insurers do not have. For example, the ACA is very specific about who may and may not be on a CO-OP's board of directors. The ACA also provided special funding for start-up CO-Ops, but that funding was cut by the Taxpayer Relief Act of 2012.

Nonprofit, for-profit, and member-owned plans are all generally subject to the same state and federal requirements for insurers and/or HMOs. As a practical matter, a payer can have any one of these structures and that choice will have little or no impact on the different types of health plans offered. In other words, all types of payer organizations compete in the same marketplace and are indistinguishable to most people.

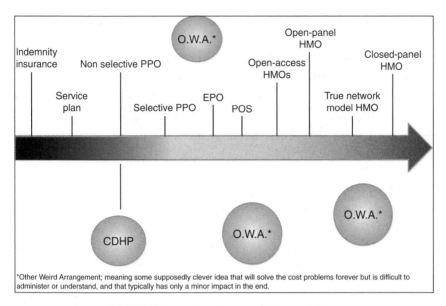

FIGURE 2–1 Continuum of Managed Care

The Continuum of Managed Care

Health insurance and managed care may be thought of as a continuum of models (Figure 2-1). These models are generally classified as follows:

- Indemnity insurance with precertification, mandatory second opinion, and case management
- Service plan with precertification, mandatory second opinion, and case management
- PPO
  - Traditional PPO
  - CDHP plan
- Exclusive provider organization (EPO)
- POS plan
- HMO
  - "Open-access" HMO
  - Open-panel HMOs
    - Independent practice association (IPA)
    - Direct contract HMO
  - True network model HMO
  - Closed-panel HMOs
    - Group model
    - Staff model

As models move toward the managed care end of the continuum, the following features begin to appear and continue:

- Provider contracts defining terms and requirements
- Tighter elements of control over healthcare benefits
- Addition of new elements of control
- More direct interaction with providers
- Increased overhead cost and complexity
- Greater management of utilization
- A net reduction in rate of rise of medical costs

Although it would be comforting to classify all payers using the models defined here, payers are anything but uniform and often offer most or all of the various types of plans other than closed-panel HMOs. The classification of health plans that follows has little to do with which party carries the actual risk for medical expense, or what the organization's ownership status is. All of these types of plans are licensed by states as health insurers except for HMOs, which are licensed separately.*

In the discussion here, various forms of provider payment and medical management approaches will be mentioned when they differ from one type of plan to another, but will not be fully described. Provider payment is the topic of the *Provider Payment* chapter, and medical management is the focus of the *Utilization Management, Quality Management, and Accreditation* chapter.

Traditional Health Insurance

Basically, two types of traditional health insurance exist: indemnity insurance and service plans. This type of plan is called traditional because it was the dominant form of coverage in the past—not because it still is. The costs of traditional health insurance rose rapidly beginning in the early to mid-1970s, such that it became very expensive compared to managed care plans and therefore could not effectively compete in the U.S. marketplace. The share accounted for by traditional insurance has now shrunk to less than 1% of the total market for healthcare coverage, although many of the companies that began as traditional insurers remain robust, as they changed along with the market.

---

* Technically, insurers are licensed while HMOs are issued a Certificate of Authority. Insurance licenses are only required for products for which the plan bears the risk. When they administer self-funded benefit plans, they are usually separately licensed as Third Party Administrators as well.

Indemnity Insurance

Indemnity health insurance protects (indemnifies) the insured (i.e., the policy holder) against financial losses from medical expenses. A person covered under an indemnity plan may receive coverage from any licensed provider. The insurance company may reimburse the subscriber for medical expenses, or it may pay the provider directly, although it has no actual obligation other than to pay the subscriber unless required to under a state's laws. Payment to physicians and other professional providers is subject to usual, customary, or reasonable (UCR) fee screens, whereas payment to institutional providers is generally based on charges. There is no contract between the insurer and the providers.

Benefits are generally subject to a deductible and coinsurance (except for preventive services as required by the ACA). Any charges by the provider that the insurance company does not pay are strictly the responsibility of the subscriber. Most plans usually require precertification of elective hospital admissions and may apply a financial penalty to the subscriber who fails to obtain precertification. Case management may also be used to help control the very high costs of catastrophic cases (e.g., a severely premature infant, a trauma case). Second opinions may be mandatory for certain elective procedures (e.g., surgery for obesity).

While traditional indemnity insurance has nearly vanished as a stand-alone product, it is still used for coverage of out-of-network services by certain types of plans. Most traditional carriers that remained in the health insurance sector have evolved to offer the other products described here, using the same insurance license.

Service Plans

Technically speaking, a service plan is not insurance, but rather a form of prepaid health care, and it applies primarily, though not exclusively, to Blue Cross and Blue Shield (BCBS) plans. At the time service plans came into being, they were controlled by the hospitals and/or physicians providing the services, but that is no longer the case. Service plans are now much more like traditional health insurers.

In service plans, relatively few restrictions are placed on licensed providers who sign a contract with the plan. This first appearance of a contract is an important milestone, and a feature of all types of plans except indemnity insurers. A service plan's provider contract typically contains certain key provisions:

- The plan agrees to pay the provider directly, eliminating collection problems with patients.
- The provider agrees to accept the plan's fee schedule as payment in full and not to bill the subscriber for any charges that exceed the

amount the plan pays, other than any deductible, coinsurance, and/or copayments.

- The provider agrees to allow the plan to audit the provider's records related to billed charges.
- Like indemnity insurance, service plans may require precertification, case management, and second opinions.

The principal advantage of a service plan over indemnity insurance lies in the provider contracts and the providers' agreement to accept the service plan's payment terms and not "balance bill" the plan's members for any charges above the amount allowed by the service plan. This, too, is a feature found in all of the other types of plans except indemnity insurance. It applies only to contracted providers, however; noncontracted providers can and do balance bill patients.

Professional fees allowed under the fee schedule represent a discount to the plan. More importantly, the plan usually obtains discounts at hospitals that indemnity plans do not. The hospitals grant these discounts for a variety of reasons, the most important of which is timely and direct payment. Some large service plans require providers to give them "most favored nation" pricing; in other words, a provider may not offer a better discount to a competitor than it does to the service plan. Such favored-nation pricing has become less common because of regulatory and legal pressure, and it is even prohibited in a number of states.

Most, but not all, service plans have evolved into PPOs, but they remain an underpinning for the non-HMO products the plans offer, as well as the basis for coverage of out-of-network benefits by other types of plans.

Preferred Provider Organizations

Although PPOs are similar to service plans, there are some important differences. A PPO typically has a smaller panel of providers than does a service plan, sometimes substantially smaller (e.g., to 30% of the total number of providers available in the area). Most PPOs have more terms and conditions for participation by providers compared to service plans, such as a requirement that physicians be board certified. PPO provider discounts are generally higher than those obtained by non-PPO service plans. The exception occurs when a large service plan has a favored-nation agreement with providers (such agreements are increasingly uncommon) or has already negotiated a significant discount. In that case, the service plan's payment terms are adopted by the PPO.

PPO networks may contract with "any willing provider" (AWP*) or they may be selective about accepting providers into the network. In the former approach, any provider who wishes to participate in the organization and who meets the conditions and agrees to the terms of the PPO's contract is offered a contract. Selective PPOs, by comparison, apply some objective criteria (e.g., location-based network need, credentials, or practice pattern analysis) before contracting with a provider. Any-willing-provider PPOs are common, particularly as numerous state laws require this arrangement, but the use of criteria-based selection still occurs, particularly with expensive or highly specialized services (e.g., for cardiac surgery). It is also being used by many insurers that offer products through the health insurance exchanges.

Precertification and case management are almost always components of PPOs, and many include some concurrent hospital stay review as well as some level of disease management. A major difference between PPOs and traditional or service plans is that failure to comply with PPOs' utilization management requirements results in a financial penalty to the provider, not the member. As with service plans, a contracting provider may not bill the member for any balance that the PPO does not pay, and that includes any payment penalties associated with the provider not complying with precertification.

A hallmark of a PPO is that benefits are reduced if a member seeks nonemergency care from a provider who is not in the PPO network. A common benefits differential is 20% based on allowed charges. For example, if a member sees a network provider, coverage is provided at 80% of allowed charges; if a member sees a provider who is not in the network, the coverage may be limited to 60% of allowed charges. If the nonparticipating provider charges more than the allowed charges, the member is responsible for all charges above what the PPO paid and what the provider charged. An example of how this works may be seen in the *Provider Payment* chapter in the table titled "Example of the Use of Maximum Allowable Charge in a PPO."

Providers agree to discount their services to a PPO because the smaller network combined with the benefits coverage differentials serve to channel patients toward participating providers. Of equal importance, this approach eliminates the risk of losing patients who switch to participating providers. PPOs are less expensive than traditional insurance, but usually more expensive than HMOs. Because they have fewer restrictions and typically contract with larger networks than do HMOs, PPOs have the largest share of the market.

---

* Not to be confused with "AWP" referring to "Average Wholesale Price" in prescription drug coverage.

Risk-Bearing PPOs

PPOs can be either risk bearing or non-risk bearing. A risk-bearing PPO combines the insurance, or payment, function with the management of the network of providers. As a risk-bearing entity, it must be licensed as a health insurer itself or owned by a health insurer and offered as one of the insurer's products.

Non-Risk-Bearing or Rental PPOs

Most payers have their own networks, but no payer—other than the federal Medicare program—has a network in place in all parts of the United States. Mid-size to large employers, however, frequently have employees who live and/or work in locations where a payer may not have a contracted network. In those areas, this potentially means the PPO may have to pay for care delivered based on full charges, and members may not have the protections found in most provider contracts. Self-funded employer groups that use third-party administrators instead of a full-service payer face a similar issue because TPAs typically do not have a network of their own.

Blue Cross and Blue Shield plans address this risk through their BlueCard program, in which a member of one BCBS plan is able to access another BCBS plan's network providers when away from home. This mechanism is based on an agreement among the Blues plans because those plans are independent, but does provide for seamless access to any Blues network.

Non-BCBS plans must take a different approach for supplementing their own networks, as do self-funded employer groups that use TPAs. The solution in both cases is to contract with one or more rental networks. A rental network comprises a network created either by the providers themselves or by a company that is not affiliated with a single payer. Some payers do rent their networks to noncompetitor payers, but that is not common. Rental networks are almost always PPO networks, rather than HMO networks (which have more requirements than do PPOs). Any PPO created by providers must not violate antitrust requirements, meaning it cannot act as a means of suppressing competition.

Rental PPOs typically charge an access fee, as well as separate fees for other services they may provide, such as utilization or case management services. Usually the rental PPO's providers send the claims to the rental PPO, which then reprices them and sends the claims on to the payer or TPA for processing. The rental PPO usually keeps a percentage of the difference between the full charges and the discount.

Depending on the state, non-risk-bearing PPOs may not need a license if they simply provide access to contracted providers. If the PPO also performs, it may need to be licensed as a utilization review organization of some type. Likewise, if it performs any other administrative functions, including prepricing of claims, it may need to be licensed as a TPA even though it does not otherwise process the claims.

In decades past, payers did not always make it clear when they contracted with rental PPOs, and there was no indicator on the member's identification (ID) card about any rental PPOs. Providers that contracted with the rental PPO but not directly with a payer would find themselves receiving the PPO payment and not the billed charges, requiring them to write down the difference. This could even happen in an area in which both a payer and a rental PPO had networks, but did not include all the same providers. At the time this was occurring, the arrangement was known as a "stealth" or "silent" PPO. Silent PPOs are now uncommon after several lawsuits were filed challenging this practice, and payers that contract with rental PPOs now typically put the logo(s) of the rental PPO(s) someplace on the member's ID card, usually on the back.

High-Deductible Health Plans and Consumer-Directed Health Plans

Each year, the Internal Revenue Service determines what the minimum and maximum deductibles need to be to qualify as a high-deductible health plan (HDHP). For 2014, the minimum deductible was $1200 for individuals and $6350 for families; the maximum allowable deductible was $2500 for individuals and $12,700 for families. In all cases, preventive services are not counted toward the deductible. HDHPs are usually associated with PPO networks, and the amounts paid toward the deductible are based on in-network costs, not out-of-network costs, just as with any other type of PPO. The maximum deductible amounts for HDHPs are the same as the maximum amount of out-of-pocket spending allowed under the ACA for all insured health plans, and fall within the coverage requirements for a bronze-level plan.

A consumer-directed health plan is an HDHP combined with a pretax savings account. A pretax account set up as part of an employer group health benefits plan is referred to as a health reimbursement account (HRA), and a pretax account applied to individual coverage is referred to as a health savings account (HSA). While they have differences, the overall concept is the same for both types of accounts.*

---

* Some other types of pretax benefits accounts exist, such as flexible spending accounts (FSAs), but those are beyond the scope of this text.

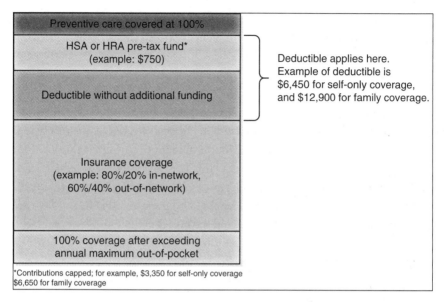

FIGURE 2-2 Example of Basic Construct of a Consumer-Directed Health Plan

In a CDHP, qualified healthcare costs (except preventive care) are paid first from the pretax account; when that is exhausted, any additional costs up to the deductible are paid out-of-pocket by the member (this gap is sometimes referred to as a bridge or a doughnut hole). The IRS also defines what is considered a qualified medical cost, but it is similar to what would be considered a medical cost in any coverage plan. To be paid from an HRA or HSA, costs must have been incurred while the account existed. A simplistic schematic of a CDHP appears in Figure 2-2.

Point-of-Service Plans

POS plans combine features of HMOs and traditional indemnity health insurance plans, so are similar to PPOs in some ways. In a POS plan, members may choose which system to use at the point at which they obtain the service. For example, if a member uses his or her PCP and otherwise complies with the HMO authorization system, minimal cost sharing is required. If the member chooses to self-refer or otherwise not to use the HMO system to receive services, the POS plan still provides insurance coverage but with higher levels of cost sharing, including a higher deductible and coinsurance instead of a copayment.

POS plans are typically based on HMOs, but even then there are two common forms they can take. The first is a POS plan with two options for cost sharing: (1) minimal cost sharing if the member chooses to stay within the HMO system and (2) significantly higher levels of cost sharing if the member chooses to go outside the HMO system. The difference between coverage for in-network services and out-of-network services is usually in the range of 30% to 40%.

The second type of POS plan is a triple-option plan in which there is minimal cost sharing when the HMO system is used, but there is also an option to use a PPO that is part of the plan, so the amount of cost sharing will be higher than when the HMO is used, but more closely follows typical PPO benefits design. In other words, cost sharing in this middle tier is less than the amount of cost sharing required for using providers who are not in either the HMO or PPO network. The differences between coverage for HMO in-network services, PPO in-network services, and out-of-network services are usually approximately 20% between the HMO level and the PPO level, and from 40% to 50% between the HMO and out-of-network levels.

Some states, such as California, require all HMOs to offer POS benefits. While POS plans were initially popular, they have become less so over the years because their costs are often higher than either PPOs (with more cost sharing) or HMOs (with more controls).

Exclusive Provider Organizations

EPOs are similar to open-access HMOs, though most are not actually HMOs. Except in the case of a medical emergency, benefits are available only when services are provided by the EPO's network providers. EPOs' management of utilization and quality is similar to the mechanisms applied by PPOs and does not involve any requirements to go through a PCP to access specialty care. EOPs are relatively uncommon, being mostly used in self-funded employer group benefits plans for a single employer or in plans offered to government employees. Commercial payers may offer their existing HMO or PPO networks to an employer to be used for that company's EPO, although an EPO can be based on a rental PPO's network as well. EPOs do not necessarily need to be licensed if the EPO serves only an employer's self-funded health benefits plan.

Health Maintenance Organizations

HMOs are unique in many ways. The majority of HMOs manage utilization and quality to a greater degree than do PPOs. Except for emergency care or when a state requires HMOs to offer POS benefits, benefits coverage in an HMO applies when services are provided by the HMO's providers in compliance with the HMO's authorization policies and procedures. Exceptions may be made on occasion when the HMO authorizes benefits for non-network services based on specific medical needs. Benefits obtained through the HMO almost always have much lower cost-sharing than is found in any other type of health plan. Payment for services received from non-HMO providers is the responsibility of the subscriber, not the HMO, unless the HMO is also a POS plan. Services delivered by contracted providers who fail to obtain proper authorization are the responsibility of the provider, who may not bill the subscriber for any fees not paid by the HMO. At least some providers in most HMO networks are paid using risk-based payment models.

Traditional HMOs currently fall into two broad categories: open panel and closed panel. These terms are no longer widely used but are helpful for understanding the different types of HMOs. A third category, the true network model, is relatively uncommon except in certain parts of the United States; that term may also be applied more broadly to open-panel HMOs. Some HMOs combine or mix different model types in the same market. Because open-access HMOs are not considered traditional HMOs, they are discussed separately from traditional open- and closed-panel plans.

Open-Access HMOs

Open-access HMOs are more like EPOs than traditional HMOs, at least regarding benefits design. In the open-access HMO model, members may access any provider in the HMO without going through a PCP. Thus, members may see any PCP or specialist in the network on a self-referral basis, as in EPOs. Unlike in EPOs, however, physicians in an open-access HMO typically share at least some level of risk for costs.

Open-access plans were popular in the late 1970s and early 1980s, especially plans sponsored by local medical societies and community physicians who saw traditional HMOs as a threat to their livelihoods. With a few exceptions, these early plans suffered substantial losses and failed. Interest in open-access plans was later revived because of consumer demands, particularly at the height of the managed care backlash. It is certainly logical for consumers to demand the following characteristics associated with open-access plans:

- Rich benefits coverage
- Low premiums and out-of-pocket costs
- Unlimited access to all providers in the community

Wanting those aspects of service may be logical but is not realistic. In reality, a health benefits plan can meet any two of those three demands, but not all three of them simultaneously.

The HMOs that currently use an open-access design assume that, because so few referral authorizations are denied, the referral requirement is not worth the cost. However, a PCP will be able to deliver routine care more cost-effectively than a specialist. Therefore, most open-access HMOs have substantial cost-sharing differences for care provided by a specialist compared with that provided by a PCP.

Open-Panel Plans

In an open-panel HMO (not to be confused with an open-access HMO), private physicians and other professional providers are independent contractors who see HMO members in their own offices or facilities. Physicians in the network typically contract with more than one competing health plan and also see non-HMO patients. A variety of payment mechanisms may be used in an open-panel HMO. The total number of providers in an open-panel plan is larger than that in a closed-panel plan but usually smaller than that in a PPO. Each member must choose a PCP, and they go first to their PCP for medical care; any other services must then be authorized by their PCP. PCPs are defined as physicians specializing in family medicine, internal medicine, and pediatrics. Women can access their obstetrician/gynecologist (OB/Gyn) directly—direct access to OB/Gyns for women is required under the ACA but was allowed by HMOs even prior to the ACA's passage—but most HMOs still require them to choose a PCP. Members may change their PCPs at designated times if they wish as long as that PCP has the capacity to take on a new patient.

Open-panel plans fall into two broad categories: IPA models, which are the most common type of HMO, and direct contract models, which are the second most common type. Although the terms IPA and direct contract model are often used synonymously, the two models are distinct.

In an IPA model, the HMO contracts with a legal entity known as an independent practice association and pays it a negotiated capitation amount. The IPA, in turn, contracts with private physicians to provide health care to the HMO members. The IPA may pay the physicians through capitation or use another payment mechanism, such as a fee-for-service scheme. The providers are at risk under this model in that if medical costs exceed the capitation amount, the IPA receives no additional funds from the HMO and must accordingly adjust its payments to the providers. Most IPAs purchase reinsurance to protect themselves financially, and some HMOs provide a similar type of protection from high costs as part of the overall contract. Finally, the scope of what IPAs do varies, with some focusing on payment terms, and others taking on many routine HMO functions involving medical management and the like.

In the direct contract model, the HMO contracts directly with the providers; there is no intervening entity. The HMO pays the providers directly and performs all related management tasks.

Closed-Panel Plans

Unlike physicians in an open-panel plan, physicians in a closed-panel plan either are members of a single large medical group or are employed by the HMO. The total number of providers in a closed-panel plan is by far the smallest of any model type. Members usually do not have to choose a single PCP but may see any PCP or any physician in the HMO; however, they may be asked to choose a primary facility to ensure continuity of care.

Closed-panel plans fall into two broad categories: group model and staff model. In a group model plan, the HMO contracts with a single medical group to provide services to members. The HMO pays the group a negotiated capitation amount, and the group in turn pays the individual physicians through a combination of salary and risk/reward incentives. The group is responsible for its own governance, and the physicians are either partners in the group or employed by the group as associates. The group is at risk in that if the costs of the group exceed the capitation amount, physician compensation is less—although the HMO generally provides stop-loss reinsurance to the group to protect it from catastrophic cost overruns. Closed-panel HMOs also contract with private physicians to provide services that the HMO's physicians do not provide.

Several types of group model HMOs exist. In one type, the HMO and medical group are distinct entities that operate as if they were partners. The largest and best-known example of this type of group model HMO is Kaiser Permanente; the HMO is the Kaiser Foundation Health Plan, and the medical groups are the Permanente Medical Groups (there are different groups for each of Kaiser's regions). In another type of group model HMO, the medical group established the HMO. An example of this type of HMO is the Geisinger Health Plan, a large and successful HMO established by the Geisinger Clinic in Danville, Pennsylvania.

Some medical groups exist primarily on paper and actually operate strictly as cost pass-through vehicles for the HMO; that is, the costs are simply passed from the medical group to the HMO, and the group does not actually bear any risk for medical expenses. This arrangement resembles a staff model plan.

In a staff model plan, the HMO directly employs its physicians. In some cases, the physicians are employed by a medical group, but it functions like a staff-based organization. Physicians receive a salary, and there is an incentive plan of some sort. The HMO has full responsibility for the management of all activities. Staff model plans run by free-standing HMOs are almost extinct now, but still exist as HMOs created by large integrated healthcare delivery systems (IDS). In this case, the IDS owns or manages the HMO, and the physicians are employed either by the IDS or by a captive medical group.

True Network Model HMOs

The term "network model" is often used to refer to an open-panel plan, but in the "true" network model, the HMO contracts with several large multispecialty medical groups for services. The groups receive payment under a capitation arrangement, and they in turn pay the physicians under a variety of mechanisms. The groups operate relatively independently. The HMO contracts with more than one group, but the number of groups is usually limited. True network models are most common in California but are also found elsewhere (e.g., in Massachusetts and New York).

Mixed-Model HMOs

Nothing in this world is pure and simple, and HMOs—like all types of payer organizations—are no exception. Many HMOs have adopted several model types, even in the same market, to attract as many members as possible and capture additional market share. Such mixed-model HMOs may offer the different models in the same products, or the models may operate independently of each other in different products.

CONCLUSION

Any understanding of health insurance and managed care requires a basic understanding of how coverage is accessed and what the basic components of coverage are. No matter which type of health plan or payer is involved, those sources and components change only in their specifics; they are always present regardless of any other features.

The means for administering coverage exists on an ever-evolving landscape of plan types with mutating definitions and operational structures. Even so, the traditional terms such as HMO and PPO retain considerable utility, including stability in the overall aspects of their operations. This characteristic should be looked on not as a hindrance toward understanding but as a mark of the exciting and dynamic nature of the industry.

The Provider Network

LEARNING OBJECTIVES

- Identify the basic elements of payer–provider contracts
- Describe service areas and access standards
- Explain basic credentialing
- Identify the basic types of contracted healthcare professionals
- Identify the basic types of contracted healthcare facilities
- Identify the basic types of contracted integrated provider healthcare delivery systems
- Describe basic contracting for ancillary services
- Discuss basic network maintenance

INTRODUCTION

The backbone of any managed healthcare plan is the provider network, which is made up of contracted physicians and nonphysician professionals, facilities, providers of ancillary and therapeutic services, and medical vendors of various types. In many cases, distinctions between provider types that were once clear have blurred over the years as new organizational models have appeared and evolved, leading to differences in how payers contract and interact with them.

This chapter explores many different aspects of provider networks. We begin by looking at basic provider contracting concepts and a few important elements common to providers in general, and then examine the most common types of providers and organizational structures:

- Professionals providing health care, with a focus on physicians
- Inpatient facilities, such as the various types of hospitals

- Ambulatory facilities, such as outpatient surgical centers
- Integrated healthcare delivery systems (IDSs), which combine facilities and professionals from an organizational and contracting standpoint

This chapter does not address provider payment, except in broad terms when such discussion is necessary in the context of the chapter. Provider payment is the subject of its own dedicated chapter in this text. One reason for separating payment from everything else is that payment is no longer as tightly linked to specific types of providers as it once was. The other—and perhaps more important—reason is the sheer complexity of provider payment models and the vast number of payment models currently in use.

CONTRACTS AND CONTRACTING

All types of payers other than the (now rare) indemnity plan rely on contracts between the plan and its network of providers. These contracts are legally binding documents that define the terms, conditions, and obligations to which both parties have agreed. In this section we consider why providers and payers might seek a contract in the first place. In addition, we examine some of the key elements found within most contracts, and briefly address contract management.

Payers usually handle provider recruiting and contracting at a local or regional level, but some types of contracting are more centralized. In recent years, many payers have actually outsourced this function, meaning the payer contracts with another company to develop and negotiate contracts with the members of its network. Some payers or health plans contract with an independent network or networks and have no direct responsibilities for managing it in any way; in some cases a health plan engages in such an arrangement for its entire network, and many do this for services provided outside of their service areas where they do not have their own contracted network.

Why Contract?

Contracts between payers and providers are voluntary on both sides, but they are also widely used. Both payers and providers have their own reasons for wanting to contract with at least some, if not all, health plans in their area. Table 3-1 provides some examples of payer and provider reasons for contracting.

Basic Elements of a Provider Contract

Typical contracts between payers and providers contain page after page of definitions, terms, obligations, and other details of the payer–provider agreement. Items that are not expected to change with any frequency are placed in the body

---

Table 3–1   Payer and Provider Reasons for Contracting

Examples of Reasons That Payers Contract	Examples of Reasons That Providers Contract
• Provide members with access to appropriate medical services and meet plan access standards required by states and by Medicare	• Have plan members be preferentially directed or steered to other contracting providers, including specialists and hospitals
• Obtain favorable pricing, meaning less than full charges*	• Ensure that the provider will not be excluded from the network of a large payer, thereby losing business to a competitor
• Define the types of clinical services the provider will provide to plan members	• Obtain favorable (higher) pricing when in a strong negotiating position*
• Define the conditions that determine whether a clinical service will be covered as a benefit and when it is not covered	• Obtain direct payment from the payer*
• Reach contractual agreement for clauses required by state laws and regulations, which may differ somewhat for different types of plans	• Ensure timely payment, meaning getting paid within a defined time period, usually 30 days or less and often 10 days or less*
	• Define rights related to disputing claims and payments

* Payment-related issues are discussed in the *Provider Payment* chapter, but are included here because payment is almost always an important element of any contract between a payer and a provider.

---

of the contract. Items that are subject to frequent changes, such as actual payment terms and dollar amounts, typically appear in appendices, so that those items may be renegotiated without having to open the rest of the contract to renegotiation. Some of the contractual terms and language will be the same for all types of providers; other terms and language will apply only to specific types of providers such as professionals or facilities. The discussion here provides broad descriptions of common elements, and some of the important but differing elements found in professional contracts and facility contracts.

Definitions

Definitions are just that—they define terms that are used elsewhere in the contract. Examples of items that are typically defined include the following:

- The type or types of health plan(s) using the contract, such as a health maintenance organization (HMO) or a preferred provider organization (PPO)
- The type or types of provider(s) to which the contract applies, such as primary care physicians (PCPs), specialist physicians, hospitals, ambulatory procedure centers, and so forth

- Plan components, such as member, subscriber, medical director, and so forth
- Routine medical services, noncovered services, and experimental and/or investigational services, some of which may be defined by reference to a plan's evidence of coverage document (described in the *Sales, Governance, and Administration* chapter)
- Services that providers are expected to provide under the contract
- Services that providers are not expected to provide under the contract
- "Medically necessary" and "emergent or urgent" medical services

Qualifications and Credentials

Participating providers must maintain a defined set of qualifications and credentials as a condition of participation, and the basic requirements are usually included in the main body of the contract. This clause may include some requirements that will not change over time, such as the provider needing to have a current and unrestricted license, as well as language requiring compliance with qualification and credentialing requirements found in an attachment or appendix.

Compliance with Utilization and Quality Management Programs

The contract contains requirements that the provider comply with the payer's utilization management (UM) and quality management (QM) programs, as well as the payer's obligations under these programs. The actual QM and UM programs are typically described in attachments or appendices to the contract to accommodate periodic changes in these programs.

Direct and Timely Submission of Claims

The provider agrees to send claims directly to the payer, not to the member. The contract also specifies when claims must be submitted, and indicates that claims submitted after that period of time will not be paid.

"Hold Harmless" and "No Balance Billing" Clauses

This important section of the contract describes the provider's agreement to accept as payment in full for medical services provided to plan members the amount that the plan determines to be appropriate. It applies to all participating providers in the same manner. For example, if a physician normally charges $100 for an office visit but the plan's allowable fee schedule is $75, then the physician agrees that under no circumstances will he or she bill the plan member for the $25 difference; in other words, the provider will not "balance bill" that difference. The provider agrees to accept payment only from the plan, except for the portion that is the clear obligation of the member, such as a copayment, coinsurance (percentages are based on the total allowed amount, not the billed amount), or deductible.

A stronger variation on the "no balance billing" clause is the "hold harmless" clause, which prohibits the provider from billing the member even in the event that the plan does not pay the fee at all.

All state and federal regulatory agencies require the "no balance billing" clause for contracts between providers and the plans for almost all forms of managed care plan. The stronger "hold harmless" clause is an absolute requirement for HMOs and a likely requirement for most PPOs and service plans. When a contract has a "hold harmless" clause, it typically includes the requirement to no balance bill; in other words, most contracts do not contain both clauses, only one or the other.

Payment

The body of the contract typically contains a short clause describing in general that the plan will pay the provider according to the contract's various requirements, then refers to an attachment or appendix for the detailed description of the method or methods of payment. The actual dollar amounts are also usually placed in an attachment or appendix because they change from time to time.

Timely Payment

The definition of timely payment may be included in the section on payment, or it may be a separate clause. It sets the requirements for how quickly the plan must pay a "clean" claim, meaning a claim that has been processed and not held until more information is submitted and that has not been rejected because the claim form was not correctly filled out.

Other-Party Liability and Coordination of Benefits

In some cases, more than one payer may be responsible for coverage of medical services. For example, two working parents may both have coverage through their employers' plans. If the couple's child receives medical care, coordination of benefits rules determine which parent's plan will be considered the primary payer and which parent's plan will be considered the secondary payer. Similarly, other party liability rules, which can vary from state to state, determine when a different type of insurance is designated as primary in terms of the health plan's coverage; for example, an automobile insurance policy may be the primary payer for medical care related to an accident.

Right to Audit

The contract gives the plan the right to conduct audits of medical records and billing data related to care provided to plan members. Audits are typically done for a specific reason, such as a concern about billing problems, but they may also be performed as part of a plan's QM program. QM audits are confined to medical records of members, usually focused on only those seen in PCPs' offices, and only for specified conditions, although they may also focus on a provider as part of an investigation of a quality-related concern.

Term and Termination

One section of the contract specifies the period over which the contract remains in effect and the circumstances under which either party may terminate it. Termination provisions have become very complex in many states. In the past, either party could terminate the contract simply by giving adequate notice—90 days' notice, for example. Some states require payers that no longer want a provider's services to furnish the provider with the reason(s) for termination, and a few states have created due process requirements that allow a terminated provider to dispute the termination. Contracts also usually specify terms under which a contract may be terminated immediately—for example, if the provider's license is suspended or restricted, or if the payer determines that a provider represents an immediate threat to the health of its members. In addition, contracts may provide for provisional participation defining a time period during which some deficiency must be resolved. For example, it takes some time for a newly trained specialist to receive specialty board certification, so the contract may allow that physician to participate as long as board certification is obtained in an appropriate amount of time.

Nondiscrimination

The nondiscrimination clause requires the provider to treat plan members no differently than the provider treats any other patients. In other words, the provider may not discriminate against plan members.

Attachments or Appendices

As mentioned, certain contract terms and specifics are subject to periodic change, so they are placed in attachments or appendices to the contract. Examples include actual payment rates and the full descriptions of programs with which the provider must comply, such as the payer's UM and QM programs.

SERVICE AREAS, AND ACCESS STANDARDS OR NETWORK ADEQUACY

The service area is a fundamental concept in managed health care. It is defined by state laws and regulations for HMOs, point-of-service (POS) plans, and managed Medicaid plans. Some states also have service area requirements for PPOs, although not all have followed this path. Federal laws and regulations define service areas for Medicare Advantage (MA) plans, but if a state's requirements are more stringent, then the state's apply.

The service area is simply the defined geographic area in which the plan provides access to primary and specialty care, hospital care, emergency care, and certain other health services. If an HMO cannot provide sufficient access to providers in a geographic area, it will not be allowed to sell its services in that area.

Health insurers typically are licensed to sell their products and services anywhere throughout the state in which they are licensed, and that permission often applies to their PPO products as well. Some states, however, require PPOs to meet access requirements for a defined service area, though they are usually are more loosely defined than are HMO standards. Most large employers have access requirements as well, though they may differ for a local HMO versus a regional or national PPO.

Service area network access standards—also called network adequacy standards—are usually defined by county, by ZIP code, or by travel time for each type of provider. Minimum access requirements for professional providers usually differ for PCPs, specialists, and behavioral healthcare providers, in recognition of the reality that it is reasonable to travel a little farther to see a specialist. HMO access requirements for PCPs count only PCPs with open practices, meaning those that are accepting new patients. Distance requirements for rural areas usually allow for fewer providers per geographic area or for greater travel time.

Medicare uses formulas to calculate the minimum number of hospitals and physicians that an MA plan must have under contract for each specialty on a county-by-county basis. While not common, a few states define access standards according to how long it takes to get an appointment; such requirements apply only to managed care plans, not the providers, and do not take into account how long it takes to get an appointment regardless of the type of coverage.

A generic example of access requirements might look like the following:*

- PCPs
  - Urban: Two within 3 miles of each ZIP code
  - Rural: Two within 30 miles of each ZIP code
- Specialty physicians (may vary by type of specialist)
  - Urban: Two within 30 miles of each ZIP code
  - Rural: Each major specialty within 100 miles of each ZIP code
- Acute care hospitals
  - Urban: Within 30 minutes of each ZIP code
  - Rural: Within 30 miles of each ZIP code
- Specialty care hospitals
  - Urban: Within 1 hour of each ZIP code
  - Rural: Within 3 hours of each ZIP code

Access standards are minimums, not maximums. Many health plans participating in the health insurance exchanges created under the ACA created products that used networks that were narrower, or smaller, than the networks used by their non-exchange products, while still meeting regulatory access requirements. The plans did this to better manage costs under the presumption that new members who obtained coverage through the exchanges would include many people who were sicker than average. However, it was initially difficult for consumers to figure out exactly which providers were in these networks and whether they were even accepting new patients. As a result, many states and even the federal government are considering redrafting network adequacy standards for exchange-based products, though no actions have been taken at the time of publication.

PHYSICIANS AND OTHER PROFESSIONALS

The typical health plan network includes many different types of clinical professionals, including many for which no access standards apply. For purposes of this chapter, such providers include many different types of licensed professional

---

* Generic examples are just that and should not be relied upon in place of any state or federal access requirements for any particular plan.

healthcare providers who hold a valid and unrestricted license in the state in which they practice, independently (meaning not under the supervision of a physician), whose services are paid for separately from any payments to a facility, and who meet the plan's credentialing requirements.

For purposes of payment, credentialing, directory listing, and so forth, nonphysician professionals who are employed by a facility or by a physician and work under supervision are typically not considered to be network providers—for example, nurses who staff a hospital, pharmacists employed by a pharmacy, and laboratory technicians. These employed professionals do not bill directly for their services, although the facility or physician may include their services as part of any overall charges.

Exhibit 3-1 provides examples of types of professional healthcare providers found in payer networks.

Primary Care and Specialty Care Physicians

Most managed care organizations divide the physician network into PCPs and specialty care physicians ("specialists"), but in reality such distinctions are not always clear. Even in the absence of a health plan design that requires enrollees to

---

Exhibit 3–1 Examples of Types of Physicians and Other Professional Healthcare Providers found in Payer's Networks

- Physicians (MD, DO):
  - Primary care physicians
  - Specialty care physicians (specialists), including hospital-based physicians
- Physicians other than MDs or DOs:
  - Podiatrists (DPM) ·
  - Dentists (DDS), orthodontists (DMD), and oral surgeons (MD)
  - Chiropractors (DC)
- Nonphysician medical practitioners who provide primary care:
  - Certified nurse practitioners (CNP or NP), including certified registered nurse anesthetists (CRNA)
  - Physician assistants (PA)
- Behavioral health and substance abuse therapists:
  - Psychiatrists (MD)
  - Psychologists (PhsD, PsyD, or EdD)
  - Psychiatric nurse practitioners (PNP) or nurse psychotherapists (NP)
  - Licensed clinical social workers (LCSW)
  - Licensed professional counselors (LPC)
  - Marital and family therapists
  - Certified alcohol and drug abuse counselors

(continues)

Exhibit 3–1 *(continued)*

- Other professionals:
  - Optometrists
  - Pharmacists
  - Physical therapists
  - Other rehabilitation therapists
  - Occupational therapists
  - Nutritionists
  - Acupuncturists
  - Audiologists
  - Respiratory therapists
  - Home healthcare providers

---

access their PCP to obtain either direct care or referral authorization for specialty care (i.e., "gatekeeper" HMOs), a great deal of the regular health care of Americans is delivered by PCPs.

Physicians specializing in family practice, internal medicine, and pediatrics are considered PCPs. General practitioners (GPs)—meaning licensed physicians who have not undergone full residency training beyond their internships—on rare occasions may also be considered PCPs in rural or underserved areas with a serious shortage of board-certified PCPs. However, the number of GPs has steadily fallen and health plans have been increasingly reluctant to contract with them.

The number of graduating physicians who choose to become PCPs is in sharp decline, as PCPs' income has lagged behind the incomes of almost all other specialties. This serious problem has the potential of being made worse by the increase in demand created under the Affordable Care Act (ACA). Nonphysician providers such as CNPs and PAs can and do provide primary care and thereby improve access, yet significant problems in accessing primary care persist in some parts of the United States.

Many obstetrics/gynecology (OB/Gyn) specialists believe that they, too, deliver primary care to their patients. They make the valid point that they are often the only physician whom a young woman sees for many years, at least in the case of generally healthy young women. Even prior to passage of the ACA, almost all plans, including HMOs, allowed direct access to OB/Gyn physicians. Under the ACA, such access is now required of all plans.

While some PCPs specialize only in general primary care, many internists are also board certified in a subspecialty—for example, pulmonary medicine or gastroenterology (pediatricians and family practitioners may have additional training as well, but subspecialties are far more common in internal medicine). Unless such a specialist restricts her or his practice to only specialized conditions or procedures (e.g., a gastroenterologist who sees mostly patients referred by other physicians), it is common to have a practice mix consisting of both specialty care and primary care patients. For that reason, and because of increasing shortages of PCPs without subspecialties, most health plans allow internists to classify themselves as both a PCP and a SCP.

For traditional HMOs, the distinction between PCP designation and SCP designation is very important because of how specialty services are authorized and paid for. In a traditional HMO in which the PCP acts as the care coordinator and must authorize any visits to a specialist (a "gatekeeper" type of HMO), the HMO cannot allow a specialist to see a member for primary care and then refer that member back to himself or herself at a later time for specialty services—in other words, to get paid first for seeing the member in the role of PCP, then to get paid a second time for seeing the same member in the role of SCP. HMOs that use a "gatekeeper" approach do not allow this form of self-referral, in which physicians refer patients back to themselves. That would not prevent other physicians from referring to that physician for specialty care, of course.

Hospital-Based Physicians

Hospital-based physicians (HBPs) occupy a unique position, and for that reason it is worth describing them separately. In this discussion, the term HBP refers only to those physicians whose practices are oriented toward care provided in the hospital; it does not include physicians who are employed by a hospital but have otherwise typical patient care practices, even if their office(s) are physically located within the hospital facility. For example, it does not include a cardiologist whose community-based private practice was acquired by a hospital, or a PCP who is employed by the hospital and sees patients at a hospital-owned annex or office building.

HBPs are typically classified into one of five specialties:

- Radiologists
- Anesthesiologists
- Pathologists
- Physicians practicing full-time emergency medicine*
- Full-time hospitalists*

---

*Full-time emergency department physicians and hospitalists may be board certified in various other specialties but are included here because payers face the same issues with all five types of HBPs.

The first three groups of specialists—those in radiology, anesthesiology, and pathology (sometimes referred to as RAPs)—are traditional types of HBPs who have been associated with hospitals for more than a half a century. These physicians must be board certified in their respective specialties. They frequently practice in a single medical group, which is typically the only group providing those services to the hospital (although exceptions exist). RAP HBPs are always associated with a facility and typically do not provide traditional office-based care, though radiologists specializing in radiation treatments for cancer may do so.

Emergency departments (EDs) have been staffed by specialists in emergency medicine for many decades now. ED physicians also may be part of a medical group with exclusive rights, or they may be employed directly by the hospital. Emergency medicine is a recognized specialty, and most, but not all, emergency medicine physicians are board certified as such. Some EDs also include physicians in other specialties such as internal medicine or general surgery on their staffs, but the care they deliver still falls into the category of emergency medicine.

Hospitalists are physicians who concentrate solely on the day-to-day management of inpatient care. In some cases, the hospitalist may concentrate solely on critical care, in which case he or she is also referred to as an intensivist. Most of these physicians are board certified in internal medicine, although other types of specialists may also become hospitalists. Until recently, there was no specific board certification for the hospitalist specialty, but that situation is now changing. The American Board of Internal Medicine has developed a Focused Practice in Hospital Medicine pilot program that is intended to lead to an internal medicine specialty board, and the American Board of Physician Specialties, which is not part of the other specialty boards, offers a hospitalist board certification program. Because this specialty is still evolving, any valid board certification is usually acceptable for credentialing purposes.

In most cases, neither a patient nor a payer has the option to select a HBP.* Moreover, because of their exclusivity, HBPs may resist contracting with a payer from which they have been accustomed to getting their full charges, since contracting may not bring them increased business. Payers, in contrast, are often reluctant to contract with hospitals or facilities if the HBPs do not also sign a contract, because the plan and its members will then be exposed to the HBPs' higher charges and balance billing.

---

* In rare instances, a hospital may have two or even more competitive groups. This model may be seen where a hospital has both an academic group and a private practice group coexisting in the same institution, or when a large multispecialty group has a significant presence and demands that its patients be seen by the group's own HBPs.

Hospitals argue that except for their employed physicians, who may include hospitalists and sometimes ED physicians, the traditional HBPs are independent physicians and not under the control of the hospital. While that is true for non-employed HBPs, the hospital is the only party with enough leverage to bring the HBPs to the negotiating table: By definition, the hospital is the only place where the HBPs practice, for all practical purposes, although some large HBP groups may serve more than one hospital system. If a hospital is not critical to include in the payer's network, a refusal by HBPs to contract with a payer may result in the payer refusing to contract with the hospital or refusing to agree to terms that the hospital wants. This negotiating tactic often proves effective because hospital executives and other physicians on staff at the hospital have various means of persuading HBPs to agree to contract. Conversely, if a hospital has no near competitors or is so important that it must be included in the network, the hospital may choose not to make the effort, or at least not for any payer with which it does relatively little business, because it knows it will get the business even without participation by its HBPs.

HBPs may also provide services in outpatient settings such as diagnostic imaging facilities and ambulatory surgery centers. As these are all elective services, a plan would most probably not contract with an ambulatory or diagnostic center unless the HBPs associated with the center also contracted with the plan.

Physicians Other Than Medical Doctors and Doctors of Osteopathy

A few types of physicians other than MDs and DOs may be in a payer's network. Unlike MDs and DOs, who are licensed to practice medicine and surgery without limitations (although MDs and DOs rarely try to practice beyond the scope of their training), these other types of physicians are licensed to practice only within the scope of their specialty. Contracting and credentialing are generally similar to what is used for MDs and DOs, though it may be somewhat less extensive.

Payers typically contract with podiatrists (DPMs) who are licensed to provide care and perform surgery for conditions related to the foot and ankle. Podiatrists are also licensed to prescribe any or most types of drugs. Chiropractors (DCs) are not licensed to prescribe drugs or perform surgery, do not have admitting privileges to hospitals or ambulatory facilities, and typically focus on issues of the spine. In some states, payers are required by law to recognize chiropractors as being in the same category as MDs and DOs for purposes of contracting and designation in the directory. Payers that do not provide dental benefits typically do not contract with dentists or orthodontists, but this practice varies widely. Plans typically contract with oral surgeons due to covering oral surgery related to medical conditions and trauma.

Nonphysician or Mid-level Practitioners

Nonphysician clinicians (NPCs) or mid-level practitioners (MLPs) include physician assistants (PAs) and certified nurse practitioners (CNPs or NPs). In addition to NPs practicing primary care, several other types of NP designations exist, each having a different focus and training—for example, advanced practice registered nurses (APRNs), nurse–midwives (NMs), nurse anesthetists (NAs), and clinical nurse specialists (CNSs).

Licensure and regulation of PAs is similar from state to state, with PAs needing to practice under physician supervision. "Physician supervision" refers to a physician being responsible for the clinical care provided by the PA, but not necessarily directly observing their practice behavior. Approximately one-third of all PAs practice in hospitals, another third practice with medical groups, and the remaining third are found in a variety of situations. All states allow PAs to write prescriptions, though some limitations may apply.

In contrast to the approach taken with PAs, states vary considerably in how they license and regulate NPs. Some states allow NPs to practice independently, without physician involvement, for defined types of services and procedures. More states require some form of physician involvement with an NP's practice. All states allow NPs to write prescriptions, but vary in the types of prescriptions that may be written and the degree of physician oversight that is required.

Health plans typically only credential and contract with NPCs who practice independently and bill for their services directly. NPCs employed by or associated with facilities and/or medical practices are not typically credentialed or contracted with separately from the facility or medical practice, and any bills for their services are part of the facility's or group's bill. With the ACA-driven demand for primary healthcare services, the number of independently practicing NPCs is likely to increase as these nurses' practices become an increasingly important portal of access for primary care.

Behavioral Health and Substance Abuse Therapists

As noted in Exhibit 3-1, many types of professionals provide behavioral health and substance abuse services. Many practice independently and may be under a direct contract with a payer, while others provide services as employees of an organization or facility that signs the contract with the health plan. A therapist may provide all types of therapy, but it is much more common for a professional to focus on either behavioral health/mental health or substance abuse therapy. Only psychiatrists, who are either MDs or DOs, may prescribe drugs or admit patients to a hospital.

Other Professionals

Other types of professionals (see Exhibit 3-1) also may be found in a health plan's network, though their inclusion varies from plan to plan and from state to state. For purposes of this chapter, all further discussion about the professional network will address only the physician network.

CREDENTIALING

Prior to signing a contract, a provider must meet the payer's credentialing standards. In reality, credentialing provides only a limited amount of information about a physician's quality and acceptability, but it does set minimum requirements for training, current certifications and licensure, and so forth, and may uncover potentially adverse actions levied against a physician. To the degree that one defines quality as meeting those standards, credentialing represents at least a baseline measurement of quality.

Each state has regulatory credentialing requirements that payers must meet to do business in the state, and those requirements may vary from state to state, though not by much. Plans that contract with Medicare must also meet Medicare's credentialing requirements, similar to the case with the states. Credentialing requirements for HMOs are usually more extensive than they are for other types of payers such as PPOs, but some payers use the same requirements for their HMO and PPO products. State regulators as well as the payer industry overall generally follow the credentialing standards developed by accreditation organizations such as the National Committee for Quality Assurance (NCQA) or URAC*; their credentialing standards are briefly discussed here, while accreditation overall is discussed in the *Utilization Management, Quality Management, and Accreditation* chapter.

The responsibility for credentialing typically resides with either the medical director or a vice president overseeing networks. Regardless of where the

---

* In the past, URAC stood for Utilization Review Accreditation Commission, but the organization's name has since been officially changed to URAC alone.

responsibility lies, the requirements are generally the same. Plans usually also establish a credentialing committee that reviews applications and credentials, and determines if a provider meets the requirements for initial credentialing or recredentialing. Some applications are held for further review while additional information is obtained, and in a few cases the provider will be denied a contract because of credentialing issues. In the event a provider appeals being denied a contract, the credentialing committee typically reviews the case. Credentialing is usually considered part of the plan's QM program, and the deliberations of the credentialing committee are usually considered a form of peer review; consequently, both are considered to be confidential, meaning not subject to disclosure.

Payers—and HMOs in particular—also usually credential nonphysician professionals who practice independently, meaning they practice without supervision by a physician and submit claims for professional services directly to the payer. Examples include psychologists and other independently practicing behavioral health providers, optometrists, chiropractors, and physical therapists. The credentialing process for independent nonphysician providers is typically similar to that used for physicians but not as extensive. Payers rarely credential nonphysician professionals if they are employed by a facility; instead, the facility takes on the responsibility to credential those providers.

The initial credentialing process is carried out prior to contracting with a new physician, prior to adding new physicians in a group or hospital already under contract, or, rarely, after an interim contract or letter of intent is signed. Medicare Advantage plans must also determine if a physician has been sanctioned by Medicare or Medicaid; as a practical matter, this is usually done even for non-Medicare plans. Initial credentialing of a physician is more extensive than recredentialing, which typically takes place every three years following initial credentialing.

The National Provider Identifier

Among the mandates included in the Health Insurance Portability and Accountability Act of 1996 (HIPAA) was use of a uniform national provider identifier (NPI). The NPI is a 10-digit number that is unique and never-ending; that is, once assigned to a particular provider, the provider will use that identifier for all transactions regardless of location, plan type, or anything else. The NPI replaced all other identifiers used by providers except for the taxpayer identification number, the Drug Enforcement Administration (DEA) number, and the state prescribing number (in those states that require one) for providers who prescribe or administer prescription drugs. The national employer identification number (EIN) is not affected either, to the extent that a provider is also an employer.

An institutional provider may, under some circumstances, obtain a separate NPI for a "subpart" if the subpart is unique (e.g., a division of a hospital system that bills Medicare separately for distinct types of services). As a practical matter, providers of all types may sometimes actually practice and bill under more than one NPI. For example, on some days a physician may practice independently, whereas on other days she or he may work as a contracted employee of another provider. These sorts of variations have made it difficult at times for a payer to actually link various services to a particular provider.

Documentation Typically Used in Provider Credentialing

Most, but not all, credentialing materials are relatively standard for physicians. In addition to the NPI, other identifiers, documents, and certifications exist. Much of this information is self-reported by physicians, but some is obtained independently by the payer or delegated by the payer to a credentials verification organization (CVO). Table 3-2 provides a few examples of the types of credentialing information and/or documents that are self-reported by physicians. For purposes of recredentialing, providers are required to update this information as necessary. Note that the examples in Table 3-2 are only a partial list of the many types of information used in credentialing by payers; for a more complete description, see the chapter titled "The Provider Network" in *The Essentials of Managed Health Care,* sixth edition (Jones & Bartlett Learning, 2013).

Credentialing information such as demographics or identifiers may be provided via a credentialing form, either on paper and submitted by mail, faxed, or entered through a secure online portal. In many cases, at least for initial credentialing, copies or images of documents must be provided, such as a copy of the license to practice medicine, a copy of the medical diploma, a copy of the face sheet of the malpractice insurance policy showing coverage effective dates, and so on.

Verification

Health plans, and in particular HMOs, must verify that a provider's credentials are valid, active, and unrestricted. Doing so requires contacting those bodies that have issued the degrees, licenses, certifications, and so forth that are required under the credentialing standards. Examples of verification measures include contacting a physician's medical school to verify that he or she received an MD, contacting the state's board of medicine to verify that the physician's license to practice is current and unrestricted, and so forth.

Table 3–2   Examples of some Types of Credentialing Information and Documentation Used in Physician Credentialing

---

- Demographics such as name, birth date, location, and so forth
- Medical license number and expiration date for each state in which the physician is licensed
- Drug Enforcement Agency (DEA) number (for prescribing controlled substances) and expiration date, as well as any state prescribing number and expiration date if a state requires it
- Standard identifiers such as the national provider identifier (NPI), tax identifier, and any other applicable legal or regulatory identifiers
- Education and training dates, locations, and degrees or certifications earned
- Specialty board certification(s) and expiration date(s)
- Participation status with Medicare and Medicaid programs
- Practice details
- Hospital privileges
- Ambulatory surgical center (ASC) privileges
- Professional liability insurance
- History of malpractice awards and settlements
- History of professional sanctions and other adverse events
- Work history and references
- Billing and remittance information
- Disclosure questions

In the past, some regulators and outside accreditation organizations required each healthcare plan to conduct primary source verification, meaning each plan had to contact each source directly, rather than relying on another party to do so on its behalf. Fortunately, the industry has evolved and now payers may rely on certain databases and accredited CVOs* to conduct much of the data collection and verification on behalf of multiple health plans, thereby reducing the burden on providers and plans alike.

The Data Bank

As a part of both initial credentialing and recredentialing, payers and CVOs routinely query The Data Bank (www.npdb-hipdb.hrsa.gov), a federal database

---

* Meaning the CVO has been accredited by NCQA or URAC as meeting the necessary standards for collecting and verifying credentials.

created by combining two other federal databases—the National Practitioner Data Bank (NPDB) and the Healthcare Integrity and Protection Data Bank (HIPDB).

The NPDB was created by the Health Care Quality Improvement Act of 1986 (HCQIA) and became operational in 1989. The HCQIA also provided for qualified immunity from antitrust lawsuits for credentialing activities as well as professional medical staff sanctions when the terms of the act are followed. To be eligible, such entities must both provide healthcare services and have a formal peer review process for the purpose of furthering the quality of health care. Information reported to the NPDB is considered confidential and may not be disclosed except as specified in the regulations.

The HIPDB was created under HIPAA as a means of combatting fraud and abuse in health care and health insurance. It holds healthcare fraud and abuse data based on required reporting and disclosure of certain final adverse actions (excluding settlements in which no findings of liability were made) taken against healthcare providers, suppliers, or practitioners that are not related to actions or events that are reported to the NPDB.

The Data Bank—that is, the combined database—holds data about malpractice awards and settlements, actions against privileges, actions limiting the scope of a provider's practice, sanctions, and healthcare fraud and abuse findings for physicians and nonphysician providers. By law, all covered entities, including hospitals, state medical boards, malpractice insurers, payers with provider networks, and others, must report any of these actions. Because of this reporting requirement, The Data Bank is the "gold standard" source of information about such events. Hospitals are required to query The Data Bank periodically, and other healthcare entities such as payers and medical group practices may query it for purposes of credentialing and recredentialing, and for peer review. Not all sanctions and disciplinary actions merit action on the part of the plan, but either a pattern of sanctions or disciplinary actions or an egregious problem, including deceiving the plan regarding such actions, typically results in the plan terminating that physician's contract.

The Universal Provider Datasource

Table 3-2 lists only some of the many sources of information and documentation used by payers in physician credentialing. New and increasingly complex sources of data are continually becoming available and being added to the credentialing process. For decades, each payer determined which additional information it would seek out for providers, but this standard was not consistent from payer to payer. It also placed an increasing burden on both payers and providers to obtain and track the growing data set.

In 2002, a coalition of payers, with the support of providers and other parties, created the CAQH* Universal Provider Datasource (UPD) as a means to improve the efficiency and effectiveness of the credentialing process. The UPD is not used by every payer, but it is used by a substantial number of them, including most of the major commercial payers and Blue Cross Blue Shield plans.

The UPD allows providers to self-report their required credentialing data to one source, either online or via fax or mail, at no cost; the cost to access the UPD is borne by the health plans, hospitals, and credentialing entities that subscribe to it. Providers maintain control of and regularly re-attest to their information in the UPD, including authorizing which organizations can access their data. Primary source verification (PSV), required as a condition of accreditation, is performed externally by a contracted CVO, by a delegated credentialing entity such as a hospital or an independent practice association, or internally by credentialing staff. CAQH also monitors data from multiple sources, including sanctions and disciplinary actions meted out by all states and the District of Columbia, the Office of Inspector General (OIG), Medicare, Medicaid, and Office of Personnel Management (OPM).

On-Site Office Evaluations

On-site office evaluations of PCPs, OB/Gyns, and high-volume behavioral health providers were once standard at the time of initial credentialing. That is no longer the case, although a few HMOs may still perform such assessments. When NCQA changed its credentialing standards in 2009, most payers stopped doing on-site office evaluations on a routine basis. Even when they did undertake such evaluations, payers typically did not conduct routine on-site evaluations of specialty physicians' offices or facilities. When on-site office evaluations were performed, they were typically limited to issues such as physical accessibility, physical appearance, and adequacy of waiting room and examining room space. Although these inspections are no longer routinely performed as part of credentialing, they may be conducted if member complaints reach a defined

---

* Formerly the Council for Affordable Quality Healthcare, this organization has formally changed its name to CAQH.

threshold—for example, a defined number of complaints or a defined level of seriousness (assuming the plan does not have good reason to simply dismiss the complaint).

Medical Records Review

In the past, as part of the initial credentialing process, the medical director of an HMO might have reviewed a sample of a physician's medical records. Such reviews are no longer performed for a variety of reasons, with the most important being the privacy requirements established by HIPAA. Under this act, plans have the right to review medical records for only their members, and then only when there is "a need to know."

Some payers perform medical records reviews for PCPs at the time of recredentialing, in which case they typically review the medical records of 5 to 10 randomly selected members who have seen that PCP within the past 3 years. Medical records reviews are not fishing expeditions, however. Rather, they are primarily structural reviews—for example, ascertaining the presence (or absence) of a medication list, a list of any known drug allergies, a list of active diagnoses, lab testing results, and the like. Such a review usually does not evaluate the actual care provided.

TYPES OF PHYSICIAN CONTRACTING SITUATIONS

Physicians contract with payers through several different types of organizations, ranging from contracting as individuals to contracting through entirely different types of providers such as integrated healthcare delivery systems. In this section, we look at a few of the common types of contracting situations involving physicians.

Individual Physicians

One common type of physician contracting situation is the direct contract, in which a physician contracts directly with the health plan and not through any third party or intermediary. This arrangement is the second most common form of HMO and is the most common model for many non-HMO plans. The major advantage of this approach is that it creates a direct relationship between the plan and the physician, which makes it cleaner and simpler to interact. The major disadvantage is that the relationship is with only one physician, such that the effort required to establish and maintain that relationship is disproportionately greater than when physicians are part of a larger organization.

Traditional Medical Groups

Traditional medical groups are legal entities, often taking the form of a professional corporation (PC) or a partnership. With this model, the physicians share office space and support services such as scheduling and billing. Groups have been growing steadily as fewer physicians go into solo practice. In some parts of the country, medical groups remain relatively uncommon, while in other areas, groups are the dominant form of practice.

Small groups (i.e., 2 to 10 physicians) usually operate relatively cohesively, but in some cases the physicians in the group are more like individual physicians sharing support staff. Medical groups can be single-specialty practices (e.g., all primary care internists or all orthopedic surgeons) or multispecialty practices.

Larger groups usually include both partners and employed physicians. In other words, some physicians jointly own the group and share in the costs and profits of the business, whereas other physicians are employed by the group but have no ownership interest. Over time, some employed physicians will be offered partnerships within the group. When both types of physicians make up a group, only the partners have the authority to sign a contract, but all physicians in the group must meet the payer's credentialing standards.

Hospitals and health systems that employ physicians sometimes do so through a captive medical group. This is common in states with Corporate Practice of Medicine (CPM) laws that prohibit a corporation (other than a PC) from practicing medicine or employing a physician to provide professional medical services; some states with CPM laws allow certain corporations such as hospitals or HMOs to employ physicians, however. For these types of medical groups, the relationship and contract go through the health system.

Most plans will refuse to contract with physicians in a group unless the entire group agrees to abide by the contract. Many payers—and HMOs in particular—will not contract with a group unless all of its members meet the payer's credentialing criteria and agree to the contract's terms and conditions. They impose this requirement because if some physicians in the group are not in the network or do not meet credentialing criteria, then members who see participating providers in that group may potentially be exposed to balance billing when the non-participating providers are covering on-call cases or seeing urgent call-in cases.

Group Practice Without Walls

Another type of medical group, known as a group practice without walls (GPWW), is usually made up of formerly independent physicians who have pooled their resources and now contract as a single medical group. These providers often continue to practice in separate offices and do not interact as frequently as physicians within a traditional medical group, but have a greater degree of financial sharing of costs and profits. As hospitals continue to acquire physician practices or hire them directly from training, many are using the GPWW as their organizational model.

Independent Practice Associations

The most common type of HMO is the independent practice association (IPA) model plan. An IPA is a legal entity that contracts with independent physicians, with the IPA then contracting with health plans. Most IPAs encompass all or most specialties, including primary care, but some single-specialty IPAs exist.

For the payer, the primary value of contracting with an IPA is that it brings a large number of physicians into the health plan at one time. Only one negotiation is required because all of the IPA physicians agree to abide by the terms settled between the IPA and the payer. The IPA may also be willing and able to accept more financial risk than a solo physician or small group could. In addition, some IPAs carry out functions such as network management, credentialing, and even medical management (both utilization and quality management) on behalf of the payer, thereby allowing for lower administrative costs. Because the ACA places limits on the percentage of premiums (for insured businesses only) that may be expended on costs for administration, sales and marketing, reserves, and surplus or profit, having the providers pick up the administrative costs for network and utilization management gives a payer more flexibility in dealing with other administrative costs.

Contracting with IPAs has two primary disadvantages. First, an IPA can function somewhat as a union, with the IPA holding a considerable portion (or perhaps all) of the delivery system hostage during its negotiations—a fact not lost on the U.S. Department of Justice. IPAs that function as anticompetitive forces may encounter difficulties with the law. Second, the plan's ability to select and deselect individual physicians is somewhat more limited when contracting through an IPA than when contracting directly with the providers. However, all physicians in the IPA must still meet credentialing standards.

Faculty Practice Plans

Faculty practice plans (FPPs) are medical groups made up of full-time academic faculty. An FPP may be a single entity, or there may be multiple FPPs for each specialty (e.g., cardiology or anesthesiology). FPPs and hospitals devoted to teaching and research can sometimes be challenging to work with from the payer's perspective.

Notably, teaching institutions and FPPs tend to be less cost-effective in their practice styles than private physicians because the primary missions of teaching programs are teaching and performing research, though teaching hospitals and faculty also care for sicker than average patients. Cost-effectiveness is a secondary goal only (if a goal at all). Some programs do emphasize managing total costs along with the use of evidence-based medical practices, however, so less efficiency is not always the case.

Another major challenge with teaching programs and FPPs is that they often provide ongoing care through multiple specialty clinics, and the specialty care provided at one site is not always integrated with the care delivered at other specialty clinics. When this is the case, the system can act like a medical pinball machine, with patients ricocheting from clinic to clinic and having each organ system attended to with little regard for the totality of care. This lack of integration can increase costs, produce continuity problems, and lead to a clear lack of control or accountability. Fortunately, academic centers have been increasing their focus on integrating and coordinating care in recent years; while integrating care remains a problem in such groups, the situation is slowly getting better.

Specialty Management Companies

Though the arrangement is not common, some companies employ and manage single-specialty physicians but are not traditional medical groups. In some cases, physician practice management companies (PPMCs) manage the specialty medical group; in this scenario, the medical group actually contracts with the payer, even though it is managed by the PPMC. In other cases, the physicians work for the specialty management company, and the company then contracts with the payer.

Specialty management companies often focus on narrow aspects of specialty care, not the specialty's usual range of services—for example, neonatal care, or emergency and critical care using non-hospital-based physicians. The physicians working for these companies obtain privileges at all hospitals in a defined service area, and are then responsible for providing care for all of an HMO's cases that fall within certain criteria. For example, they may care for patients in the neonatal intensive care unit, or patients seen in the emergency department who must be evaluated for possible hospital admission.

Management Services Organizations

Management Services Organizations (MSOs) may be physician-only organizations, but more often they either include a hospital or are run by one. In most cases, MSOs function in a similar way. Rather than dividing the discussion into two parts, MSOs are discussed in the section titled Integrated Delivery Systems.

HOSPITALS AND AMBULATORY FACILITIES

In the past, recruiting hospitals into a new plan's network was a primary area of focus. In today's market, payers are usually past the point of adding new hospitals to their networks; instead, network maintenance and periodic renegotiation of existing contracts is the primary focus. Also, as markets matured, hospitals merged or acquired other hospitals, resulting in larger multihospital systems and fewer independent hospitals. Ambulatory facilities, in contrast, have grown in both number and scope.

The approach taken toward hospital and facility network development and maintenance will be affected to some degree by the type of health plan. An HMO is more likely to have a smaller network than a PPO, for example. In past decades, HMOs often contracted with a limited number of hospitals to obtain significant discounts in return for channeling patients to those facilities, but that dynamic eroded in the face of market demand for broad networks. As costs have escalated, however, interest in narrower networks has resurfaced, particularly for products sold through the health insurance exchanges.

Types of Facilities and Contracting Situations

A payer may have many different types of facilities in its contracted network. Hospitals may be for-profit or nonprofit, owned either by investors or the community. Hospitals also vary in their focus, including general acute care, tertiary care, or single specialty. Ambulatory facilities are even more widely varied. They include ambulatory surgical centers, facilities focused on specific types of procedures such as endoscopy centers, dialysis centers, urgent care centers, and so forth. They may be owned by a health system, by the physicians who use the facility, or by a for-profit company; alternatively, they may be jointly owned by different types of parties.

Community-Based Single Acute Care Hospitals

Once the dominant type of hospital, community-based single acute care hospitals (i.e., nonprofit hospitals that are not part of a larger system) have been in a slow decline in the United States for decades, with some of these facilities closing and many more merging with larger health systems. Though they can be found in most parts of the country, only rural areas have mostly independent single acute care hospitals, but many have closed for economic reasons and others are being acquired by expanding health systems.

Contracting with rural free-standing acute care community hospitals can be difficult if there are no viable alternatives. They are also far less likely to negotiate payment terms beyond the most basic forms. Fortunately, rural hospitals are also among the least expensive inpatient facilities, as they have fewer high-tech services and tend to be located in low-cost areas. A payer may agree to a minimal discount to obtain agreement on the rest of the contract's terms, if a particular hospital is necessary to have in its service area.

Single independent hospitals surrounded by larger competitors are usually receptive to contracting as a response to competitive pressures. In the past, large systems sometimes exerted their negotiating leverage by insisting on exclusivity, at least in the geographic area they served, leaving smaller acute care hospitals out in the cold. More recently, antitrust concerns have diminished this practice to some extent.

Multihospital Systems

Consolidation in the U.S. hospital industry has been significant. From the mid-1990s through the mid-2000s, the total number of hospitals decreased as struggling hospitals closed. That trend was reversed by mid-decade, however, as new hospitals were built to meet increasing demand. Nevertheless, the growth in capacity did not occur through the creation of new free-standing acute care hospitals, but rather through expansion of large multihospital systems (MHSs), primarily through mergers and acquisitions of previously independent hospitals. By 2006, there were more hospitals in MHSs than there were free-standing hospitals in the United States, and that trend continues apace.

Hospital consolidation has had a profound impact on the hospital networks of health plans. As hospitals have merged into regional MHSs, thereby eliminating competition, they have wielded their greater market power to negotiate significant increases in payment rates. Large MHSs also typically require that all hospitals in their system be included in all products a payer sells as a condition of contracting with the system's flagship hospitals.

MHSs have also been buying the practices of community physicians as well as hiring physicians who are looking for practice opportunities. These physicians are not the traditional HBPs, but rather PCPs and specialists working in high-volume specialties. Their inclusion within MHSs has provided even greater negotiating leverage for the MHSs as well as increases in physician fees.

For-Profit Hospitals

For-profit hospitals account for only about one-third of all hospitals in the United States. For-profit hospitals range from free-standing individual facilities owned by the physicians who use them, to national hospital corporations that own and operate facilities in multiple locations. Some are built as new facilities, while others are nonprofit hospitals that are acquired by for-profit hospital companies. In a few locations, for-profit hospital companies have achieved the type of market dominance attained by nonprofit MHSs.

Because national companies are organized much like any other business, individual hospitals have less local autonomy than do nonprofit hospitals and MHSs. Negotiating and contracting are more likely to be done at a national level when the payer is also national or a multistate regional health plan. National hospital companies also usually have a strong regional management structure, so local or state health plans, and sometimes multistate health plans, are more likely to contract at that level. In all cases, however, contracting by the hospital company is supported by its national-scale resources, such as its legal department.

Free-standing individual for-profit hospitals, which are often owned at least in part by the physicians who use them, are addressed in the next section on specialized hospitals.

Specialized Hospitals

Some hospitals specialize in providing care to only certain types of patients. They can be classified into two broad categories: hospitals that provide care for patients with serious complex conditions, and hospitals that provide care for patients with less intense and/or chronic conditions. In some cases, a specialty hospital is owned by the specialty physicians who use it—an arrangement that has been associated with higher utilization of the hospital's services.

Children's hospitals are an example of hospitals that focus not just on providing care to children, but on providing care to patients with complex conditions. Women's hospitals, focusing on conditions specific to women, and obstetrics in particular, are less common than they once were, but are otherwise similar, as are other types of specialized facilities such as eye and ear hospitals. Examples of hospitals providing less intense or chronic care include rehabilitation hospitals and hospitals providing psychiatric care or substance abuse treatment.

Hospitals specializing in very complex care usually have few, if any, competitors that can provide the same degree of specialized care. As a result, health plans will usually be able to obtain a contract, but payment terms are typically high. Hospitals providing chronic or long-term care are much more likely to agree to favorable rates if they also admit patients with Medicare and Medicaid, but are less likely to negotiate if they serve only private-pay patients.

Physician-Owned Single-Specialty Hospitals

Physician-owned hospitals account for slightly fewer than 10% of all hospitals in the United States, and are found in most, but not all, states. The physicians who use the facility may own the entire hospital, or they may have an ownership interest that is shared with nonphysician owners such as a management company. They are typically focused on a type of specialty that is associated with a high volume of procedures, such as interventional cardiology (catheterizations, pacemakers, and so forth), orthopedics, eye surgery, and so forth.

Physician-owned hospitals typically do not have emergency departments and are not equipped to handle patients with multiple and severe medical conditions. As a result, they are often criticized by leaders of community and teaching hospitals, who accuse them of "skimming" off the most lucrative cases, meaning they admit only healthy patients who require fewer resources for their care and who also have private insurance or Medicare coverage. In addition, studies show a strong relationship between physician ownership and high utilization rates, with some physician-owners performing substantially more procedures than physicians in the same specialty who have no ownership interest.

The Medicare Modernization Act of 2003 (MMA) froze the ability of physicians to self-refer to *new* single-specialty hospitals in which they had an ownership interest (existing ones were not included), but that restriction expired in August 2006 and development of new hospitals resumed. The ACA, however, limited expansions of the number of operating rooms, procedure rooms, and beds in physician-owned facilities, and prevented any facilities that were not certified as Medicare participants by December 31, 2010, from caring for Medicare-covered patients. The ACA also now requires physician-owned hospitals and the physician-owners to disclose that ownership structure to patients.

Commercial payers differ widely in their approach to negotiating with physician-owned single-specialty hospitals. Some avoid these facilities because of concerns about overutilization. Other payers choose to contract with them because of they offer prices significantly lower than the typical general hospital, and are often willing to accept capitation conditions from HMOs. When a payer does contract with a single-specialty hospital, the general and tertiary hospitals in the network may seek an increase in their own payments, because presumably those patients not treated at the single-specialty hospital will be sicker and require more resources for their care.

Government Hospitals

Some hospitals may be controlled by local and state governments or by the federal government. County-run community hospitals differ little from any other nonprofit acute care hospital. State-run hospitals sometimes focus on specialized care, such as long-term psychiatric care, although many of those facilities have closed over the years.

Hospitals run by the federal government include those managed by the Department of Veterans Affairs, the Department of Defense, the U.S. Public Health Service, and the Indian Health Service. In the past, they often did not contract with commercial payers because they did not depend on those sources for revenue. While these facilities usually billed commercial payers when one of their patients had coverage, most of their patients lacked such insurance. This situation has been changing because actually getting paid by a commercial payer is usually easier if a contract exists, but with coverage expansions under the ACA we may see even more contracting by government hospitals.

Subacute Care: Skilled or Intermediate Nursing Facilities

In addition to contracting with acute care hospitals, payers usually contract with at least one subacute facility (i.e., a skilled or intermediate nursing facility) and/ or rehabilitation facility within the service area. Subacute facilities are well suited for prolonged convalescence or recovery cases (e.g., a patient requiring prolonged traction, a frail patient requiring prolonged intravenous antibiotics for a deeply seated infection, or a patient requiring prolonged stroke rehabilitation), if home therapy is not appropriate for some reason, because the cost for a bed-day in a subacute facility is much less than the corresponding cost in an acute care hospital. In other cases, a patient may be able to be cared for at home, but it is still more cost-effective to deliver the therapy in the subacute facility due to more favorable pricing achievable through economies of scale.

Hospice

Hospice is a broad term referring to healthcare services provided at the end of life. Such services may be delivered within an inpatient facility, an ambulatory facility, or a program that has no facilities of its own. In most cases, the contract between a payer and the hospice organization will be similar to the contracts that apply to subacute care facilities or home care.

Ambulatory Surgical Centers and Other Ambulatory Facilities

In the context of payer network contracting and management, *ambulatory facilities* refers to the various types of facilities in which physicians and others do procedures or provide specialized services, but not the offices where physicians and others see patients in the normal course of their practice (e.g., a physician's office). Facilities in this context are separate from the physicians, and they bill separately from any professional charges.

Those in which outpatient surgery and other invasive procedures are performed are often referred to as ASCs. The number of ASCs has been increasing over the years, as have the number of procedures performed in ambulatory facilities overall. Similar to single-specialty hospitals, these facilities are typically equipped to handle only routine cases, though many can accommodate patients who require general anesthesia. Some are owned by health systems, often as a for-profit subsidiary; others by physicians; and still others by independent for-profit or nonprofit organizations not associated with a health system. Payers view physician-owned ASCs in much the same way they regard physician-owned single-specialty hospitals.

Unlike the case when hospitals become consolidated into MHSs, there is usually greater competition between ambulatory facilities. Health systems, particularly MHSs, typically require a payer to contract with their ambulatory facilities as a condition of contracting overall. A demand to exclude competing ambulatory facilities may be seen as anticompetitive, however, so payers often contract with multiple facilities. This approach allows payers to obtain more favorable pricing, which is important because simply changing the site of care from an inpatient setting to an outpatient setting does not, in itself, necessarily reduce costs.

ASCs are not the only types of ambulatory facilities, just as not all ambulatory facilities provide surgical services. Nevertheless, ASCs are specialized in regard to

---

Exhibit 3-2   Examples of Nonsurgical Ambulatory Facilities

- Dialysis centers
- Chemotherapy centers
- Birthing centers
- Community health centers
- Diagnostic imaging centers
- Endoscopy centers
- Lithotripsy centers
- Occupational health centers
- Pain management centers
- Radiation oncology centers
- Surgical recovery centers
- Women's health centers

the services they offer. Exhibit 3-2 provides some examples of common types of nonsurgical ambulatory facilities.

Retail Health Clinics

Retail health clinics, also called convenient (or convenience) care clinics (CCCs) are essentially small clinics, usually associated with a retail operation such as a grocery store or pharmacy. They are typically staffed by employed nonphysician primary care providers such as NPs and PAs. The majority are operated by a small number of for-profit retail chains, although some may be operated by physician groups or hospital chains or even as stand-alone clinics. Charges typically include professional services, which are not billed separately as they are in most other facilities.

Retail clinics provide basic primary care services for common minor health-care problems as well as routine preventive health care and screening. The level of care provided in retail clinics is usually much lower than that provided in physician's offices; in turn, most retail clinics have contracts with commercial payers and with Medicare. Because it costs the payer or employer less when the patient visits a retail health clinic visit for a minor condition than when the patient visits a physician's office for the same condition, some health plans even reduce the amount of cost sharing incurred by a member for a CCC visit.

Physicians, particularly PCPs, have mixed attitudes toward retail health clinics. On the one hand, their use may ease some capacity pressures on a very busy practice. On the other hand, those visits may be regarded as lost revenue by PCPs (or EDs—although EDs are so overcrowded these days that the CCC visits are seen as welcome relief to most). Physicians also worry that use of retail health clinics does not provide for continuity of care, may not provide adequate-quality care, or may lead to missing a serious condition, although such issues have never been found to be significant problems.

Urgent Care Centers

Urgent care centers might at first appear to be similar to retail clinics, but they are not. They more closely resemble a hybrid of a low-level ED and a PCP practice. Such facilities are staffed by physicians as well as nurses and nonphysician providers. They are able to provide a relatively wide scope of care, including performing minor procedures, wound treatment, casting of broken bones, and so forth.

Like ASCs, urgent care centers may be owned by health systems, by a medical group, or by independent for-profit or nonprofit organizations not associated with a health system. Most operate as for-profit entities, even when they are owned by a nonprofit hospital. Free-standing, private, for-profit urgent care centers often do not accept private insurance because doing so means discounting their charges, but this has been changing as competition increases and payers are more willing to direct members toward contracted facilities. Urgent care centers run by health systems usually include them in their overall contract. HMOs, in particular, may contract with one or two of these facilities in a community so as to provide an alternative to the emergency room. Some payers, especially closed-panel HMOs, may run their own urgent care centers.

Credentialing of Hospitals and Ambulatory Facilities

Hospital and facility credentialing refers to facilities meeting applicable state licensure and accreditation standards, as well as participation with Medicare and Medicaid. Payers do not credential facilities the same way that they credential physicians and other professionals for several reasons, the most important of which is that payers simply do not have the resident knowledge to adequately assess the many types of facilities in a community. Conversely, state licensure agencies and facility accreditation organizations do have the necessary expertise, knowledge, and experience to properly evaluate facility performance against industry standards.

Likewise, payers do not typically contract with or credential the nonphysician professionals who work at facilities—for example, nurses, pharmacists, CRNAs, PAs, technicians (e.g., radiology, lab, pharmacy), and so forth. The facility is responsible for that task, and state requirements as well as the standards of the facility accreditation organizations include those criteria.

States typically carry out the inspections and initial evaluations of new facilities, after which they accept accreditation by recognized facility accreditation organizations as meeting state and industry standards and requirements. Hospital accreditation is usually carried out by The Joint Commission (TJC, formerly the Joint Commission on Accreditation of Health Care Organizations [JCAHO]), though there are also other acceptable accreditation organizations. For community hospitals, this is usually sufficient and no further credentialing is done.

Ambulatory facilities are credentialed in similar fashion, though the accreditation agency may be an organization other than TJC. For example, the Accreditation Association for Ambulatory Health Care (AAAHC) focuses on ambulatory facilities such as ASCs, endoscopy centers, and dialysis centers.

Examples of acceptable accreditation organizations other than TJC and AAAHC include the following:

- Healthcare Facilities Accreditation Program (HFAP), focusing on osteopathic hospitals
- Det Norske Veritas (DNV), focusing on hospitals
- American Association for Accreditation of Ambulatory Surgery Facilities (AAAASF) Accreditation Program, focusing on ASCs
- Community Health Accreditation Program (CHAP), focusing on community services such as home health, hospice and similar programs
- Accreditation Commission for Health Care (ACHC), focusing on community services similar to those accredited by CHAP

In some cases, a health plan will establish further criteria that are applicable to certain types of care—for example, cardiac surgery or bariatric surgery (for morbid obesity). Examples of such criteria include the following:

- A minimum number of cardiac bypass operations each year
- A percentage of patients who achieve the defined outcomes following obesity surgery
- A staffing ratio of nurses and physicians for an intensive care unit
- Participation in National Cancer Institute protocol studies

A hospital that meets the appropriate criteria for a defined set of procedures would be considered a "center of excellence," and the health plan would, at a minimum, selectively refer those types of cases to the hospital and provide higher levels of coverage. In some cases, especially with HMOs, the plan may provide benefits coverage only when a center of excellence is used for certain procedures.

INTEGRATED DELIVERY SYSTEMS

An integrated delivery system (IDS), sometimes called an integrated healthcare delivery system,* may comprise any of several provider organizational structures involving different types of providers. To be considered an IDS, it must have some type of legal structure for purposes of managing health care and contracting with payers, including contracting with a health plan that the IDS owns and operates. IPAs are essentially physician-only IDSs, but by common usage, IPAs are not considered IDSs. Most IDSs include hospitals and physicians, although

---

* Regardless of what term is used, the "h" is not used in the acronym.

they may include other types of providers as well. This section describes the most common types of IDSs with which payers contract, as well as IDSs that may perform managed care functions on behalf of either a payer or an employer, including a health plan owned by the IDS.

Finally, considerable overlap exists between the different types of IDSs—even more so than between different types of payers. In some cases, these differences are nearly indistinguishable, and the IDS itself may not use any particular label. IDSs also change and evolve over relatively short periods of time. One might even say that the word "evolve" applies less to IDSs than does the term "mutate."*

Independent and Hospital-Employed Physicians in IDSs

In the context of this text, the term "employed physicians" refers to physicians employed by the hospital or MHS, not to HBPs or to physicians employed by a medical group. This includes physicians who are not employed directly by the MHS, but rather through a captive medical group that is owned, controlled, or otherwise exclusively affiliated with the MHS.

Two basic types of physician contracting are used in IDSs:

- IDSs may be primarily made up of a hospital system and independent private practitioners. This model has been in slow decline over the past several years.
- IDSs may be primarily made up of an MHS that employs a large number of physicians other than HBPs. This model is rapidly growing.

The two types are not mutually exclusive, and it is common to see both in the same system. Nevertheless, the dynamics are different in each of these models, even when they coexist. Over the past 10 years, the number of physicians employed by hospitals and MHSs has been steadily increasing compared to the number of independent physicians. In many cases, an MHS may employ more than 1000 community-based physicians, and double that number is not unheard of.

Some types of IDSs involve mostly or only independent physicians, and a few involve mostly or only employed physicians. Most, however, support both types of relationships between hospitals and physicians. When the IDS includes substantial numbers of each type of provider, tension may arise if the independent

---

* The author, trained not only in medicine but also in biology, fully understands that evolution requires mutation, but trusts that the reader gets the point.

Table 3–3   Common Types of IDSs and Their Relationships with
Independent and Employed Physicians

Type of IDS	Relationship to Independent and Employed Physicians
Physician–hospital organization (PHO)	Used almost exclusively with independent physicians. The physicians may participate as individuals, medical groups, GPWWs, or some combination. Physicians may also participate solely through an IPA.
Management services organization (MSO)	Used primarily with independent physicians, but may be used when physicians are indirectly employed or otherwise exclusive to the IDS. An MSO can also be combined with a GPWW or an IPA.
Foundation, GPWW, and captive medical groups	Used primarily for physicians employed indirectly due to state laws prohibiting the employment of physicians by nonphysicians, or used when an MHS wishes to keep services by employed physicians separate from other services. A GPWW may also be used for physicians employed by an entity other than a hospital. All of these models may be combined within an MSO.
Patient-centered medical home (PCMH)	Originally conceived as geared toward independent physicians, it can apply now to both independent and employed physicians, including both at the same time.
Accountable care organization (ACO)	Can apply to both independent and employed physicians, including both at the same time, and will mirror the distribution of independent and employed physicians who provide care at the hospital system. Some IDSs may choose to focus the ACO primarily on their employed physicians, however.
Vertically integrated system	Can apply to both independent and employed physicians. Unlike in the past, however, this model is now far more likely to be used primarily with employed physicians.

physicians come to believe that the IDS favors its employed physicians. As the number of employed physicians continues to grow, this type of tension is increasing as well. Table 3-3 lists common types of IDSs and summarizes how they relate to independent and employed physicians.

Independent Physicians in IDSs

IDSs involving mostly independent physicians may face federal scrutiny for potential antitrust violations such as price fixing. That risk is lower if physician payment involves some level of financial risk sharing as discussed in the *Provider Payment* chapter, and/or the IDS includes substantial clinical integration as discussed in the *Utilization Management, Quality Management, and Accreditation* chapter.

IDSs that include independent physicians also may not be able to use a single contract or signature page with a payer; that is, a separate contract or signature page may be required for each independent provider. Also, many states will not allow health plans (especially HMOs) to enter into contracts with any entity that does not have the power to bind the provider. In most cases, this issue is addressed by having a master contract between the IDS and the payer that contains the terms and conditions; the contracts between the payer and each independent provider are then relatively short and serve to legally bind the provider to the terms and conditions in the master contract.

Employed Physicians in IDSs

The employed-physician type of IDS first appeared in the mid- to late 1990s, when hospitals acquired PCP practices as a response to the growth of managed health care, and HMOs in particular. In most, but not all, cases, such moves were followed by serious financial losses, as physician productivity plummeted. Many hospitals then divested their physician service lines, sending the PCPs back out into their own practices. Beginning in the early 2000s, hospitals once again began to employ physicians. Now, however, they are employing both PCPs and specialists, and are doing so in steadily increasing numbers. These physicians may not be direct employees of the hospital system, but rather be employed through one of the other models described in this section.

When a hospital employs a sufficiently large number of PCPs and specialists, it substantially increases its negotiating leverage, particularly as payers face increasing demands for access because of the ACA. This increased leverage means the MHSs with large numbers of employed physicians should be able to obtain higher prices from commercial payers.

There is potential value to payers in such systems as well:

- The employed-physician type of IDS helps meet a payer's access needs for PCPs and other physicians.
- Such a system features more efficient management, including greater electronic data exchange.
- The IDS has the ability to invest in and effectively use electronic medical records (EMRs).

- Working with payers on new models of care and new payment structures is encouraged in the ACA.
- The IDS can work with payers to create smaller "private label" network products.

Physician–Hospital Organizations

PHOs are organizations that, at a minimum, allow a hospital and at least some of its independent physicians to negotiate with payers. PHOs are considered the easiest type of integrated system to develop, although managing them successfully is anything but easy.

PHOs may do little more than provide a negotiating vehicle, although this can potentially create an antitrust risk if the arrangement gives the appearance of being used to fix prices. The weakest form of PHO is the messenger model. With this approach, the PHO analyzes the terms and conditions offered by a payer and transmits its analysis results and the contract to each physician, who then decides on an individual basis whether to participate. More commonly, the PHO has a limited amount of time to negotiate the contract successfully—90 days, for example. If that deadline expires without agreement on a contract, then the participating physicians are free to contract directly with the payer; if the PHO successfully reaches an agreement with the payer, then the physicians agree to be bound by those terms.

PHOs also may actively manage the relationship between payers and the PHO's physician participants, or they may provide other administrative services. The "PO" portion of a PHO need not always be individual physicians, but rather might be an entirely different model; for example, a GPWW or an IPA (though not both) could represent the physician portion of the PHO. There is little reason to use a PHO with employed physicians, regardless of how the MHS employs them.

In the mid-1990s, PHOs were formed primarily as a defensive mechanism to deal with an increase in managed care contracting activity. Even then, it was not uncommon for the same physicians who joined the PHO to be under contract with one or more managed care plans. Since then, fewer PHOs have been created, and while existing ones continue to operate, the popularity of this type of IDS is declining rapidly.

Management Services Organizations

MSOs, like PHOs, often include a hospital or an MHS and at least some of the independent physicians affiliated with the hospitals, although some MSOs have no direct affiliation with a hospital. These organizations are identified as

IDSs here—even though some are not affiliated with a hospital—because they work in more or less the same way regardless of the presence or absence of a hospital affiliation.

Like PHOs, MSOs provide a vehicle for negotiating with payers. But the defining element of MSOs is that they provide services to physicians. MSOs can be owned and managed in a variety of ways:

- The MSO may be owned by a hospital, and managed either by the hospital or by another company under contract.
- The MSO may be owned by the MSO's physicians themselves, and managed either directly or by another company under contract.
- The MSO may be owned and managed by an independent company that is not affiliated with a hospital, and that may also purchase the independent physicians' practice assets and contracts with those physicians on a long-term basis.

In its simplest form, an MSO operates as a service bureau, providing basic practice support services to physicians. These services include such activities as billing and collection, administrative support, and electronic data interchange. Independent physicians contract with the MSO, but usually have no obligation to practice exclusively under the MSO unless the physicians are employed or the MSO has purchased their practices. In this model, and especially when the MSO is owned and operated by a hospital, the MSO must receive compensation from the physicians at fair market value, or the hospital and physicians could incur legal problems. The MSO should, through economies of scale as well as good management, be able to provide those services at a reasonable rate.

An MSO may also be considerably broader in scope. In addition to providing all the services described earlier, the MSO may actually purchase many of the assets of the physician's practice. For example, the MSO may purchase the physician's office space or office equipment (at fair market value), and employ the office support staff of the physician as well. Physicians who sell their practice assets to an MSO also sign long-term contracts with the MSO for ongoing services offered at fair market prices.

Some MSOs go beyond practice management and incorporate functions such as QM, UM, provider relations, and member services. In some cases, MSOs with these extended functions also contract with HMOs to accept global risk and are able to both manage utilization and negotiate favorable pricing from hospitals and referral specialists. An MSO model may be used with employed physicians, in which case it is really a subsidiary function of an MHS.

Foundations, Group Practice Without Walls, and Captive Medical Groups

In a foundation-model IDS,* a hospital creates a not-for-profit foundation, purchases physicians' practices (both tangible and intangible assets), and then puts those practices into the foundation. This model is usually selected when a legal or regulatory barrier prevents the formation of another type of arrangement—for example, when state CPM law prohibits a hospital from employing the physicians directly or using hospital funds to purchase the practices directly. More common in the past than today, foundations of this sort are now mostly confined to a few states.

The GPWW model as applied to physicians alone was discussed elsewhere in this chapter, but is included here because an IDS may use a GPWW model in similar fashion, with the GPWW serving as a captive medical group for the health system's employed physicians. This is usually the case when a hospital purchases physicians' practices but does not relocate the physicians from their existing offices, similar to what occurs with an MSO. In some cases, the IDS may actually have walls, providing the office space where the employed physicians practice; in this case, the physician model is not really a GPWW but rather a captive medical group. All of these arrangements work in more or less the same way in an IDS.

The foundation owns and manages the practices, but the physicians become members of a medical group that has an exclusive contract for services with the foundation; in other words, the foundation is the only source of revenue to the medical group. The physicians sign long-term contracts with the medical group that contain non-compete clauses. Despite this close relationship, to qualify for and maintain its not-for-profit status, the foundation must prove that it provides substantial community benefit, and it must be governed by a board that is not dominated by either the hospital or the physicians.

Patient-Centered Medical Homes

PCMHs are a concept much like the original vision for HMOs—that is, organizations focusing on prevention and maintenance of health. Whereas HMOs

---

* A second form of foundation model does not involve a hospital. In that model, the foundation is an entity that exists on its own and contracts for services with a medical group and a hospital. This type of arrangement dates back to the early days of HMOs, when many open-panel plans were not formed as either foundations or IPAs. Instead, in this model, the foundation held the HMO license and contracted with one or more IPAs and hospitals for services.

provide these services for all of their members, PCMHs focus on those individuals with one or more significant chronic illnesses—for example, a person with symptomatic congestive heart failure and diabetes. People with significant multiple chronic illnesses are at high risk for developing medical complications and incurring frequent hospitalizations, and they account for a very high percentage of total healthcare costs. According to the U.S. Agency for Healthcare Research and Quality (www.ahrq.gov), as of 2014:

- Five percent of the U.S. population accounted for almost half of the country's total healthcare expenses.
- The 15 most expensive health conditions accounted for 44% of total healthcare expenses.
- Patients with multiple chronic conditions cost up to seven times as much as patients with only one chronic condition.

Except for individuals involved in existing disease management (DM) programs described in the *Utilization Management, Quality Management, and Accreditation* chapter, the care for people with multiple chronic conditions is often not coordinated. Many of these patients receive care from multiple specialists, are prescribed different drugs by different doctors, and may have little or no follow-up or continuity of care.

PCMHs were conceived originally as "primary care medical homes" in which a patient's PCP served to coordinate all of a patient's care, again much like the original HMOs but without a "gatekeeper" requirement. Although many still refer to PCMHs as primary care medical homes, the acronym PCMH now more often stands for patient-centered medical home, a change in terminology that reflects the shift in focus to the patient and the embrace of a broader range of approaches. Currently, the most effective PCMHs rely on an organized team of providers. These teams may be led by physicians, but more often the physicians are team members, with the teams being led by other clinicians. Team members also include other types of providers such as NPs, PAs, pharmacists, and medical social workers.

Payer contracts with PCMHs usually do not supersede existing network contracts or replace any parts of the network, but rather add to the ongoing system. PCMH contracts may be limited to PCPs in some markets, but more often the contracts are reached with IDSs. Contracts with PCMHs also typically use payment models, as discussed in the *Provider Payment* chapter, that support the twin goals of improved outcomes and lower costs.

The Centers for Medicare and Medicaid Services (CMS) gave PCMHs a boost prior to passage of the ACA through pilot programs designed to see if these models could be successfully applied to traditional fee-for-service (FFS) Medicare. The ACA boosted their profile even more by addressing these IDSs directly, including allowing PCMHs* that meet other state requirements to offer coverage directly through the health insurance exchanges (see the *Sales, Governance, and Administration* chapter), although these organizations must still meet all applicable state requirements for health insurers or HMOs. Accreditation organizations have also developed standards for PCMHs. However, the studies showing positive results from their adoption have mostly come from medical groups or IDSs that were already experienced in providing cost-effective care, and it remains unknown how well this concept can be expanded or if it will work on a long-term basis.

Accountable Care Organizations

"Accountable care organization" is term coined by the Medicare Payment Advisory Commission (MedPAC), adopted by CMS, and incorporated into the ACA. For Medicare, it describes an organized group of providers that coordinates the care for designated beneficiaries in the traditional Medicare FFS program. An ACO is similar in many ways to a PCMH, in that it focuses on patients with significant chronic conditions and high costs. As used for FFS Medicare, however, it has a more narrowly defined organizational structure under federal law.

Many different types of provider organizations may be eligible for designation as ACOs, although some restrictions apply. All provider members of an ACO must demonstrate meaningful commitment by either contributing financially, providing services, and/or being subject to the ACO performance standards. In addition, CMS requires ACOs to meet other standards in governance, management, and so forth. An ACO must also have at least 5000 traditional Medicare beneficiaries "assigned" to it by CMS. An ACO can be structured as an IDS working mostly with independent physicians, its employed physicians, or both; or it could be structured as a physician-owned entity that may or may not include hospitals.

As defined in the ACA, CMS contracts with Medicare ACOs only for the traditional FFS Medicare program, and does so in a relatively uniform way. Commercial payers may also contract or even partner with ACOs, but in the commercial sector there is no consistency between different payers or with CMS

---

* Though Section 1301 [42 U.S.C. 18021] of the ACA still refers to them as Primary Care Medical Homes.

regarding definitions, organizational structures, payment methods, or much else relative to ACOs, other than the focus on members with significant chronic illnesses. Like PCMHs, accreditation organizations have developed standards for ACOs that accommodate both Medicare ACOs and commercial ACOs.

Medicare ACOs are initially paid by CMS through normal Medicare FFS payments, but are also subject to a specific payment model called "shared savings" that includes some shared risk for medical costs. This payment model means the ACO is accountable for reducing or at least meeting cost goals set by CMS for selected high-cost Medicare beneficiaries, although those beneficiaries are not "locked in" to the ACO and may seek care from any qualified provider; shared savings is discussed further in the Provider Payment chapter.

To test the ACO concept, CMS had begun an ACO pilot program prior to passage of the ACA. That pilot program was still under way when the ACA was passed, but the new law included language requiring CMS to press ahead with ACOs even though it was not clear if they would achieve their goals. As with PCMHs, it is unknown how well the ACO concept can be expanded or if it will work on a long-term basis.

Vertical Integration

Vertical integration refers to a concept once thought to be the future of the healthcare sector in the United States: physicians, hospitals, and insurance or benefits administration all gathered together within a single entity. The thinking was that by bringing these elements under the same umbrella, all incentives would be aligned and efficiencies would prevail. This concept looks almost identical to the early group- and staff-model HMOs, but the focus of vertical integration was more on the hospital and its associated providers that were still primarily paid through traditional FFS.

Many IDSs attempted to vertically integrate in the 1990s and early 2000s. While some succeeded, most ended in failure and loss. Some of the reasons for the failures included the following problems:

- A lack of management experience
- A lack of understanding about how to manage, or even account for, financial risk
- Conflicting financial incentives from being paid mostly through FFS or other traditional means that rewarded higher utilization and prices instead of lower ones

- Conflicting personal incentives as executives at hospitals tried to maximize bed-days and revenue, while executives at the IDS's payer organization tried to reduce them but with only tepid internal support
- Independent physicians' perception of the IDS payer as a means of reducing what they perceived as HMO interference, resulting in higher utilization
- Enrollment of a higher than normal percentage of people familiar with the IDS because they had serious chronic illnesses, resulting in a sicker than normal risk pool without enough premium income to cover costs

Large and well-managed medical groups were often able to succeed, as did some strong regional MHSs that approached the payer aspect with as much seriousness as existing successful payers. Unfortunately, this tack often resulted in strained relations with the independent physicians, at least initially.

There is renewed interest in vertical integration by IDSs—in particular, those with large numbers of employed physicians. They certainly face challenges similar to what they encountered in the past, but should have a greater chance of success for the following reasons:

- IDSs are much larger now, allowing them to market their services more broadly.
- An IDS may choose to create a Medicare Advantage plan instead of an ACO because of MA's greater financial potential.
- There are more executives with payer experience that an IDS can bring in.
- Computer and other support systems are much better.
- Utilization management support tools and general knowledge have improved considerably.
- IDSs with a large panel of employed PCPs and specialists, when there is strong and capable physician leadership, can function much like a group- or staff-model HMO.

At the same time, commercial payers have made considerable improvements in their practices and are much more experienced overall. They tend to have far more financial stability, larger market shares, and more knowledge and experience in marketing and sales than their earlier-generation counterparts.

Rather than compete, some IDSs and payers are partnering to create narrow-network products in which the IDS has more responsibility and shares more in the financial performance of the organization. Other IDSs are creating their own licensed payer organizations, but contracting or even partnering with an existing commercial payer to provide all of the administrative and specialized services. It is not possible here to predict the overall success or failure of any of the new vertically integrated approaches.

ANCILLARY SERVICES

Ancillary services are unique in that they are seldom sought out by a patient unless ordered by a physician. They are broadly divided into diagnostic and therapeutic services.

Examples of Diagnostic Ancillary Services

- Laboratory;
- Imaging, such as routine radiology (X-rays), nuclear imaging, computed tomography (CT), magnetic resonance imaging (MRI), and the like
- Electrocardiography
- Other cardiac testing, such as stress testing and cardiac nuclear imaging
- Any other types of diagnostic testing

Examples of Therapeutic Ancillary Services

- Home care
- Generalized rehabilitation and habilitation
- Focused rehabilitation such as cardiac or post-stroke rehabilitation
- Physical therapy (PT)
- Occupational therapy (OT)
- Speech therapy
- Other long-term therapeutic services

Pharmacy services are a special form of ancillary services that account for a significant portion of overall healthcare costs, and are discussed in the chapters titled *Provider Payment* and *Utilization Management, Quality Management and Accreditation.*

Contracting for Ancillary Services

Ancillary services are often provided by free-standing facility-based companies, although they are also provided by hospitals. Ancillary care provided in the course of an inpatient stay or an outpatient procedure is included in the overall facility services, and is not traditionally counted as ancillary services for purposes of separate contracting.

Because ancillary services are elective and non-urgent, payers may contract with a limited number of ancillary providers, often through a national or regional chain. They also rely far more heavily on favorable pricing terms to manage the cost of ancillary services than they do on managing utilization. Hospitals also provide non-urgent outpatient ancillary services, but typically have higher prices than do free-standing ancillary services providers.

Some diagnostic services companies do not require a physician order to provide ancillary services, such as a free-standing cardiac testing company or a company offering "comprehensive" testing to consumers. Testing performed without a physician's order is seldom, if ever, covered by health plans.

Physician-Owned Ancillary Services

In some cases, ancillary services providers are owned by the same physicians that order their use, a practice called self-referral. Self-referral represents a unique and significant problem in health insurance and managed health care because compelling evidence shows that physicians who have an ownership interest in some kind of ancillary service will use it far more often than will physicians without an ownership interest.

From a contracting perspective, it is neither practical nor desirable to completely restrict physicians' ability to use appropriate services or equipment that they own to deliver routine care within their specialty. For example, orthopedists cannot properly care for their patients if they cannot take X-rays in their offices. Of course, it is also too costly to ignore this potential conflict of interest completely. Payers, therefore, use different contracting and payment approaches to try and reduce its impact.

Payers' credentialing of ancillary service providers is similar to the credentialing used for facilities. That is, payers rely on state licensure and, in some cases, external accreditation or certification. Some payers such as HMOs may also evaluate an ancillary services provider on the basis of geography and access needs, ability to produce reports on quality, and so forth.

NETWORK MAINTENANCE

Network maintenance is an important function for any payer, and for HMOs in particular. Recruiting and credentialing new providers is an ongoing activity, but more focus is typically placed on maintenance of the existing network.

Maintenance includes activities such as recredentialing, resolving claims or other problems, managing access to providers, managing network issues that affect members' experiences, and managing the overall relationship between the providers and the payer. Many plans differentiate between network management for facilities and network management for the professionals.

How plans approach network maintenance is continually changing. For example, the increase in self-service capabilities via the web allows provider staff to handle many routine tasks such as checking eligibility, submitting authorizations, checking on claims status, and reconciling submitted and paid claims. For issues not addressed through self-service, most routine network maintenance relies on the provider's office staff. But physicians in particular should not be neglected, and regular two-way communication with network providers is important, as are communications channels that provide for physicians to directly contact a plan medical director. In addition, bringing network physicians into projects, and paying them fair market value for their professional time and effort, is both beneficial and helps the plan achieve its goals.

CONCLUSION

One of the hallmarks of managed health care is the existence of a provider network, and this applies now to nearly every form of health insurance as well. Payers depend on their networks to deliver medical care to their members; even closed-panel HMOs depend to some degree on a network of private physicians and hospitals. A payer's network is an asset and a critical part of its overall ability to succeed over the long term.

Provider Payment

LEARNING OBJECTIVES

- Understand the difference between payment and reimbursement
- Explain the most common forms and variations of payment for physician services, including their strengths and weaknesses
- Explain the most common forms and modifiers of payment for facility-based inpatient and outpatient services
- Describe the common forms of payment that combine facility and physician payment
- Identify the basics of pay-for-performance arrangements for physicians and for facilities
- Discuss the basics of the shared savings program under the Affordable Care Act
- Explain the most common forms of payment for ancillary services and pharmaceuticals

INTRODUCTION

The reason for broadly referring to health insurers, managed care organizations (MCOs), and benefits administrators as "payers" is because that is what they do: pay clinical care providers, clinical support services, and drug and device manufacturers for medical services and goods. Of course, payment is not the only thing they do, but it is a key element of their primary function of managing healthcare benefits coverage.

It is obvious that payers do not pay—and never have paid—all types of providers in the same way. What is not so obvious is the astonishing number of different ways in which such payments are made, along with the continual introduction of new and increasingly complex approaches to payment being introduced. Payment models have been blurring and blending for decades, and they continue to do so. In short, payers, consultants, and policy makers seem to be endlessly creative in terms of how to pay providers and how they attempt to use payment methods to change provider behavior in ways that will lower costs, or at least slow the rate of increase in those costs. Providers are no less creative about payment, but not always in an effort to reduce costs.

Provider payment is not magic, of course, and no payment model alone will be able to solve the problem of health cost inflation. Nevertheless, certain methods of provider payment are less likely to cause cost inflation, and that alone is a worthy goal. More importantly, payment can be a tool in which the financial incentives of providers and payers become aligned, which in turn supports medical management of utilization. This is important because overall costs are the product of a simple equation: cost = price × volume.* In health care, this equation can be seen as equivalent to total healthcare cost = provider payment × medical utilization. To manage the cost of health care, both of these factors—provider payment and medical utilization—must be addressed.

In this chapter, we will look mostly at the common methods used to pay physicians as well as hospitals and facilities. As we discuss these methods, we will consider how payment methods are modified on a case-by-case basis, an issue that affects hospitals more than physicians. We will also examine payment methods that include some level of risk and reward sharing based on overall cost goals, which affects physicians more often than it affects hospitals. Other methods combine physician and hospital payments, including some new forms under the Affordable Care Act (ACA), and may or may not include some form of risk sharing. We will briefly look at payment for ancillary services and drugs as well. Note that our focus here is mostly on payment models used by commercial payers. Medicare and Medicaid payment methods are described, but not in great depth and often in the context of methods also used by commercial payers.

Before we examine different methods of provider payment, we discuss the difference between "payment" and "reimbursement" and why it is important. We also consider the electronic transaction and code set requirements that apply to most payment models, and briefly address the distinction between risk-based and

---

* The equation may be simple, but it is simple in much the same way that "$e = mc^2$" is simple—meaning it is not so simple when you look at the details.

non-risk-based provider payment. Once that stage is set, we can explore some of these common forms of provider payment:

- Payment of physicians and other professionals
- Payment of hospitals and ambulatory facilities
- Combined or bundled payment of physicians and hospitals
- The Medicare Shared Savings Program
- Pay for Performance (P4P)
- Payment of ancillary services
- Payment of pharmaceuticals (also discussed in the *Utilization Management, Quality Management, and Accreditation* chapter)
- Payment reforms under the ACA

IT'S PAYMENT, NOT REIMBURSEMENT

On the two sides of the payment coin (so to speak), payment models either counter or take advantage of the natural inclination of most individuals, including physicians, and executives of hospitals and health plans, to maximize their income, at least up to a point. That brings us to this singular and important point: Provider payment is payment; it is not reimbursement.

Reimbursement means being made whole for actual out-of-pocket expenses on a dollar-for-dollar basis—for example, being reimbursed by an employer for out-of-pocket business travel expenses. Reimbursement works the same way for everyone (not counting expense account padding, which is a minor form of fraud); in other words, out-of-pocket travel expenses are reimbursed the same way for a corporate vice president as they are for a sales trainee. For that reason, reimbursement does not influence behavior other than by making a person more willing to travel as part of employment because the employee knows doing so will not cost him or her any money.

Payment, in contrast, makes up a person's wages or salary, or any type of work-related bonus. It is not the same for everybody. Wages and salaries typically vary based on training, education, and skill levels; how much an employer wants or needs to hire someone based on what that person can do; and the negotiating strength of both parties. In this sense, payment most definitely drives behavior, from basic compensation to productivity and achievement bonuses. This is also the case in provider payment.

Why is it important to make the distinction between provider payment and provider reimbursement? While it might seem to be a minor difference in vocabulary, it is not: Referring to payment *as* payment helps us see it as payment, which in turn helps us better understand its impact. Thinking of provider payment as reimbursement reduces our awareness of how payment affects personal and organizational behavior, along with its impact on costs, and even why payment methods and amounts vary so much. Furthermore, it can cause us to subconsciously think of payment as being more fair and neutral than it really is—that is, as being above such tainted motives as profit or personal enrichment; a comforting fiction, but a fiction nevertheless.

That is not to say that all healthcare providers are driven primarily by money.* They are not; they are usually far more motivated by the desire to help sick patients, improve health, treat disease, and relieve suffering. Within that context, however, payment still influences behavior. Sometimes direct behavior is affected, such as when payment concerns consciously or subconsciously motivate some doctors to perform high-paying procedures or tests when they also derive income from the facility or testing device itself. Payment also influences behavior on a larger scale. For example, specialists are paid more than primary care physicians (PCPs)—usually a lot more. In turn, medical students have increasingly chosen to become specialists instead of PCPs, resulting in too many specialists but a shortage of PCPs in the United States, the very opposite of what society needs right now.

Payment methods are not by themselves necessarily good or bad, although some align better than others with the goals of managing costs and improving outcomes. Even when they are better aligned, payment methods alone will not succeed in achieving those desired outcomes. At best, payment incentives will support management of utilization and quality; at worst, they will work against those ends. As the songwriter Randy Newman put it, "It's money that matters."†

STANDARDIZED CODE SETS AND TRANSACTIONS UNDER THE HEALTH INSURANCE PORTABILITY AND ACCOUNTABILITY ACT

Although the Health Insurance Portability and Accountability Act of 1996 (HIPAA) was initially drafted as a means of allowing individuals to keep their health insurance under certain circumstances, this law's biggest impact, in

---

*The same can be said for executives for that matter, but executive payment is not the topic of this chapter.

† Randy Newman. "It's Money That Matters." *Land of Dreams*. Reprise/Warner Bros.; 1988.

addition to its privacy and security requirements, has been its requirements mandating "covered entities," including payers, providers, and their business associates,* to comply with standards included in the section of HIPAA titled "Administrative Simplification." These standards, which went into effect in 2004 and are regularly modified, apply to the following areas:

- Electronic transactions
- Code sets
- Electronic funds transfers
- Identifiers
- Privacy
- Security

Because electronic transactions, code sets, and electronic funds transfer are related, directly or indirectly, to provider payment, they are addressed here. The national provider identifier (NPI) is discussed in the chapter titled *The Provider Network*, and other identifiers are discussed in the *Sales, Governance, and Administration* chapter, as are privacy and security requirements.

Electronic Transaction Standards

Prior to HIPAA, each payer had its own requirements for common types of electronic transactions such as submitting claims. HIPAA mandated that all covered entities use the same standardized transactions. The HIPAA requirements apply only to a subset of business transactions; for example, they do not apply to medical records or communications between providers.

Technical Standards

HIPAA requires certain specific organizations to periodically update the transaction standards, and the covered entities typically have a year or more to make the necessary changes to their information technology (IT) systems. Transactions other than pharmacy claims are subject to the X12 (sometimes referred to as X12N) standards developed by the American National Standards Institute (ANSI). For pharmacy claims, the designated standards are those of the National Council for Prescription Drug Programs (NCPDP). The ANSI X12 standard transactions are listed in Table 4–1.

---

*Business associates (BAs) are companies working for payers or providers that have access to the medical and/or claims data or any personal information about patients or members.

Table 4–1   Electronic Transaction Standards Required Under HIPAA

Type of Transaction Standard	ANSI X12 Transaction Standard
Eligibility for health plan benefits	270—Request 271—Response
Health claim status	276—Request 277—Response
Electronic funds transfer and remittance advice	835
Health claims or equivalent encounter information; includes coordination of benefits information	837p—Professional 837i—Institutional 837d—Dental
Health plan enrollment/disenrollment	834
Health plan premium payments	820
Referral certification/authorization	278—Request and Response
Health claims attachments (this standard had not been fully defined or finalized at the time of this text's publication)	275

Source: Federal Register for 45 CFR Part 162.

Transaction Implementation Policy Requirements Under the ACA

Electronic transactions standards are highly technical, and they actually support a degree of flexibility in regard to how certain data fields are defined and used. HIPAA set requirements for the electronic transaction standards, but did not specify how those standards were to be implemented. Payers did all not use the same approach, which created some incompatibilities. The ACA amended HIPAA to address this inconsistency and directed the U.S. Department of Health and Human Services (DHHS) to develop implementation standards and prohibit payers from creating their own.

DHHS had addressed three of those implementation standards at the time of this text's publication. Health plans will be required to submit documentation that demonstrates compliance with the adopted standards and operating rules for these three types of electronic transactions:

1. Eligibility for a health plan
2. Healthcare claim status
3. Healthcare electronic funds transfer (EFT) and electronic remittance advice (ERA) transactions

At the time of this text's publication, however, only proposed rules had been issued for these three implementation standards, not the final rules. Additional implementation standards will follow.

Code Sets

Almost all provider billing involves the use of standardized codes—that is, numbers and letters that represent a particular service, procedure, diagnosis, treatment, medical device, drug, or the like. Some types of codes are used by all providers, but more often the codes are specific to certain types of providers.

HIPAA made the use of certain diagnostic and procedure codes mandatory only for electronic transactions between covered entities, but as a practical matter these codes are used even when paper bills are submitted by mail or fax if for no other reason than payers will not pay a bill that does not use them, regardless of how the payer received it. There are some other code sets that HIPAA does not require all covered entities to use, but that may be required by Medicare or be commonly used by commercial payers. Table 4–2 lists the code sets required under HIPAA, and Table 4–3 identifies commonly used code sets that are not required under HIPAA.

Table 4–2   Code Sets Required Under HIPAA

Code Set	Type of Usage
Current Procedural Terminology, Fourth Revision (CPT-4)	Procedure or type of service by physicians and other professionals for inpatient and outpatient care.
Healthcare Common Procedural Coding System (HCPCS)	Many different types of codes used by many different types of providers.
Until October 1, 2015: International Classification of Diseases, Ninth Edition, Clinical Modification (ICD-9-CM)	Used to report diagnoses in all clinical settings. Volumes 1 and 2 are used by most types of providers and include services not covered under the CPT-4 codes. Volume 3 is used by facilities to report procedures.
Beginning October 1, 2015: International Classification of Diseases, Tenth Edition, Clinical Modification (ICD-10)	Used to report diagnoses in all clinical settings. ICD-10 replaces Volumes 1 and 2 of ICD-9-CM, and ICD-10-PCS replaces Volume 3.
National Drug Codes (NDC)	Used for drugs and biologics.
Code on Dental Procedures and Nomenclature	Used for dental procedures and services.

Table 4–3   Commonly Used Code Sets Not Mandated by HIPAA

These codes are not necessarily used directly for billing, and are usually created through the use of other codes and supplemental information.

Diagnosis-related groups (DRGs)	For inpatient care, but no longer used by Medicare and being phased out by commercial payers that used it.
Medicare severity-adjusted DRGs (MS-DRGs)	For inpatient care; used by Medicare and many commercial payers; replaces DRGs.
Other types of DRGs	See Table 4–10.
Ambulatory payment classifications (APCs)	Used for ambulatory facilities by Medicare and some commercial payers.
Ambulatory Payment Groups (APGs) and Enhanced Ambulatory Patient Groups (EAPGs)	Proprietary ambulatory facility code sets related to APCs and used by many commercial payers and state Medicaid programs. EAPGs have largely replaced APGs.

Electronic Funds Transfers

As of 2014, HIPAA requires payers to use electronic funds transfers if a provider requests it. HIPAA does not require a provider to accept EFTs. However, a payer can make the use of EFTs a condition of participation in its network, which Medicare does for its traditional program. The standards for EFTs are set by the banking industry, not HIPAA.

Risk-Based Versus Non-Risk-Based Payment

Provider payment can be risk based or non-risk based, and may be used with different types of providers. Risk-based payment means that the provider shares some portion of financial risk for overall costs, such that higher than budgeted costs can result in payment reductions while lower than budgeted costs can result in higher payment. This serves to align the financial goals of the provider with those of the payer and/or employer. Non-risk-based payments do not align those goals, and higher costs generally equate to higher provider payments, so that there is no provider incentive to reduce costs. Most methods of provider payment do not contain any financial risk. Both types of payment can also be affected by modifiers that can change the method or the amount of payment depending on various factors.

Any payer, including a health maintenance organization (HMO), may use any type of non-risk-based payment. In contrast, only HMOs may use risk-based payment, and until the ACA was passed, exceptions to this rule were very limited. The ACA, however, created a new type of integrated healthcare delivery system (IDS) called an accountable care organization (ACO) for the traditional Medicare program. Medicare ACOs are required to move toward a "shared savings" payment model that includes shared risk, and many commercial payers are also using shared savings with ACOs, albeit in different ways.

PHYSICIAN PAYMENT

Many different methodologies are used to pay physicians. These payment methods may differ based on a number of factors or combinations of factors, including the following:

- The type of health plan or payer
- Benefits design
- Physician location
- Physician specialty
- Physician organizational structure
- Negotiating strength of either party
- State and federal laws and regulations

Physician payment methodologies are anything but uniform, and the *same* payer may pay the *same* physicians in the *same* locations for the *same* procedures using *different* methods of payment and/or *different* payment amounts for *different* products or plan designs.*

Medical and payment policies may also be combined. For example, a second surgeon attending an operation is typically paid half the fee paid to the primary surgeon. In the same markets, payers may use different payment methods, and the same payer may use different payment methods in different geographic regions. In short, it is nearly impossible to know how, and how much, physicians are paid by any one commercial payer in any one market.

To make things even more confusing, the payment methodology used by a payer often differs from how individual physicians are compensated. Most medical groups and IDSs that employ physicians pay them a salary with bonus incentives. Independent physician associations (IPAs) are often paid through capitation, but the IPA's physicians are paid through some form of fee-for-service

---

* If you are not confused yet, the author suggests you reread this sentence.

(FFS) arrangement. These and other examples show how payment methodologies by payers do not always directly affect individual physicians.

Like provider payment in general, most physician payment is not risk based. Nevertheless, a considerable number of HMOs still use risk-based physician payment, although this practice varies by region. Exhibit 4–1 lists common non-risk-based physician payment methodologies, and Exhibit 4–2 lists common risk-based physician payment methodologies.

Exhibit 4–1   Non-Risk-Based Physician Payment Used by All Types of Payers

- Fee for service
    - Straight charges
    - Usual, customary, or reasonable (UCR) fee allowances
    - Percentage discount on charges
    - Fee schedule
    - Relative value scale (RVS)
    - Resource-based relative value scale (RBRVS)
    - Percent of Medicare RBRVS
    - Special fee schedule or RVS multiplier
    - Facility fee add-on
- Case rates and global fees

Exhibit 4–2   Risk-Based Physician Payment Used by HMOs

- Capitation
    - Variation factors
        - Age and sex
        - Level of illness ("acuity")
        - Other
    - PCP only
        - With a withhold
        - Without a withhold
    - Pooled versus individual risk
    - Specialist
    - Global
    - IPA
    - Contract capitation
- At-risk FFS
    - Fee percentage withhold
    - Budgeted FFS

Non-Risk-Based Physician Payment

All types of payers, including HMOs, may use physician payment methods that do not share financial risk with the physicians. Even HMOs that use risk-based payment also use non-risk-based methods for at least some participating physicians, with the exception of HMOs that globally capitate an IPA. Nevertheless, even these HMO exceptions typically use FFS to pay for emergency or authorized care from out-of-network providers, and capitated IPAs frequently pay their physician members through FFS. There are some no-risk forms of payment other than FFS, and even though FFS may be the predominant form of physician payment, there is more than one way to implement it.

Fee for Service

FFS is used by all type of payers for at least some services. This payment method is simple on its surface but complex in how it is actually realized. On the surface, a physician bills for services based on procedure codes, meaning what service(s) or procedure(s) were performed. The complexity is just below the surface and comes from the number of codes, the differences among them, the fees a physician charges for each code, other codes that are added to the bill, and more. Many believe that FFS is one of the most important drivers of cost inflation because it rewards physicians for doing more, for charging more in general, and for doing procedures with higher charges compared to less costly options. There is much truth to this statement, but like so many things in health care, it is not as simple as it sounds. Even so, this concern is one reason why there are so many different ways of paying physicians, including different methods of FFS payment.

Fee Schedules; the Maximum Allowable Charge; and Usual, Customary, or Reasonable Fees All providers, including physicians, may charge whatever they want to charge, at least to commercial payers and individuals not covered under one of the entitlement programs. As a result, charges vary widely from one provider to the next. Charges also usually differ by specialty and by location. Nevertheless, even different physicians in the same specialty and in the same community may have different charges. Physicians are prohibited from sharing information about their fees with competing physicians because this could lead to price fixing. As a result, fees charged for any procedure may vary by as much as 500% or even more between physicians, though most are within a somewhat narrower range.

Payers cannot simply pay whatever any provider charges. If they did, providers would continually inflate their fees. To address this issue, payers use fee schedules for processing claims and determining coverage. A fee schedule is simply a list of the maximum amounts that will be allowed—the maximum allowable charge—for each type of service for purposes of benefits coverage and claims payment. For nonemergency services, there is typically no coverage for charges higher than the maximum, though how that affects plan members depends on each member's use of the plan's provider network and other requirements. As a side note, a physician's charges might potentially be below the maximum allowable payment, but that situation has become extremely rare.

Payers use fee schedules not only to pay in-network providers, but also for benefits coverage of charges from nonparticipating physicians for nonemergency care in those plan types that offer out-of-network benefits coverage. We can illustrate how this approach is used by considering the example of a member covered under a preferred provider organization (PPO).

Most PPO benefits use fixed copayments for in-network physician visits and percentage coinsurance for out-of-network physicians, but they may use coinsurance even for in-network physician services for procedures. Most PPOs also apply different deductible amounts to in-network services versus out-of-network services. To keep matters simple, however, in Table 4–4 we will ignore any deductible and copayments, instead using only coinsurance to look at how the maximum allowable charge is used for in-network and out-of-network coverage.

In this example, the amount of coinsurance paid by the member for in-network care is calculated as a percentage of the maximum allowable charge or in-network fee, not the full charge. That is because the coinsurance is a percentage of the total cost of the service when it is rendered by a network provider, and is therefore limited by the No Balance Billing clause in the provider contract. This level of protection is not available for charges from out-of-network providers.

Payers may use any of several ways to determine what the maximum allowable charge should be for covered claims from noncontracted providers. The historical method is known as the UCR. Where once it was defined as "usual, customary, *and* reasonable," it is now often defined as "usual, customary, *or* reasonable." The definition of "reasonable" is in the eye of the beholder, however, and payers often determine that certain services are grossly overpriced for reasons discussed below.

The traditional approach to determining prevailing fees is to collect data for charges by CPT-4 and HCPCS codes in a defined region (e.g., a city); calculate the 10th, 25th, 50th, 75th, and 90th percentiles; and then choose which percentile represents a reasonable prevailing fee, which traditionally was the

Table 4–4   Example of the Use of Maximum Allowable Charge in a PPO

	In-Network Benefit: 80% Coverage	Out-of-Network Benefit: 60% Coverage Based on Maximum Allowable Charge
Fee charged by physician	$200.00	$200.00
Maximum allowable charge	$150.00	$150.00
Amount paid directly to participating physician	$120.00 (80% of $150.00)	$0.00[1]
Amount paid to member[1]	$0.00	$90.00 (60% of $150.00)[2]
Amount paid by member	$30.00 (20% of $150.00)[3]	Directly to the provider: $200.00 Net cost to the member: $110.00 ($200.00 minus the $90.00 covered by the PPO)[4]

[1] Unless required by state law, health plans do not directly pay noncontracted providers, except for emergency care in some cases. The member is responsible for paying the provider, and the covered amount is sent by the plan to the member.

[2] There is no coverage for charges higher than the maximum allowable charge.

[3] Contracted providers agree to not balance bill the member for any difference between the PPO's maximum allowable charge fee schedule and their full charges.

[4] Benefits coverage is limited to a percentage of the maximum allowable charge, not a percentage of whatever a provider charges. Because they do not have a contract with the PPO, out-of-network providers are not required to limit how much they charge and may pursue payment in full. The member must pay the provider the entire amount but receives a check from the PPO for the amount that is covered.

90th percentile.* Unfortunately, this approach drives price inflation: When enough providers raise their fees to a higher level, that also increases the average charges—resulting in higher payment amount, which in turn encourages providers to raise their fees once again. In a similar way, physicians charging less than the maximum allowable charge will raise their charges so they can collect more and not "leave money on the table."

A small number of physicians take this to an extreme and charge fees that are 10 to 20 times higher than average, which can drive the percentiles very high. Payers once used statistical techniques to reduce the impact of excessively high physician charges on the UCR calculation, but a lawsuit by the Attorney General

---

*A percentile means the percentage that charge the same or less than an amount. For example, if the 10th percentile is $50.00 and the 90th percentile is $500.00, then only 10% of physicians charge $50.00 or less, while 90% of physicians charge $500.00 or less.

of New York stopped that practice. Therefore, payers typically combine UCR data with other sources of fee information (often Medicare payment rates) to determine the maximum allowable charge for each code. Increasingly, payers no longer use UCR data at all, but instead simply base their maximum allowable charges on Medicare fees, increased by a fixed percentage.

Even though it might appear that a physician can earn more money by not contracting with any payer and charging full fees, it is not always easy to collect that money. Indeed, sometimes those fees are never collected at all, although some states now require payers to pay even noncontracted providers directly. In most cases, being in a network means getting paid directly, thereby avoiding at least some problems with collection. Patients are also more likely to see in-network physicians, and those physicians are also less likely to lose patients because of cost differences. For these and other reasons, we end our look at payment to noncontracted physicians here, and turn to the common methods payers use to pay contracted providers.

Discounts on Charges   Payment using a simple discount on charges has been used by both HMOs and PPOs. The advantage associated with this approach is that it is extremely easy to implement. Most physicians will gladly accept a discount on fees if it ensures rapid and direct payment and being listed in a plan's network directory. But the relentless upward pressure on fees remains in full force, and the discount system does nothing to reduce the rate of cost inflation. Because of this, payment through discounted charges is relatively uncommon.

Relative Value Scale and the Resource-Based Relative Value Scale   The use of a relative value scale (RVS) is widely used in FFS. Each procedure or billing code, as defined in CPT, has relative values associated with it called relative value units (RVUs). The plan pays the physician on the basis of a fixed dollar amount multiplied by the value of the RVUs. This allows a payer to update a fee schedule simply by changing the fixed dollar amount rather than having to recalculate each fee separately. Nevertheless, a simple RVS that reflects UCR fees will also reflect the higher prices associated with procedures compared to office visits. This factor explains why the simple UCR-based RVS has given way to the resource-based relative value scale (RBRVS).

The most well-known RBRVS is the one used by the Centers for Medicare & Medicaid Services (CMS) for Medicare. For each CPT-4 code, three different RVUs are added together to make up the overall value:

1. The amount of work and the amount of resources invested by the physician in training

2. The cost of the practice, including the cost of personnel, supplies, and so forth

3. The cost of malpractice insurance

Table 4–5 provides an example of a hypothetical calculation of the allowed fee for a routine office visit (CPT-4 Code 99213) using an RBRVS scale.

Most payers use Medicare's RBRVS as the basis for their fee schedules, often by simply adjusting the value of the multiplier by some percentage (e.g., the Medicare rate plus 10%). However, the Medicare RBRVS is not the only scale in use because it does not cover all procedures, so commercial payers may also license an RBRVS scale from an external source. Both may be used depending on the types of services provided, and payers may use other schedules for services not typically addressed by an RBRVS.

The value of the multiplier is usually the same for all physicians in the network in the same general area, but large medical groups and hospitals with a large number of employed physicians may negotiate a higher rate. This can make claims processing more complex and add to administrative costs, but it is increasingly common as the marketplace changes.

Variation Based on Location of Service   Because the facility costs make up part of the total cost of a procedure, many health plans pay attention to where a procedure is performed. For example, the same procedure performed in a hospital facility is often far more expensive than when it is performed in a free-standing ambulatory surgical center, due solely to the differences in what each type of facility charges (unless the plan has negotiated equivalent charges for each type of location). To lower total costs, the plan may reduce the fees paid to the

---

Table 4–5   Illustration of Hypothetical RBRVS Payment Calculation for CPT-4 Code 99213 ("Routine Office Visit")

Step 1	Step 2
Calculate total RVUs for CPT code 99213: • Work RVU = 0.97 • Practice expense RVU = 0.99 • Malpractice insurance cost RVU = 0.07	Multiply total of RVUs by the fixed-dollar amount conversion factor: • Total RVUs = 2.03 • Hypothetical conversion factor = $35.00
• Total RVUs (0.97 + 0.99 + 0.07) = 2.03	• Allowable payment amount (2.03 × $35.00) = $71.05

physician if the procedure is performed in a hospital or other high-cost location, but increase the fees paid if the physician uses a low-cost facility.

Add-on Facility Fee

Another increasing trend is inclusion of an add-on facility fee, in which a hospital that runs the clinics or offices used by their employed physicians bills the payer a separate fee. This fee is actually a payment to a facility, not a physician, but is included here because payments to physicians practicing in their own offices include all the costs associated with providing care, and no extra fee is paid for office space or support. An add-on facility fee is rarely offset by a lower physician charge. When payers contract with hospitals that charge an add-on fee, they typically negotiate that fee out of the payment and require the participating hospital to not balance bill the member. When the payer does not have enough negotiating leverage to do so, or if the system is not in the payer's network, however, members may find themselves facing an unexpected additional cost that is usually not covered in their benefits.

Electronic Visits

Electronic visits, also called e-visits or online visits, comprise a clinical interaction between a physician and a patient that takes place via electronic communications other than normal phone calls, not on a face-to-face basis. Electronic visits must comply with HIPAA's privacy and security requirements, as discussed in the *Sales, Governance, and Administration* chapter. This compliance is usually ensured by using a specialized form of secure e-mail, a structured and secure application, or a live video interaction. Some payers now pay physicians for providing care via e-visits, although the fee is usually less than that charged for a standard office visit. The member may be required to pay the usual copayment based on plan design, but this practice is not uniform. There is also no uniformity of fees or coding for such visits, but eventually that will change.

Case Rates

A case rate is a single payment that includes all professional services delivered in a defined episode of care. Common examples of case rates include obstetrics, in which a single fee covers all prenatal visits, the delivery itself, and at least one postnatal visit; and certain surgical procedures, in which a single surgical fee pays for preoperative care, the surgery itself, and postoperative care. Case rates are similar to FFS in that they are event based, but they reduce the ability to unbundle charges (charge separately for items once included in a single charge) or to churn visits (see patients more often than is necessary). A case rate may be subject to additional outlier fees if significant complications occur, in which case payments are typically based on a discounted charges.

Price Transparency

The term *price transparency* or *pricing transparency*, sometimes also referred to as *cost transparency*, refers to making information about the cost or price of healthcare services available to consumers. Information about physician pricing usually consists of how much the plan pays contracted physicians for certain things (e.g., office visits, delivering a baby), and in some cases, what the local prevailing charges are. The availability of such information allows consumers to understand how much more they will have to pay if they see noncontracting physicians. As yet, most health plans that post information (if they do so at all) are not posting pricing information specific to individual physicians, but rather using aggregate type of data.

Some also believe that making fees transparent will lead to lower fees due to competition. This has not been proven, however, and there is equal reason to believe that it will increase fees as providers with lower charges play "catch-up."

Risk-Based Physician Payment

Capitation is the most well-known type of risk-based payment, but risk-based FFS is also common, and both may be used in the same HMO. Because of concerns in past decades about risk-based physician payment—especially capitation—potentially incentivizing a physician to withhold necessary services, state laws typically allowed only HMOs to capitate providers. At least initially, this same concern was one of the reasons HMOs were required to have more stringent rules about utilization and quality management than other types of plans. Ultimately, the concern about capitation leading to poor quality of care proved to be unfounded.

Capitation

Capitation is prepayment for services on a per-member per-month (PMPM) basis. In other words, a physician is paid the same amount of money every month for every member in his or her patient panel regardless of whether that person actually receives services, and regardless of how extensive those services are. It is important to keep that point in mind because the capitation payment rate is not the same as the payment rate for office visits. Capitation is paid whether the member comes in or not, and the same amount is paid even if the member sees the doctor only once in a year. Capitation provides a predictable amount of income. Equally important, it is "prepaid," meaning the physician does not need to send bills or try to collect money after the fact. When physicians do have to collect money owed to them for past services, they are rarely able to collect it all; capitation eliminates that risk.

Capitation is used by many HMOs that also use a PCP "gatekeeper" system in which a member selects a single PCP or primary care group for services, and the PCP manages the member's access to specialty care. Because of this, utilization and costs can be attributed—directly or indirectly—to that PCP. Not all HMOs that have PCP "gatekeeper" systems use capitation, but over two-thirds of them do. HMOs that use capitation, other than HMOs that capitate a large IPA or medical group with both PCPs and specialists, typically capitate PCPs more often than they capitate specialists.

Capitation paid to a large physician organization does not necessarily mean that the individual physicians in the organization will be compensated through capitation. For example, a large medical group may be capitated, but the individual physicians may be paid via salary with productivity bonuses. Likewise, an HMO may capitate an IPA for all professional services, but the IPA might then pay its physician members through a mix of FFS and capitation or even entirely through risk-based FFS.

This variety of options illustrates that how a health plan pays its contracted physicians and how the physicians themselves are personally compensated are not always identical. Most physicians contract with multiple payers, each of which uses different forms of payment. Even the same payer may pay physicians differently based on product design; for example, it may use capitation for its HMO product but use FFS for its PPO. Employed physicians and physicians in larger medical groups are also typically compensated through a salary plus bonus (usually based on productivity), not directly through health plan payment.

"Lock-in Requirements" and Scope of Covered Services   One key requirement if capitation is to work is that members must be "locked in" to a particular provider and not covered for nonemergency services obtained from another provider of the same type under most circumstances. Plan types in which members are free to access any network provider make it difficult at best to attribute costs and utilization to any one physician.

The other key requirement for successful capitation is that the contract with a capitated physician must define which services are included and which services are not included. Excluded services are also referred to as "carve-outs" because they are carved out of the capitation payment. Services typically included are such things as preventive services, outpatient care, and hospital visits. Certain services require more definition than other things; for example, selected diagnostic testing (e.g., office urinalysis or electrocardiograms) may be included in the capitation, but for other lab testing the patient might be sent to a free-standing outside reference lab. This concept applies to any type of medical service a physician may provide.

Calculation of Capitation Payments   The actual amount of dollars paid in capitation varies by product design and based on a few other factors. Product design affects the total amount of payment because any copayments paid by members are not included in calculating the overall payment. For example, if a patient sees the PCP 4.5 times per year and each office visit is approximately $60.00, then the total capitation for each member would be 4.5 × $60.00 = $270.00 per member per year (PMPY), or $22.50 PMPM.*

That $22.50 is not the monthly capitation payment, though. It would be only if the HMO paid for the entire office visit, but members typically pay a copayment for each visit. In this example, we will assume that the copayment is $20.00. The calculation, then, must deduct the copayment amount from the total visit cost—in this example, $60.00 − $20.00 = $40.00. The capitation payment then uses $40.00 per visit instead of $60.00, so the calculation comes out to $40.00 × 4.5 = $180.00 PMPY, or $15.00 PMPM. If the PCP has 100 members, the monthly capitation payment would then be $15.00 × 100 = $1500.00. Because most HMOs offer benefits plans with different copayment levels, the calculation is based on the mix of copayment amounts actually in place for the capitated physician's panel of members.

Other factors affecting capitation amounts include age, gender, and geographic location. From birth to about 18 months of age, infants are seen by their doctor quite often, but then they are seen increasingly less frequently. Young adults also differ, with young women seeing their doctors more often than do young men. In fact, men typically do not use more medical services for many years, but by middle age they use more than women of the same age. Location has an impact related to cost of living and a doctor's costs to maintain office space, hire personnel, and so forth.

---

*All numbers used to show how capitation works are made up and do *not* represent accurate visit costs, utilization rates, or capitation rates.

HMOs that offer point-of-service (POS) products face difficulties when calculating capitation rates. Capitation is usually calculated based on the capitated physician providing all appropriate services for a defined panel of members, while a POS plan also provides benefits for services provided by a PPO provider (in a triple-option POS plan) or an out-of-network provider. As a consequence, some services will not be provided by the capitated physician, so the usual way of calculating capitation will overpay that provider. If a capitated medical group or IPA is large enough, the HMO can base the capitation rate based on an average amount of out-of-network services. In contrast, if capitation is based on individual physicians or small groups, that method is not reliable. This has led some HMOs that offer POS plans to abandon capitation and revert to FFS payment, which can be used regardless of benefit design.

Withholds and Physician Risk Pools   Some HMOs that capitate PCPs apply additional forms of capitation-related PCP financial risk and reward through withholds and capitation risk pools for nonprimary care. Close to half of all open panel HMOs use withholds, but only one-quarter of all closed panel HMOs do. Withholds and risk pools may be used with individual physicians, medical groups, or IPAs, but the example that follows will look only at its use with PCPs.

A withhold is simply a percentage—for example, 20%—of the primary care capitation that is withheld every month and used to pay for cost overruns in referral or institutional services. For example, if a physician is capitated at $20.00 PMPM, a 20% withhold would be $4.00. Each month, the PCP would receive the capitation minus the withhold amount; in this example, the monthly payment would be based on $16.00 PMPM. The withhold money is held by the plan and used at year's end to pay for cost overruns for services allocated to the risk pool or pools, though less commonly it may be applied to cost overruns for the entire HMO; any remainder is returned to the PCP. The amount of money allocated to risk pools is calculated the same way that capitation is calculated and is an average of the expected costs for the services to which the risk pool applies.

HMOs typically calculate both the capitation payment rate and the withhold amounts so that lower than expected costs results in an actual bonus compared to FFS, not just the avoidance of a loss in payment. They also use "stop-loss" methods, meaning that particularly costly cases do not deplete the risk pools all by themselves. The larger the medical group or IPA is, the less it needs stop-loss protection, but it is still used even if the amount is different.

Risk-Based Fee for Service

Capitation is only one type of risk-based HMO physician payment. Another option uses FFS payments, typically through the use of withholds, but sometimes by the application of mandatory fee reductions or "budgeted" FFS. When withholds are used, the same approach is applied as for capitation; rather than withholding a percentage of the capitation payment, however, a percentage of each fee is withheld. This option may be used for PCPs only, or for all physicians in the HMO or IPA. Budgeted FFS is an across-the-board reduction in the fee schedule when costs exceed a target, but this is less commonly used than are withholds and risk pools.

Pay for Performance

Pay for Performance (P4P) refers to financial incentives aligned with the practice of evidence-based clinical care and is based on incentives rather than being risk-based. P4P programs began in HMOs, but are now widely used by many types of payers as well as Medicare. Medicare's shared savings program is also a form of P4P, but because it combines physician and hospital payment, it is discussed later in the chapter.

P4P programs typically apply to PCPs, but may involve specialists as well. The focus with P4P arrangements is on the following factors:

- Common conditions
- Conditions for which physicians vary in how they treat cases
- Conditions for which there are good evidence-based medical guidelines
- A payer's ability to measure performance using data it has on hand, such as medical and pharmacy claims data

For example, patients with diabetes should have their eyes checked regularly because these individuals have a higher than average risk of blindness. The payer can use its claims data to see if diabetic patients are visiting an eye doctor to have the test performed. In some cases, data from focused PCP medical chart reviews may also be used for P4P purposes.

The financial incentive for providers is usually based on target percentage compliance with several such measures. The higher the compliance rate, the higher the incentive payment. There will also be a minimum compliance rate below which there is no incentive payment. Physician P4P programs usually look at the performance of groups of physicians because there are usually only a small number of measures that any individual physician may be able to report. Exceptions include common process measures for certain individual physicians in primary care—for example, immunization rates.

PAYMENT OF FACILITIES

Facilities refer to hospitals, health systems, and ambulatory procedure facilities—in other words, to the physical facilities in which care is provided and that bills for its services.

The Chargemaster

All of a hospital's or ambulatory facility's charges are listed in its chargemaster. The typical hospital chargemaster contains between 25,000 and 50,000 separate billing codes and associated charges,* as well as codes that modify the charges for various reasons. The chargemaster is used to generate the complex bills that hospitals now create, and is usually the basis for how hospitals determine their prices regardless of which payment methods are used by the payers it contracts with.

Chargemasters are a bit like snowflakes: No two are alike, and the charges and even codes in each chargemaster may differ from facility to facility. Chargemaster charges also typically have only a passing relationship with actual costs. There are several reasons for this disconnect, including the difficulty in tracking costs, challenges with associating those costs with individual cases, and the need to include nonclinical but necessary costs, such as the cost of building maintenance or the cost of bulk-purchased gauze dressings, or wages and salaries paid to clinical and nonclinical personnel. Except in the case of a pass-through cost—an implanted device, for example—the chargemaster reflects only a relative difference in the amount of resources used, and costs are spread to all the charge codes.†

Another important reason why chargemasters differ is that hospitals, like all providers, are free to charge whatever they want in their chargemasters, at least for private-pay patients and commercial payers. Maryland is currently the only exception to this rule; in that state, an independent commission sets rates for each hospital that are used by all public and private payers, including Medicare. Everywhere else, hospitals typically adjust their chargemasters every year by making a

---

*Some large teaching hospitals and health systems may have more than 100,000 different chargemaster codes. Ambulatory procedure facilities typically have far fewer.

† This is what accounts for anecdotes such as a $25.00 charge for an over-the-counter pain pill.

small number of adjustments to charges for specific services and then increasing all of the remaining charges by a percentage amount applied across the board.

Carve-outs and Outliers

Before describing the different common methods of facility payment, it is important to recognize that the amount actually paid for any particular case may be modified in two ways: carve-outs and outliers. These factors are different and are not mutually exclusive.

Carve-outs

Hospitals typically seek to carve expensive surgical implants, devices, or drugs out of the payment method and pass their full costs through to the payer, often with a markup. Because of the high costs of some devices and drugs, this practice may or may not be unreasonable, but carve-outs also eliminate any incentive for the hospital to negotiate prices with its own vendors or to get physicians to agree to use only the products from a single device manufacturer. Payers seek to limit the number of carve-outs to provide that incentive, and to better control case costs. This is particularly the case when the volume of the implantable device or the expensive drug is high, and therefore predictable. Carve-outs can affect any type of payment to facilities other than payment based on full charges.

Outliers

Outliers or outlier cases refer to extra payments allowed if a patient's costs exceed certain thresholds. Outliers can affect any type of payment method other than payment based on charges, including discounted charges. This practice is also not an unreasonable protection, but it is worth noting that cases are classified as outliers based on "costs," which in turn are typically based on the hospital's chargemaster. As a consequence, price increases in the chargemaster result in more cases being considered outliers. Payment for outlier cases is typically a combination of the original payment plus discounted charges beginning at the point where the outlier threshold was crossed. Depending on the type of payment and the negotiated terms, as many as one-third or more of all inpatient cases may be classified as outliers.

Types of Facility Payment

As with physicians, there are a few dominant forms of payment, but experimentation has produced many variations on those common approaches and created some entirely new methodologies. Table 4–6 lists the most common facility payment methodologies. Sometimes only one method is used, but the same payer will often use different payment methods or amounts for the same hospital for different products—for example, HMO, PPO and Medicare Advantage products. Except when charges or discounted charges are used for all services, outpatient facility payments differ from inpatient payments. Most facility payment methods are also subject to modifiers that alter the payment on a case-by-case basis; Table 4–7 lists the most widely used payment modifiers.

Charges

There are several ways in which charges may be used as the basis for payment to facilities, including discounted charges and a sliding scale discount on charges. Charge-based payment is also combined with non-charge-based payment under certain circumstances. Payment terms directly related to charges are the least desirable payment method because they are highly vulnerable to price inflation.

Table 4–6   Facility Payment Methods

Facility Payment Method	Inpatient	Outpatient
Straight charges	X	X
Discounted charges	X	X
Per diem	X	
Diagnosis-related groups (DRGs)—old method	X	
Medicare severity DRGs (MS-DRGs)—new method	X	
Percentage of Medicare allowable	X	X
Case rates—facility only (may be bundled with professional)	X	X
Capitation (HMOs only)	X	X
Ambulatory surgical center (ASC) rates under the Medicare Hospital Outpatient Prospective Payment System (HOPPS)		X
Ambulatory payment classifications (APCs)		X
Ambulatory Payment Groups (APGs) and Enhanced APGs (EAPGs)		X
Other	X	X

Copyright P.R. Kongstvedt Company, LLC. Used with Permission.

Table 4–7 Hospital Payment Modifiers

Facility Payment Modifier	Inpatient	Outpatient
Volume-related sliding scale—applicable to all but full charges or capitation	X	X
Carve-outs—applicable to:		
• Discount on charges	X	X
• Per diem	X	
• DRGs and MS-DRGs	X	
• Percent of Medicare	X	X
• Case rates	X	X
• Capitation	X	X
• APCs and APGs		X
Credits—applicable to all types of facility payments	X	X
Differential by service type—applicable to per diem	X	
Differential by day—applicable to:		
• Discount on charges	X	
• Per diem	X	
Outlier or stop-loss—applicable to:		
• DRGs and MS-DRGs	X	
• Percentage of Medicare	X	X
• Case rates	X	X
• Capitation	X	X
• APCs, APGs, and EAPGs		X

Copyright P.R. Kongstvedt Company, LLC. Used with Permission.

Straight Discount on Charges

A straight percentage discount on charges is a contract in which the facility submits its claim in full and the plan discounts it by the agreed-to percentage, which is considered payment in full other than any applicable cost sharing by the member. This type of arrangement is not infrequent in markets with low levels of managed care penetration such as rural markets, but is very uncommon in markets with high levels of managed care.

To address price inflation, a payer will usually require a provision such that no single charge from the chargemaster exceed a certain degree of inflation from year to year for purposes of payment. The payer cannot tell the facility what it can charge others, however. In other words, the facility is free to raise chargemaster fees as much as it likes, but the payer's exposure is limited to a certain percentage increase.

Of note, the discount on charges method is commonly used in hospital-based outpatient and emergency department services, even when a payer uses another payment methodology for inpatient care.

Sliding-Scale Discount on Charges

Sliding-scale discounts are another payment option, especially in markets with low managed care penetration but some level of competitiveness between facilities. With a sliding scale, the percentage discount reflects the facility's total volume of admissions and outpatient procedures. Table 4–8 shows a simplified hypothetical example of a sliding scale.

Per Diems

Unlike straight charges, a negotiated per diem is a single charge for a day in the hospital regardless of any actual charges or costs incurred. It applies only to inpatient cases and is very common. For example, the plan pays $2500 for each day regardless of the actual cost of the service. Per diems are predictable and provide savings for shorter lengths of stay, unlike some other types of payment such as diagnosis-related groups.

Flat per diems means a single per diem rate is negotiated and applied to any type of inpatient day. In other words, the payment for a day in the intensive care unit is the same as for a day for a routine medical patient. Because of the high differences in costs, service-specific per diems are more common in acute care hospitals.

Service-specific per diems refer to multiple sets of negotiated per diems based on service type; examples include different per diems for medical–surgical care, obstetrics, intensive care, neonatal intensive care, rehabilitation, and so forth. Service-specific per diems also minimize the need to negotiate outlier provisions.

Table 4–8   Simplified Hypothetical Example of a Sliding-Scale Discount

Total Number of Bed-Days per Year	Percent Discount off Charges
0–200	10%
201–300	15%
301–400	20%
401 and greater	30%

Per diem differential by day in hospital refers to the fact that most hospitalizations are more expensive on the first day. For example, the first day for surgical cases includes operating suite costs, the operating surgical team costs (nurses and recovery), and so forth. This type of payment method is generally combined with a per diem approach, but the first day is paid at a higher rate. For example, the first day may be paid at $4000 and each subsequent day is $1200.

Sliding-scale per diems, like sliding-scale discounts on charges, are based on total volume.

Diagnosis-Related Groups and Medicare Severity [Adjusted] Diagnosis-Related Groups

DRGs, which were initially developed for Medicare, are broadly referred to as inpatient prospective payment. They provide a flat payment per admission and apply only to inpatient cases. DRGs place responsibility on the hospital to manage the inpatient stay. Savings from shorter stays are kept by the hospital and do not go to the payer, whereas longer stays usually do not cost the payer more unless it is an outlier. DRGs do pay more for outlier cases, and the number of cases being classified as outliers has continually risen. To deal with this trend, Medicare changed from DRGs to MS-DRGs to better incorporate severity of illness and complications into the payment system.

DRGs and now MS-DRGs are sorted into major diagnostic categories (MDCs), each of which represents a system in the body. Within each MDC, DRGs are assigned by a "grouper" program based on the mix of diagnoses, procedures performed, age, sex, discharge status, and presence of complications or comorbidities (i.e., medical problems in addition to the one that resulted in the admission). In other words, DRGs are created through the submission of other code set data and supplemented by additional information.

As seen in Table 4–9, several forms of DRGs exist, and two are being phased out or have already been phased out (phased-out DRG types appear in *italics* in the table). The reason for the different types of DRGs is that DRGs, and now MS-DRGs, were and are intended for use by Medicare and, therefore, do not have the same types and levels of detail needed for commercial populations of members representing all ages; for example, they do not cover childbirth or neonatal care. Medicare uses only MS-DRGs, which are also used by many commercial payers. Many commercial payers supplement MS-DRGs with another type such as APR-DRGS that cover a broad range of patients. DRGs and all-patient DRGs (AP-DRGs) have been phased out and do not comply with ICD-10, so any

Table 4–9   Types of DRGs

Type of DRG	Acronym	Developer
Medicare	DRGs or CMS-DRGs	3M[1] for CMS
Medicare severity	MS-DRGs	3M for CMS
All patient	AP-DRGs	3M
All patient refined	APR-DRGs	3M and NACHRI[2]
All patient severity adjusted	APS-DRGs	OptumInsight[3]
Department of Defense	Tricare DRGs	3M

[1] 3M is a private corporation.

[2] National Association of Children's Hospitals and Related Institutions, a nonprofit association of children's hospitals.

[3] OptumInsight, formerly known as Ingenix, is a subsidiary of United Health Group.

commercial payers still using them will need to transition to the new system before ICD-10 becomes a required code set under HIPAA.

Some commercial payers negotiate rates based on a percentage markup of whatever Medicare would pay for similar services. Such rates may vary from as low as Medicare plus 5% to as high as Medicare plus 60%, and the percentage often varies by type of product such as Medicare Advantage, HMO, and/or PPO. For cases that must use a DRG type other than MS-DRGs, a similar calculation is applied, but in those cases the other DRGs do not necessarily come with pricing attached; consequently, payment terms may need to be described in more detail.

Facility-Only Case Rates

Facility-only case rates are a flat payment for a defined service. They differ from DRGs in that they may apply to both inpatient and outpatient services. Case rates for inpatient cases also differ from DRGs in that are typically used at the same time that another payment method is also applied.

An example of a common type of facility-based case rate is for obstetrics, with the payer and facility negotiating a flat case rate for a normal vaginal delivery and a flat rate or case rate for a cesarean section, or a blended rate for both. Case rates for specialty procedures at tertiary hospitals are also common—for example, for coronary artery bypass grafts, heart transplants, and certain types of cancer treatment. Inpatient cases other than those subject to case rate payment are paid through another method such as per diems. Case rates are also used for defined types of outpatient procedures, such as screening colonoscopies and cataract surgery.

Capitation

Facility capitation, like HMO capitation of physicians, refers to the approach in which an HMO pays the facility on a PMPM basis to cover all institutional costs for a defined population of members. Unlike physician capitation, it is not common for an HMO that capitates one or more hospitals to capitate all hospitals in its network. The payment may be adjusted based on the age and sex of the population, but not always if the capitation covers a large enough group of members. Severity-adjusted capitation is still relatively uncommon, but is starting to be used by some HMOs for Medicare members. Capitation can be used for inpatient as well as outpatient services.

Hospital capitation contracts typically define both carve-outs and outliers. Outlier provisions also lower the amount paid under capitation because costs not included under capitation are excluded from the capitation calculation. Some capitated hospitals may also purchase commercial stop-loss or reinsurance to cover a portion of high-cost inpatient cases.

Ambulatory Payment Classification and Ambulatory Patient Groups

Although the discount on charges method is often used to pay for hospital-based outpatient services, it is not the only method. Furthermore, free-standing ambulatory facilities are more likely to agree to payments using methods other than discounted charges. Two classification systems are commonly used in the payment of ambulatory procedures or encounters: Ambulatory Patient Groups (APGs) and the newer Enhanced Ambulatory Patient Groups (EAPGs),* and ambulatory payment classifications (APCs).

APGs, EAPGs, and ACGs are to outpatient services what DRGs are to inpatient services, although they are calculated differently. APGs were developed by 3M as a forerunner of APCs, and the two are quite similar. APGs have subsequently been updated as EAPGs. Under these payment methods, the thousands of different procedures are grouped into hundreds of different treatment groups.

---

*Ambulatory Patient Groups and Enhanced Ambulatory Patient Groups are registered trademarks owned by 3M.

Such a group includes all ancillary costs, but certain items are carved out, such as particular drugs, the cost to acquire transplanted tissue, and so forth. Payments may also be adjusted for geography and complexity of the procedure.

Penalties and/or Refusal to Pay

As discussed in the chapter titled *The Provider Network*, hospital contracts, like payer contracts with providers, include provisions for financial penalties or conditions in which the plan will not be required to pay some or any portion of a hospital claim and the hospital may not balance bill the member. Two other payment-related penalties may also be used: one applying to avoidable readmissions, and the other to costs associated with serious reportable events (SREs), also called "never events."

A provision of the ACA requires CMS to reduce Medicare payments to hospitals that have a higher than expected rate of avoidable readmissions. An avoidable readmission is defined as a readmission to the hospital less than 30 days after discharge for certain clinical conditions such as heart failure or pneumonia. Penalties are applied to only a percentage of hospitals, and no hospital is expected to have no readmissions. Commercial payers are beginning to implement similar programs, but unlike Medicare, commercial payers must negotiate the specific terms of such arrangements.

Medicare and most commercial payers refuse to pay anything for the cost of avoidable complications that occur in a facility or for any care associated with an SRE. An SRE is defined as a serious health or safety error, or a criminal violation that takes place in a hospital, such as the amputation of a wrong limb or a serious error in prescribing or administering a drug. What is considered to be an SRE is defined and regularly updated by a nonprofit organization called the National Quality Forum.

COMBINED PAYMENT OF HOSPITALS AND PHYSICIANS

Payment for both physician and facility services may be combined rather than paying for each type of service separately. Several approaches are possible, but the three most common methods, listed in order to the amount of financial risk, are as follows:

1. Bundled payment, also called package pricing, global payment, or (less frequently) case rates
2. Shared savings
3. Global capitation

Bundled Payment

Bundled payment, also called package pricing and global payment,* refers to use of a single fixed fee covering all facility and professional services related to a particular episode of care or procedure. It differs from facility-only case rates by including physician payment. A bundled payment might cover multiple types of procedures, or a different bundled payment might be set for each type of procedure. Like capitation, the services covered by the bundled payment must be well defined. Unlike capitation, bundled payments are paid only for services provided, not month in and month out. Like facility-only payments, bundled payments are typically subject to modification by outliers and/or carve-outs.

Successful bundled payment contracts all have one thing in common: The hospital and physicians have a predetermined way of dividing the payment, and all involved providers agree to those terms. The payer is not involved in this internal arrangement. When bundled payment contracts fail, it is typically because this aspect of the deal—that is, the splitting of the payment—is not solid. Academic medical centers with a unified faculty practice plan, very strong multispecialty medical groups with an affiliated medical center, and health systems with a large panel of employed physicians are best able to implement such schemes.

The ACA specifically requires bundled pilot programs for FFS Medicare, and was testing four different models at the time of this text's publication.† Confusingly, the first of those four models applies only to facility payment and does not include physician services; the other three models do include physicians' fees, however. The first model provides for a type of shared savings if costs are lower than set targets. The second model applies to an episode of care, defined as a hospital admission and all post-discharge services for a defined period such as 30, 60, or 90 days. The third model applies only to services provided after discharge for a defined period. The fourth model is similar to the FFS mechanism used by commercial payers.

Shared Savings

In the past, shared savings referred to a payment method in which cost targets were set for an episode of care, and savings were shared between the payer and

---

*Just to keep things confusing, the term "global fee" is sometimes used to refer to a specialist case rate that does not include facility payment. The term must therefore always be taken in context.

†Actually, only three models were being implemented at the time of publication, but the fourth had been designed and, therefore, is included here.

the provider. The term may still be used this way, but the ACA includes a require-ment that Medicare implement a shared savings payment method that is broader, which has essentially replaced its earlier meaning. It is applicable to ACOs in the traditional FFS Medicare program and is called the Medicare Shared Savings Program (MSSP). The MSSP program is a kind of hybrid payment model, com-bining FFS with some elements of risk-sharing and Pay for Performance (P4P), which is discussed later in the chapter.

Under the MSSP, both savings and losses relative to targets are shared, and the targets are based on the costs of care for a defined set of individual Medicare ben-eficiaries over a three-year period. This program is one of the few exceptions to provider risk sharing that does not involve an HMO, which is a major difference between the MSSP and a P4P program that is based on incentives. Commercial payers have also been piloting shared savings programs, but their implementation is far from uniform and the results are not yet known.

In the Medicare program, for purposes of measuring performance, an ACO must have at least 5000 assigned beneficiaries covered under traditional FFS Medi-care.* Which beneficiaries are assigned to the ACO is determined by CMS, not by the ACO. CMS assigns beneficiaries based on whether they receive primary care from an ACO-participating PCP or whether the majority of charges come from ACO participants. Assignment in this case simply means the member is attributed to the ACO for purposes of measuring performance. Assigned beneficiaries are not "locked in"; that is, they are not restricted to using only ACO providers. Beneficia-ries can see any provider they want with no benefits differential.

The goal of the MSSP is to reduce overall costs, particularly the costs associ-ated with individuals who have significant or multiple chronic conditions. CMS calculates overall cost benchmark targets for the group of beneficiaries assigned to the ACO by using their actual incurred costs in the immediate past. In other words, benchmark cost targets are not based on the overall costs of all beneficia-ries in the same area, but rather are specific to the assigned beneficiaries. Bench-mark targets are also adjusted for other factors such as medical cost inflation.

From a day-to-day payment perspective, ACO providers are paid under traditional Medicare terms: FFS for physicians, MS-DRGs for hospitals, and APCs for ambulatory facilities. ACO performance against the benchmark tar-gets, however, determines whether the ACO participants receive a portion of the

---

*In other words, Medicare beneficiaries enrolled in a Medicare Advantage plan cannot be attributed to an ACO as well, although beneficiaries covered under traditional FFS who are also enrolled in a Medicare Part D prescription Drug Plan can be.

shared savings as an additional bonus or whether they will share in the losses and repay a percentage of what they were paid initially. ACOs may elect to share only savings in the first three-year period, although the amount of bonus will be less, but all ACOs must share both savings and losses after that point.

Global Capitation

Global capitation means HMO payment of a single entity for all medical services, although some costs, such as pharmacy charges, are often carved out. Said another way, global capitation is the near-complete transfer of risk to providers. It requires a single entity to accept the single capitation payment and manage all care. Global capitation in past decades led to significant losses by health systems that were unable to manage the risk, and since then it has been uncommon in most parts of the United States, though it has not disappeared entirely. Global capitation may actually have begun increasing recently as some health systems have started their own health plans to "cut out the middleman."

Global capitation, like bundled pricing, requires the hospital and physicians to have predetermined policies about how the payment will be shared, and payment methods should be aligned. For example, paying physicians using FFS creates potential losses for a globally capitated IDS unless the physicians are part of an experienced IPA. Hospitals and health systems with large panels of employed physicians are at least potentially well positioned to accept global capitation. Adequate reinsurance is a requirement.

PAY FOR PERFORMANCE

There is some overlap between P4P programs focused on hospitals and those focused on physicians, at least in regard to the clinical conditions under review, but the actual measures tend to be different. P4P programs for hospitals measure results for individual hospitals or health systems, whereas physician programs usually look at the performance of groups because there are usually only a small number of measures that any individual physician may be able to report. The exception to this scenario is Medicare, in which process measures (e.g., did the physician write the prescription, even if the patient did not fill it) for individual physicians are used.

P4P programs are dependent on a variety of data collection approaches, which can lead to inaccuracies if they are not managed properly. Consequently, leading payers maintain openness to improvements in methodologies for data collection.

Unfortunately, with the exception of California, the programs currently in place vary—an issue that creates difficulty for providers that are required to report data to multiple programs.

PAYMENT FOR ANCILLARY SERVICES

Ancillary services are broadly divided into two major categories and one minor one. One major category is diagnostic services, such as laboratory testing, imaging studies, cardiac studies, and the like. The other major category is therapeutic services, such as physical or occupational therapy. The minor category is transportation, including ambulance and scheduled medical transportation.

Many ancillary services are among the first to be "carved out" of provider networks to take advantage of cost reductions based on economies of scale through volume increases to the contracting provider. This concept applies to any type of plan, but for HMOs in particular, carving out an ancillary service allows an HMO to more easily use a risk-based payment approach such as capitation. It is also reasonable to require plan members to travel farther for nonurgent ambulatory ancillary services. Depending on the type of payer, strict limits on benefits coverage may be applied, except in the case of emergency care, even for those plans that offer coverage for both in-network and out-of-network services.

Unlike physician services, ancillary services are typically limited to a small subset of providers, which allows for greater leverage in negotiating payment and service terms. In certain areas, however, there may be little competition between ancillary service providers—for example, in a rural area or a very small town—in which case the payer has less negotiating leverage. Ambulance services are another area where there is typically little competition, plus ambulances are frequently summoned on a nonelective basis, both of which have an impact on payment policies.

Types of Payment for Ancillary Services

There are no particular types of payment applicable only to ancillary services, although some are less suitable than others. A brief description of common payment methods follows.

Discounted Fee for Service or a Fee Schedule

Many routine diagnostic ancillary services, such as laboratory testing, are high-volume services. In such cases, it is not difficult to obtain substantial discounts, usually in the form of a fee schedule. Even so, most payers prefer payment methods other than FFS.

Flat Rates

Similar to per diem payments to hospitals, flat rates simply mean that the ancillary provider is paid a fixed single payment rate regardless of the resources used in providing services. For high-volume services such as laboratory testing or routine radiology, a fixed fee may be negotiated that does not change regardless of what is ordered.

For therapeutic ancillary providers, case rates can be tiered, similar to differing per diem rates based on the type of service in a hospital. For example, when home health care includes high-intensity services such as chemotherapy or other high-technology services, the plan may pay different case rates depending on the complexity of the specific case.

Capitation

In HMOs or plans that have absolute limitations on out-of-network benefits, ancillary services are frequently capitated, albeit only if members have acceptable access to the ancillary services providers. HMOs with out-of-network benefits such as a POS plan may still capitate payments and provide no coverage for non-emergency services from a noncontracted provider. The benefit to the provider of the ancillary service is a guaranteed source of referrals and a steady income. Capitation also removes the fee-for-service incentives that may lead to overutilization of provider-owned services.

Certain types of ancillary services are easier to capitate than others. If an ancillary service is highly self-contained, then it is easier to capitate. For example, physical therapy usually is limited to therapy given by physical therapists and does not involve other types of ancillary providers. Home health care, by comparison, often comprises a combination of home health nurses and clinical aides, durable medical equipment (DME), home infusion and medication delivery (which includes the cost of the drug or intravenous substance as well as the cost to deliver it), home physical therapy, and so forth. A number of plans have successfully capitated home healthcare services, although those have tended to be larger plans with sufficient volume of members to be able to accurately predict costs in all of these different areas. Other plans have been able to capitate only parts of home health care—home respiratory therapy, for example—but have had less success in other forms. In those cases, a combination of capitation and fixed case rates is useful. For instance, capitation may be applied to basic home health care, but case rates paid for a course of chemotherapy.

In some cases, a single entity accepts capitation from the plan for all of a particular ancillary service and then serves as a network manager. Services are then provided by the organization's providers, if it has them, and by participating ancillary services providers under a subcontract with the network manager. The subcontracted providers are paid through sub-capitation, some form of FFS, or case rates; the network manager, however, remains at risk for the total costs of the capitated service.

PAYMENT FOR PRESCRIPTION DRUGS

Prescription drug benefits are usually administered not through a payer's usual claims system, but rather through a pharmaceutical benefit manager (PBM) that may be owned by a payer or may be an independent company contracted by a payer or an employer. There are actually two types of pharmaceutical providers: (1) pharmacies that dispense standard types of prescription drugs (the most common type) and (2) specialty pharmacies and compounding pharmacies for unique types of drugs. Pharmaceutical providers are described in the *Utilization Management, Quality Management, and Accreditation* chapter.

Standard Methods of Payment

The usual method of paying pharmacies combines a fill fee and the ingredient cost. The fill fee is an amount that the PBM pays the pharmacy for filling a prescription regardless of the drug prescribed. For example, a PBM may pay a pharmacy $2 for each prescription filled. The ingredient cost is the cost of the drug itself. It is not easy to determine the ingredient cost because the price that one pharmacy or pharmaceutical chain pays for a drug may not be the same as the price that another pharmacy pays. For example, nationwide chains are able to obtain lower prices (through their wholesale distributors) than small community pharmacies can obtain. It is common for the PBM to use a standardized listing of drug prices to determine the cost of a drug. This standardized price is called the average wholesale price (AWP), and a PBM commonly pays for a drug based on a percentage of AWP (e.g., 95%).

Coverage of pharmaceutical therapy is almost always tiered. In other words, a lower copayment is required for preferred drugs, whereas progressively higher copayments are required for non-preferred drugs. The list of drugs covered in the various tiers is called a formulary. In a closed formulary, there is no coverage under most conditions for drugs not included in the formulary. In an open formulary, all prescribed drugs are covered to some degree, but nonformulary drugs are subject to a higher level of coinsurance.

Rebates

PBMs and large payers, as well as some large employer groups, frequently negotiate a rebate from drug manufacturers. This approach does not apply to every drug, of course, but rather to drugs that are relatively widely prescribed and for which multiple good alternative therapies exist. For example, if six different drugs are available to treat individuals with high cholesterol levels, the PBM or payer may negotiate with the manufacturers of one or two of those agents to obtain rebates based on the inclusion of those drugs in a favorable tier in the formulary.

Reference Pricing

Reference pricing is a payment methodology that is most often used in the following circumstances:

- For specialty and compounding pharmacy drugs
- When there are no alternatives to a particular drug that is being used to an increasingly greater extent
- When a manufacturer is able to bypass the usual distribution channels and control how its product is obtained
- When a drug must be administered by a physician or in a facility that adds on high administration and markup fees

What all of these situations have in common is very high costs, and at least some limits on the ability of a payer or PBM to negotiate prices. Reference pricing may also be used to pay for medical devices.

With payment through reference pricing, coverage is based on either the best price a payer has obtained from any source or the price charged by the manufacturer to the providers who administer or provide the treatment. In other words, coverage is not based on whatever is being charged to the payer. As a practical matter, for drugs with no alternatives, the best price available may not differ tremendously from the price available anywhere else, but not always. For administered drugs subject to high add-on fees, coverage is based on the best price available to the payer or PBM, plus a set administration fee—for example,

6% of the cost of the drug, and no more—which reduces the high profits that add-on fees bring.

NEW MODELS OF PAYMENT UNDER THE PATIENT PROTECTION AND AFFORDABLE CARE ACT

The ACA addresses some approaches to payment for FFS Medicare, and possibly Medicaid, by specifically calling them out. Examples that have been discussed already include the following:

- No payment for SREs
- Payment reductions for hospitals with higher than average avoidable readmissions
- Bundled payments
- MSSP for ACOs

The ACA has even more provisions focusing on payment reform in Medicare. One major provision in this act created the new Center for Medicare and Medicaid Innovations (CMI), now called the Innovation Center. The Innovation Center is charged with testing, evaluating, and expanding different payment methodologies in Medicare and Medicaid. The ACA specifically describes 20 possible models for testing, but does not restrict the Innovation Center to only those options; it directs the Center to look at other approaches as well.

The Innovation Center has piloted, is now piloting, or will pilot various payment methodologies. Some are variations on payment methodologies described elsewhere in this chapter but focused on specific outcomes, costs, provider types, and so forth. Other Innovation Center approaches to payment do not fit neatly into the specific payment methodologies discussed in this chapter. It is not known which, if any, of the new payment methods that the Innovation Center is testing or considering will be adopted by Medicare for broad use, so little more can be said other than to make two observations:

- Because Medicare accounts for such a high percentage of the total payments to hospitals and most physicians, any changes it makes in payment methodologies will affect private payers, often in unknown or unpredictable ways.
- Where CMS goes, private payers often follow.

CONCLUSION

Provider payment is payment; it is not reimbursement. Payment has the potential to affect behavior, whereas true reimbursement does not. Consequently, to the greatest degree possible, payment methodologies should align the financial incentives and goals of the health plan and the network providers who deliver the care. Capitation for HMOs, P4P for all types of payers, and shared savings represent attempts to achieve that alignment in ways that traditional FFS does not.

Any payment methodology is a tool, however, and like any tool it has limitations. Consider the following analogy: A hammer is the correct tool for pounding and removing nails but is a poor choice for cutting wood. Likewise, if payment methodologies are used without at least a modicum of skill and forethought, their application will likely result in a painful self-inflicted injury. Also, while a hammer is certainly handy, other tools must be used to successfully build something. Payment may similarly be a powerful and often effective tool, but it can be truly effective only in conjunction with other managed care tools: utilization management, quality management, network contracting, provider relations, and the many other activities undertaken by a well-run managed healthcare plan.

Utilization Management, Quality Management, and Accreditation

LEARNING OBJECTIVES

- Recognize the different approaches to managing wellness and prevention
- Identify the basic metrics and measures used to assess costs and utilization in health plans
- Describe the basic components of utilization management for medical services, including prospective, concurrent, and retrospective review
- Explain the basic concepts underlying disease and case management
- Describe the basic components of quality management, including structure, process, and outcome
- Understand the purpose and scope of external review and accreditation of managed care plans

INTRODUCTION

The term "managed care" derives from the practice of managing certain aspects of medical services, specifically medical costs and quality. To be sure, these aspects are also managed by providers, but in their capacity of actually providing healthcare services. The only types of payers that directly provide healthcare are group and staff model health maintenance organizations (HMOs), including large integrated healthcare delivery systems (IDSs) that are also licensed as HMOs or insurers, but they provide coverage and care to only a very small fraction of the U.S. population. The vast majority of people are covered by health benefits plans that do not themselves provide care, but rather manage healthcare benefits coverage. As discussed in the *Health Benefits Coverage and Types of Health Plans* chapter, health plans manage what will be paid for, how much will be paid, and under which circumstances benefits will or will not be paid.

One of the key goals for utilization management (UM)* in a health plan is managing costs. The overall cost of health care is calculated as the result of two variables: price multiplied by volume. The *Provider Payment* chapter addresses the challenge of managing the first variable, price, by adopting various payment mechanisms. In this chapter, we look at means to manage the other variable, volume, through UM. We also consider two related types of specialized UM that focus on high cost and/or medical conditions—namely, case management (CM) and disease management (DM).

Quality management (QM) is also a focus for payers such as HMOs, point-of-service (POS) plans, and preferred provider organizations (PPOs), often referred to collectively as managed care organizations (MCOs). Several other terms are used as alternatives to QM, such as quality assurance (QA) and quality improvement (QI); some sources also use the word "total," as in "total quality management" (TQM). For our purposes, they all essentially mean the same thing. Thus, to avoid confusion, only the acronym QM is used in this text.

Accreditation programs assess an MCO's policies, procedures, and performance in a number of areas, with much of that assessment being focused on UM, CM, DM and QM, as well as network management, member services, and other member-centric functions. The heavy emphasis placed on UM, CM, DM and QM in accreditation is the reason it is addressed in this chapter.

For UM, QM, and accreditation purposes, the privacy requirements established in the Health Insurance Portability and Accountability Act (HIPAA) and various state privacy laws set limitations on access to medical and personal health information. As a practical matter, only medical records and information for the plan's members may be accessed, and even they must be accessed for a clear reason. In turn, a plan's UM, QM, DM, and CM programs must be carried out according

---

* The terms "utilization review" (UR), which is an older term; "utilization management" (UM); and the less frequently used "care management" (CM) also refer to the practice of managing the utilization of medical services. To avoid confusion, only the acronym "UM" is used in this text.

to the plan's policies and procedures; they cannot be "fishing expeditions" in which plan personnel dig through any records they like just to see what they contain.

Finally, the functions described in this chapter as part of MCOs' core operations. Nevertheless, a provision of the Affordable Care Act (ACA) of 2010 places limits on the medical loss ratio (MLR) for all insured businesses, meaning the total percentage of the premium that must be spent for medical benefits and not operations, sales, governance, profit, and so forth. Under the ACA, the costs of providing wellness and prevention and the costs to perform QM are usually *not* considered to be administrative costs; in contrast, the costs to perform UM, CM, and DM, as well as credentialing and network management, *are* considered administrative costs and are included in the MLR limits. This consideration has prompted some payers to contract with organized provider groups or systems such as accountable care organizations (ACOs) to both provide care and manage utilization. With such a strategy, the costs to perform UM are shifted into the category of medical care services. For purposes of this chapter, however, all of these functions are addressed at the level of a health plan.

PREVENTION AND WELLNESS

Preventive healthcare spans both the management of utilization and of quality. Dr. Paul Elwood coined the term "health maintenance organization" in the 1970s to highlight the idea that HMOs were dedicated to providing preventive services and maintaining health. At the time, preventive services were not covered by most health insurers, and it was many years before coverage of prevention became the norm. Under the ACA, first-dollar coverage of preventive services is mandatory, meaning no cost sharing is allowed when such services are provided by network providers, regardless of any other required cost sharing.

Unsurprisingly, prevention is aimed at preventing certain diseases or conditions. Childhood immunizations are the most common form of prevention, but this type of care also includes other services such as adult immunizations, Pap smears, mammography, and screening for high cholesterol, high blood pressure, diabetes, and other common chronic diseases. Wellness programs are another form of prevention, directed at helping members to change their lifestyles and develop healthy habits—for example, weight loss, smoking cessation, and exercise programs.

Health risk appraisals (HRAs) are a self-administered assessment tool used to quickly make an overall assessment of a new patient's medical condition and risk factors. Many or most payers have automated HRAs on their websites that also provide feedback, serving to encourage a member to make better health choices. Examples of such feedback might include the value in potential added "life-years" from losing weight, stopping smoking, or having routine screening tests done.

Different types of HRAs may be focused on specific groups of members, such as commercial, Medicare, or Medicaid members. Some advanced Medicare Advantage (MA) plans go beyond data-gathering forms and physical exams and actually send a nurse, clinical social worker, or home aide to the residence of a new Medicare member. Once there, they may do a nutritional assessment, check for compliance with prescribed medications, and look for simple interventions that could save problems later, such as providing an inexpensive bathmat to prevent the member from slipping in the tub and breaking a hip.

MEASURING UTILIZATION

Many different types of measurements or metrics are used when managing utilization and the cost of medical services. Most payers use metrics based on a standard set of calculations; depending on the type of payer, those measures may be refined even more. The most commonly used ones are described here.

Some measurements are completely straightforward. For example, the average length of stay (ALOS, or just LOS) is just what it sounds like for inpatient hospital stays. Other measures and metrics take into account the number of plan members (also referred to as covered lives) as a third element to make sense of the numbers. For example, an average of 500 hospital inpatient admissions per month is a high number of admissions for a small 20,000-member plan, but a low number of admissions for a 500,000-member plan. Time must also be taken into account in usable ways, which means a per-day, per-month, or per-year basis depending on the type of measurement.

In health insurance and managed care, many statistics are given on a per-member per-year (PMPY) or per-member per-month (PMPM) basis. These metrics refer to the average number of times something happens or the average cost of something, spread across the entire membership over the course of a year or a month. As an example of PMPY, a typical commercial (non-Medicare/Medicaid) HMO may report physician encounters, or visits to physicians, as being 3.4 visits PMPY, meaning that, on average, members saw a physician 3.4 times per year. Obviously, some members will see the physician more often, whereas other members will see a physician less often.

Utilization and/or cost for a particular type of service may also be reported on a PMPM basis, meaning that the total utilization and cost for all of that type of

TABLE 5–1   Hypothetical Example Showing Calculation PMPM Costs for Outpatient Procedures

Total membership in the month	100,000
Total number of outpatient procedures in the month	7000
Average cost per outpatient procedure that month	$1500
Total cost of outpatient procedures that month (in whole dollars)	$10,500,000
Total month's whole-dollar cost is divided by total membership to calculate the PMPM cost	$105 PMPM

service during a month is divided by the total number of members in the plan that same month, regardless of whether each member received care (and most do not). A hypothetical example is shown in Table 5–1 for a commercial HMO, using the following assumptions:

- The HMO has 100,000 members for a particular month.
- On average, 7000 outpatient procedures are performed on the HMO's members in a particular month.
- The average cost per outpatient procedure paid by the HMO is $1500 (procedure costs vary widely, even for the same procedure, so the average cost is used in this example).

A similar form of measurement is per 1000 members; that is, instead of the average based on each member, the data are averaged based on every 1000 members. Per-thousand metrics are most often used for inpatient bed-days, inpatient admissions, and ambulatory procedures; an example is bed days per 1000 (sometimes abbreviated as BD/K). Utilization per thousand is an annualized metric, meaning it is measured based on a year. For example, an admission rate of 55 admissions per thousand means that 55 out of every 1000 plan members are admitted during the course of a year. But while per-thousand metrics are annualized, they may be used for any period of time.

The standard formula to calculate utilization per thousand is relatively straightforward and will be illustrated by looking at bed-days per thousand. The exact same formula is applicable to calculating admissions and ambulatory procedures per thousand. It may be calculated for any chosen period (e.g., a single day, month to date, a quarter, or year to date). Because the measure is always annualized, the calculation

Table 5–2   Sample Calculations of Bed-Days per Thousand (BD/K)

Calculation of BD/K for a Single Day	Calculation of BD/K for Three Weeks into the Month to Date (MTD)
Assume: • Current hospital census: 300 • Plan membership: 500,000 • Days being measured: 1	Assume: • Total gross hospital bed-days: 6382 • Plan membership: 500,000 • Days so far in MTD: 21

Step 1: Gross days
    300 ÷ (1 ÷ 365)
    = 300 ÷ 0.00274
    = 109,500
	Step 1: Gross days
	    6382 ÷ (21 ÷ 365)
	    = 6382 ÷ 0.0575
	    = 110,925.24

Step 2: Days per 1000
    109,500 ÷ (500,000 ÷ 1000)
    = 109,500 ÷ 500
    = 219 (rounded)
	Step 2: Days per 1000
	    110,925.24 ÷ (500,000 ÷ 1000)
	    = 110,925.24 ÷ 500
	    = 222 (rounded)

Result: The BD/K for that single day is 219.	Result: The MTD BD/K is 222.

of bed-days per thousand uses the assumption of a 365-day year as opposed to a 12-month year to prevent variations that are due solely to the length of a month.

The formula is $[A \div (B \div 365)] \div (C \div 1000)$, where:

- **A** is the gross (meaning the total) number of bed-days (or admissions or ambulatory procedures) in the time period;
- **B** is the total number of days in the time period being measured, such as:
  - a single day,
  - number of days, month to date,
  - number of days in a month,
  - number of days, year to date, or
  - 365 days (i.e., one year); and
- **C** is the average plan membership in the period being measured.

This calculation may be broken into steps. Table 5–2 illustrates the calculation for bed-days per thousand using two separate methods.

MEDICAL NECESSITY AND BENEFITS COVERAGE DETERMINATIONS

The fundamental role of any payer is to manage healthcare benefits coverage. In practical terms, that means determining what will and will not be covered and under which circumstances. Coverage decisions are not the same as medical care decisions made by a doctor and a patient. Indeed, with the exception of closed-panel HMOs, managed healthcare plans make *only* coverage decisions. They do not actually provide the care, prevent it from being provided, or prevent it from being sought out by the member. A statement like "My HMO would not authorize my care," really means the HMO would not authorize coverage or payment for a particular medical service, not that the HMO somehow has the power to order doctors around. This is not to say that denial of coverage cannot create a substantial barrier to costly medical services—it does, though not an absolute one. Some people do pay for their care out of their own pockets; costly cosmetic plastic surgery is a common example.

Medical Necessity

"Medical necessity" and "medically necessary" are broad terms used by payers for a very specific purpose as part of the process for benefits coverage determinations, and both terms mean the same thing. Medical necessity is a factor in coverage determinations when medical goods or services may or may not be covered depending on certain criteria. It is not a factor for services that are specifically excluded from coverage, and it is typically not a factor for many types of routine services such as care from a primary care physician (PCP).

Medical necessity as applied to benefits coverage policies and determinations is often difficult for members and providers to understand. A provider or member may consider a medical service to be necessary, yet that service may not be considered medically necessary as applied to benefits coverage. This conflict arises because the service must still meet the definitions, exclusions, and coverage requirements of the benefits plan.

The specific wording used to define medical necessity often varies somewhat from plan to plan, but its meaning is similar in most plans. Medical necessity in commercial health benefits plans is typically defined by broadly describing the medical goods or services that may be justified as reasonable, necessary, and/or appropriate, based on evidence-based clinical standards of care. Medical necessity definitions also typically describe the types of services that are excluded from coverage because they are not considered to be medically necessary. Examples of the types of services that may be excluded include:

- Services that are primarily for the convenience of the patient or physician
- Services that are more costly than an alternative service or sequence of services at least as likely to produce equivalent results
- Custodial care or care that is essentially assistance with acts of daily living

- Experimental or investigational care, except in defined circumstances
- Care not considered medically appropriate by generally accepted standards of medical practice

Most of the coverage exclusions on this list also mean that some medical services, drugs, or devices may be covered for one member but not another depending on each member's specific clinical circumstances as defined by evidence-based clinical guidelines. In some cases, it is more a matter of providing the proper clinical information to the health plan than it is not meeting clinical criteria. In other cases, something is not covered simply because a less expensive alternative has not been tried, but it will be covered if the less costly alternative does not work, or work well enough, or cannot be tolerated.

Use of Evidence-Based Clinical Guidelines for Coverage Determinations Based on Medical Necessity

Coverage decisions involving medical necessity are made with input from many possible sources, but the primary source is typically the treating physician and, in the case of HMOs using PCP gatekeepers, the PCP. For example, a treating physician may be asked to provide clinical justification about why a very costly test is being requested when a less costly test will provide much the same information. In some cases, however, UM managers and medical directors will also review cases based on condition-specific medical necessity coverage guidelines.

Medical necessity coverage guidelines are not arbitrary, but rather typically rely on evidence-based medical guidelines that take precedence over differing community-based practice standards or even the opinion of the treating physician. Payers do so because of several limitations associated with physician practice behaviors, such as the following:

- Physicians cannot easily keep up with all changes in medical knowledge.
- There are significant regional variations in physician practice behavior that are unrelated to clinical conditions.
- There is a lack of consistency in adopting evidence-based medical practices.
- Some physician practice behaviors are habits, not medical judgment, and often change over time as a result of payment policies.
- Some physicians will adopt medical interventions not yet shown to be effective through randomized controlled medical studies.

Evidence-based clinical criteria and guidelines are based on formal medical studies and clinical trials that compare different approaches to care, with their results being published in peer-reviewed medical journals.* Some guidelines may be absolute—for example, no coverage for experimental or investigational treatments administered outside of a qualified research institution, or no coverage for a procedure that is not considered effective. Many (even most) other guidelines are relative, meaning they take into account an individual patient's medical condition. For example, most inpatient procedures are done on the day of admission, but a frail elderly person with kidney and heart failure is likely to need to be properly hydrated or otherwise attended to so that already risky surgery is not made riskier.

Larger payers may have internal working groups that create the evidence-based clinical guidelines and change them as medical science advances. The Centers for Medicare & Medicaid Services (CMS), the federal agency in charge of Medicare, also has extensive guidelines it uses for the Medicare program. The Agency for Healthcare Research and Quality (AHRQ), a federal agency related to CMS, provides access to a wealth of evidence-based clinical studies through its database. Commercial vendors also license guidelines that are continually updated and that payers can load into their computer systems to use for UM and claims processing. Hospitals may likewise license these guidelines for their own internal UM programs. Finally, payers typically make the guidelines accessible on a self-service basis to all of their providers through a web portal.

BASIC UTILIZATION MANAGEMENT

Basic UM usually refers to the routine functions used to manage the cost of the most widely used medical services. Basic UM, which is considered distinct from DM and CM, encompasses prospective, concurrent, and retrospective review (Figure 5–1). Prospective review addresses utilization before it occurs. Concurrent review addresses utilization as it occurs. Retrospective review, which takes place after the fact, includes reviewing utilization patterns or specific cases after utilization has occurred.

Prospective Utilization Management

Prospective utilization management includes demand management, referral management, and precertification of costly or facility-based elective medical goods or services. Some include prevention in this category as well, a topic we looked at earlier.

---

* Not all types of medical studies are useful. The most useful are called "randomized" trials that compare two options head to head. The least useful are case studies.

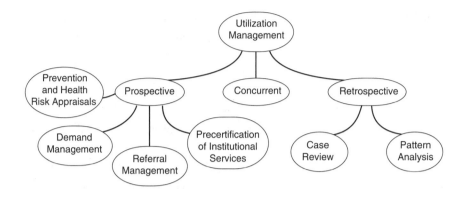

FIGURE 5–1 Components of Utilization Management

Demand Management

Demand management is intended to influence the future demand for medical services, but differs from prevention in its focus on acute or near-term care. The most popular demand management methods include providing a round-the-clock nurse advice line so that members can access a trained nurse 24 hours a day, 7 days a week, by calling a toll-free number. The advice lines rely heavily on clinical protocols. Many payers that have advice lines have seen a decline in emergency department utilization. Closely related to this practice are the outreach programs used by most DM programs.

Referral Management

Referral management, sometimes called referral authorization or preauthorization, is principally confined to HMOs (and POS plans for their highest coverage levels) that use a PCP gatekeeper model. In this model, a member's PCP determines which medical services are truly necessary, coordinates the provision of these services, and thereby reduces unnecessary utilization. The provision of care by any healthcare professional other than the PCP must be authorized by the PCP.

An authorization requirement allows the PCP to determine if a health problem or condition requires treatment by a specialist. If it does, the PCP authorizes a referral to a network specialist. Referral authorization is seldom open ended, but may authorize a specific number of visits (e.g., one to three) or a course of treatment (e.g., chemotherapy is fully authorized for the entire course of treatment).

The ACA requires all types of payers to allow direct access to obstetricians/gynecologists (OB/Gyns), including gatekeeper-type HMOs, though this had long been the practice of most HMOs even prior to the ACA's enactment.

However, HMOs vary as to whether an OB/Gyn may also authorize a referral to another specialist.

It is rare for an HMO to become involved in a PCP's referral authorization process other than to capture the authorization data to process the claim properly. The PCP is expected to exercise proper clinical judgment without the HMO's intervention. The HMO typically provides the PCP with periodic reports containing data on referral rates and costs, as well as reports on the PCP's capitation pool or withhold if that is appropriate (see the *Provider Payment* chapter).

Precertification of Institutional Services

Prospective management of institutional services, both inpatient and outpatient, is a staple of almost all types of payers. It is usually referred to as precertification, though occasionally it is also called preauthorization. The process is simple: Someone calls the MCO to request authorization for an elective admission or outpatient procedure, the MCO checks the request against clinical criteria and determines whether the facility is in the contracted network, and the MCO either does or does not authorize coverage of the procedure. In the case of an inpatient admission, the MCO usually assigns an expected length of stay as well.

Clinical criteria for authorization are commercially available, or an MCO may develop its own criteria. Likewise, maximum allowable LOS guidelines are commercially available, but an MCO may modify those guidelines to suit the local area. Most MCOs now use computerized programs that enable them to determine quickly whether the clinical criteria are met and to capture pertinent data.

In indemnity insurance plans or to access the out-of-network benefits in PPOs and POS plans, failure to obtain precertification results in the member facing an economic penalty. For HMOs and to access the in-network benefits in POS and most PPOs, the burden of responsibility falls on the provider, and it is the provider who faces an economic penalty for failure to comply with precertification requirements. Contracts between payers and providers also frequently contain provisions requiring the facility to verify authorization as well so as to avoid a payment penalty. The type of financial penalty can vary from a coverage reduction for PPOs to denial of payment by HMOs.

The ACA requires all payers to cover emergency care without preauthorization at an in-network level of benefits if it meets a "prudent layperson" standard. This means emergency care is covered when a member experiences acute symptoms for which an average person with an average knowledge of health and medicine believes that not getting care could result in harm. This provision applies regardless of whether emergency care is provided by in-network or out-of-network providers.

Concurrent Utilization Management

Concurrent UM refers to UM activities performed while care is being provided. It is used primarily for hospital inpatient care, where it is sometimes called continued stay review. Concurrent UM may also be used for certain types of long-term outpatient care such as an extensive period of physical therapy. In both cases, it is typically used for long and potentially costly cases, and less so for routine cases.

Concurrent review is performed for purposes of benefits determinations, not to interfere directly with care. If the hospital stay will exceed the previously authorized days, the UM nurse will collect clinical data and compare them to clinical guidelines for a particular condition or procedure, thereby determining whether the case meets those guidelines for continued coverage. The reviewer then either authorizes the additional days or denies coverage for them. Rather than deny coverage outright, however, the UM nurse is more likely to work with the physician and the hospital's own utilization review and discharge planning department to obtain any necessary additional documentation and help facilitate the patient's discharge.

Payers with many hospitals in their network often perform concurrent review via telephone, working through hospitals' UM nurses to find out the status of cases. HMOs that more actively manage utilization will often send a UM nurse to the hospital to obtain more detailed and timely information and more actively manage the case. The process is otherwise the same as just described, but communications and information exchange are better than when only the telephone is used. Some large organized medical groups may use a hospitalist for this purpose as well (see the chapter titled *The Provider Network*).

When UM nurses determine that continued stay criteria have not been met for a particular case but the attending physician disagrees, the UM nurses rarely confront the attending physician directly. Instead, they refer such cases to a medical director. The medical director may call the attending physician to discuss the case, after which they make a determination regarding authorization for further coverage. If the medical director denies continued coverage authorization, the denial may be appealed, as described briefly in this chapter and in more detail in the *Sales, Governance, and Administration* chapter.

Discharge Planning

Discharge planning is a function of concurrent UM, but it can also be an important element of case management. Routine discharge planning involves working with a hospital's discharge planning department to facilitate discharge by arranging follow-up services such as physical therapy, scheduling follow-up appointments, and so forth. It is also common to contact a recently discharged patient to see how well the individual is doing, including asking the patient specific questions related to any procedures and answering any questions the newly discharged patient or his or her family may have.

In recent years, a more specialized form of discharge planning has grown in importance as Medicare and many commercial payers have begun to focus on preventing avoidable readmissions. An avoidable readmission refers specifically to a patient who is readmitted to the hospital within 30 of discharge for either the same problem or a complication related to the original problem; it does not include being admitted for a completely different problem. CMS now sets goals for the rate of avoidable readmissions for each hospital based on specific types of cases; those goals then can affect overall payments to the hospital. Many commercial payers have followed suit. As a result, hospitals have developed more intense discharge planning and follow-up programs for these types of cases that more closely resemble case management.

Retrospective Utilization Management

Retrospective UM refers to UM or UM-related activities that take place after care has been provided. Retrospective UM can be classified into two broad categories: case review and pattern analysis.

Case Review

In case review, past cases are examined for appropriateness of care, billing errors, or other problems. If an error or irregularity is found in a particular case, the payer may adjust payment or at least investigate the case. Case review also may occur if a member seeks coverage after services have been provided without prior authorization or precertification.

Pattern Analysis

Pattern analysis involves using utilization claims data to determine whether patterns exist. Because the scope of claims data is so massive, computers are required to perform this analysis. Those computers, however, must be told what to look for and which data to use. A payer cannot simply dump all data into the system and hope the computer can figure out what to analyze. Identified patterns may be provider specific; for example, a physician may have an abnormally high procedure rate. Patterns may also be plan-wide; for example, there may be an unanticipated increase in cardiac testing costs. After a pattern is identified, the reasons underlying it must be investigated so that corrective action may be taken.

Payers often seek to improve how they share retrospective data with the network providers to allow the providers to compare themselves with their peers and modify their own practices as appropriate. Such an element may be part of a pay-for-performance program, for instance. It is also used in data transparency programs in which MCOs provide comparative data about healthcare cost and quality to members.

APPEALS OF COVERAGE DECISIONS

Prior to the ACA, almost all payers were required to provide a mechanism for members to appeal a denial of coverage, whether it was before services were received (preauthorization or precertification) or after services were provided but were then not paid for by the payer. The ACA made these requirements standard for all types of payers. There are two formal types of appeal reviews, which are discussed in more detail in the *Sales, Governance, and Administration* chapter:

- Internal review, in which physicians in the same or a related specialty and who work or consult with the health plan but who were not involved in the denial decision, review relevant material and either uphold the denial or overturn it
- External review, in which neutral third-party physicians review the case and either uphold or overturn the denial

DISEASE AND CASE MANAGEMENT

Although the majority of healthcare plan members have routine medical needs, some have serious chronic medical conditions—for example, severe diabetes, acquired immunodeficiency syndrome (AIDS), or certain heart conditions—that require a great deal of expensive medical care. Likewise, certain acute cases—such as an individual who is involved in a severe motor vehicle accident or a very premature newborn—are expensive. In fact, a large majority of any payer's total medical costs are incurred by a small percentage of its members or beneficiaries, regardless of the type of coverage program. Payers address this issue through disease management and case management programs.

Case management and disease management are similar in that they are designed to address the medical needs of members requiring very expensive care. By paying particular attention to these members, the payer is able to lower costs while improving outcomes and quality. While the two types of programs are similar, there are some distinctions between DM and CM, as seen in Table 5–3.

Almost all payers have a case management program, which is also sometimes called a large case or a catastrophic case management program; most, but not all, also have a DM program. Many payers use outside companies to conduct their DM activities because a large company that focuses only on DM is better able to stay current with advances in treatment options and make the necessary investments in information technology (IT) to support these specialized clinical functions. It is less common for payers to outsource CM, but that occurs as well. The largest payer companies typically provide both DM and CM through internal resources.

Case Management

Case management of catastrophic or chronic cases, whose costs often exceed routine costs by several orders of magnitude, has the potential to deliver substantial savings. In this type of UM, trained nurses coordinate aspects of care such as rehabilitation, home care, health education, and the like, thereby improving outcomes and reducing expenses. CM differs from DM in two main ways: It includes acute cases, such as trauma and premature birth, and it includes chronic conditions that are not part of the DM program, such as rehabilitation after a stroke.

An intense form of case management has recently emerged in response to CMS's avoidable readmission program, as well as new programs involving ACOs. This more intense type of case management usually involves a team consisting of different types of professionals rather than a single case manager.

Disease Management

Disease management is a form of CM that focuses on a handful of selected conditions and works proactively with each patient to manage the course of the disease and avoid the need for hospitalization in the first place. The usual result is greater continuity, lower overall costs, and better outcomes compared to unmanaged cases. What sets DM programs apart is their focus on specific common chronic conditions such as diabetes and heart disease—conditions that are both widespread and manageable.

DM programs use many different approaches intended to improve outcomes, or at least slow down the effects and complications associated with those conditions. This is accomplished not only through more intense monitoring, but also by improving patients' ability to care for themselves by improving medication

TABLE 5–3   Differences Between Case Management and Disease Management

Traditional/Catastrophic Case Management	Disease Management
Emphasis is on single patient	Emphasis is on a population with a chronic illness
Early identification of people with acute catastrophic conditions (known high costs or known diagnoses that lead to high costs in the near term)	Early identification of all people with targeted chronic diseases (20–40) whether mild, moderate, or severe
Acuity level of catastrophic cases is high; acuity level of traditional cases is high to moderate	Acuity level is moderate
Applies to 0.5%–1% of commercial membership	Applies to 15%–25% of commercial membership
Value relies heavily on price negotiations and benefit flexing	Value stems from member and provider behavior change that results in improved health status
Requires plan design manipulation (e.g., adding more home care visits)	Requires plan design changes that reward enrollment in DM and shrink drug copayments
Primary objective is to arrange for care using the least restrictive, clinically appropriate alternatives	Primary objective is to avoid hospitalization *and* modify risk factors, lifestyle, and medication adherence to improve health status
Episode is 60–90 days	Intervention is 365 days for most conditions
Site of interaction is primarily hospital, hospice, subacute facility, or health and home care	Site of interaction includes work, school, home, and physician office
Driven by need for arrangement of support services, community resources, transportation	Driven by nonadherence to medical regimens
Outcome metrics are single-admit LOS and cost per case	Outcome metrics are annual cost per diseased member and disease-specific functional status and gaps in care

Source: Chapter 8 "Fundamentals and Core Competencies of Disease Management" by David W. Plocher in The Essentials of Managed Health Care, Sixth Edition (Kongstvedt editor) 2013 Jones & Bartlett.

compliance, instilling better eating and exercise habits, promoting self-monitoring, and facilitating greater understanding of their own medical problems.

Just as with the newer intensive discharge and case management programs for ACOs, the hallmark of a disease management program is the inclusion of numerous types of health professionals, not just physicians. For example, a clinical pharmacist may play a more active role in treating childhood asthma than the pediatrician—for example, by teaching the child how to use inhaled steroids. Likewise, a dietitian may be of great service to patients with a severe heart condition by teaching them how to maintain a good diet and avoid unhealthy habits.

DM and traditional CM programs must have multiple ways of identifying which members might be good candidates. Individuals with clinical conditions who would benefit from greater interventions may be identified by nurses or hospitals during utilization review, through computer programs that analyze claims for diagnoses and for the types of drugs being prescribed, through abnormal laboratory results, through HRAs, or through sophisticated data modeling programs that seek to predict which members may be deteriorating clinically. In addition to identifying these members, it is important to determine which level of intervention would be most appropriate. This process is illustrated in Figure 5–2.

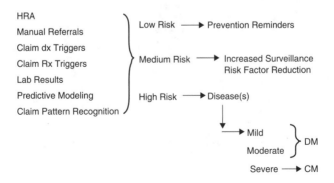

Population Triage

Case Finding Data Supplied to Single Call Center

FIGURE 5–2 Identification of Candidates for Case Management or Disease Management

UTILIZATION MANAGEMENT OF ANCILLARY SERVICES

The two common groups of ancillary services are diagnostic services and therapeutic services.* Ancillary services are not personally provided by physicians and, though hospitals provide such services, they are not classified as hospital or facility services except when included as part of an inpatient stay or ambulatory procedure. Examples of diagnostic ancillary services include laboratory testing, electroencephalography, cardiac testing, and imaging studies such as radiology, nuclear testing, computed tomography (CT), magnetic resonance imaging (MRI), positron emission tomography (PET), and so forth. Examples of therapeutic ancillary services include cardiac rehabilitation, non-cardiac rehabilitation, physical therapy, occupational therapy, and speech therapy (but not behavioral health services).

Except for certain types of services and situations as described shortly, managing pricing and payment terms for ancillary services is generally more important than managing their utilization. Active management of overall utilization of ancillary services is usually done only by those MCOs that actively manage most aspects of care, such as an HMO. Active management makes use of several approaches (Figure 5–3). Notably, excessive ordering of ancillary services by some

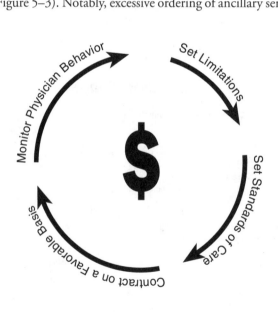

FIGURE 5–3   Methods for Managing Ancillary Service Costs

---

* Medical transportation services make up a small and unique third group that does not neatly fit into this category and that is beyond the scope of this text.

physicians can often be reduced through practice profiling and feedback, as well as direct discussions between the medical director and these physicians. Some HMOs may include the cost of ancillary services in the capitated risk pools, and many MCOs include it in the pay-for-performance (P4P) programs.

Precertification is often used for costly diagnostic services, and for imaging services in particular—for example, CT, MRI, and PET scans. High overall costs may be mostly due to high prices, but they are more often due to higher than average utilization, or a combination of both pricing and utilization. Utilization as a primary driver has been associated with the number of available scanners— that is, the more scanners there are, the more often scans are ordered. It has also been associated with physician ownership, which is discussed below.

Precertification may be used with therapeutic services, but usually simple notification is enough for certain types of conditions—for example, extended physical therapy following rotator cuff shoulder surgery. Therapeutic services requiring multiple treatments are typically authorized for a set number of visits, and concurrent review is used if the therapist believes additional treatments are required.

As is the case for UM in general, medical necessity criteria typically form the basis for any coverage determinations, unless benefits are simply limited by the schedule of benefits or not covered at all. Medical necessity for ancillary services is addressed in the same way as for other clinical services coverage determinations, by applying evidence-based clinical appropriateness criteria to individual cases.

A potential area of concern involves a physician or physicians with an ownership interest in a diagnostic scanner or facility. Physician ownership of costly diagnostic devices or facilities is strongly associated with higher utilization of those resources by their owners.

The recent trend of hospital consolidation and physician employment has also been associated with higher trends in both pricing and utilization. With this model, hospital-employed physicians are directed to refer patients to hospital-owned facilities and diagnostic centers rather than lower-cost free-standing imaging centers.

Coverage and UM for specific therapeutic ancillary services is frequently affected by state-mandated benefits for insured individual or group policies (but not self-funded plans). For example, many states require coverage of treatments for autism, a condition for which treatment approaches vary widely.

Coverage and UM for therapeutic services has been made even more confusing for commercial insured policies under the ACA. Prior to the ACA, insurers usually limited coverage to rehabilitative services. The ACA's 10 essential health benefits, however, expanded this coverage to include "rehabilitative *and habilitative* services and devices" [emphasis added by author]. Unlike rehabilitative services, which focus on regaining functionality lost after an illness or injury, habilitative services help people learn or maintain functional skills rather than regain them. The ACA does not further define habilitative services, however, leaving it to the states to clarify this point. At the time of this text's publication, only half of the states had addressed it at all, doing so in different ways.

MANAGEMENT OF PHARMACEUTICAL BENEFITS

Prior to HMOs, coverage of prescription drugs was uncommon. When it became law in 1965, traditional Medicare provided no benefits coverage for drugs, whereas traditional Medicaid always has. Under the 1973 HMO Act as well as state HMO laws, HMOs were not required to cover drugs, although most did. Over time, drug coverage by all types of commercial plans became the norm, although it was always a "rider," meaning an add-on type of policy that was treated separately from the rest of the coverage. The main exception for most types of plans (other than Medicaid, in which no exception was needed) was for injectable drugs such as insulin or intravenous antibiotics for which coverage was typically included under a "major medical" policy that included the physician's bills and outpatient care.

The Medicare Modernization Act (MMA) of 2003 created a prescription drug benefit called Medicare Part D that older Medicare-eligible adults could purchase as a Medicare Advantage Part D plan (MA-PDP) stand-alone product or as part of a broader Medicare Advantage (MA) plan, but it remains voluntary. The ACA, on the other hand, now requires qualified commercial health plans to cover prescription drugs as one of the 10 essential health benefits, not as a rider.

Even before the ACA included drug coverage as an essential health benefit, greater levels of prescription drug coverage by private health insurers, HMOs, self-funded benefits plans, and private MA and MA-PDP plans fueled rising costs related to this type of therapy. This trend is evident in Figure 5–4, which shows total expenditures for prescription drugs from 1970 to 2010, and in Figure 5–5, which shows the costs and the sources of payment for these drugs.

Similar drugs may be equally effective in treating the same condition, and several different types of drugs may sometimes be used for the same condition

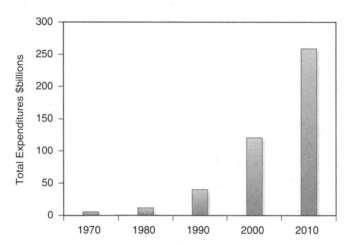

FIGURE 5–4 Total Expenditures—Prescription Drugs, 1970–2010

Data compiled by author from National Health Expenditures data released in January 2012 by the Centers for Medicare and Medicaid Services.

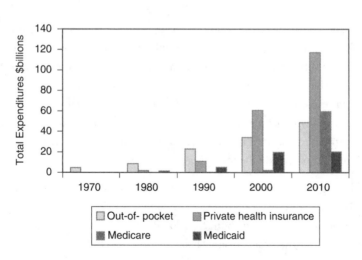

FIGURE 5–5 Sources of Payment for Prescription Drugs

Data compiled by author from National Health Expenditures data released in January 2012 by the Centers for Medicare and Medicaid Services.

as well. Examples of factors typically affecting treatment options include the following:

- Some drugs are much less costly than other drugs that may be used for the same condition.
- Some drugs are no longer covered by a patent and may be manufactured as generic medications, whereas others are still under patent protection and are available only as brand-name drugs.
- Brand-name drugs are marketed heavily to doctors as well as through direct-to-consumer advertising.
- Some drugs may be equally effective as others in most cases, but some people may not respond as well to them.
- Some drugs may be equally effective as others, but not as convenient to take.
- Some drugs may be effective, but have fewer or greater side effects than other options.
- Potential serious side effects may be more of a risk for some drugs compared to others.
- Some drugs are commonly prescribed as "off-label," meaning they are prescribed to treat clinical conditions not included in the list of specific conditions for which the drug is approved by the U.S. Food and Drug Administration (FDA) for use.

Before describing how the cost of the drug benefit is managed, it is important to emphasize that prescription drugs may ultimately help lower overall healthcare costs. Prescription drugs are an increasingly important aspect of health care overall, but they are critical to DM—that is, to managing the care of individuals with multiple chronic conditions and to preventing avoidable readmissions. Many chronically ill people end up in the emergency department or are admitted to the hospital because of problems related to taking their medicines. Examples of such problems include the following:

- Having to take a large number of different medicines, leading to confusion and difficulty keeping track of them
- Lack of understanding about how to take the medicines or what roles they play, despite medical personnel believing they had fully informed the patient
- Forgetting to take all or some medicines
- Taking medicines at doses or intervals other than what was prescribed
- Stopping one or more medicines for a variety of reasons, including side effects, real or perceived

- Multiple prescriptions written by multiple physicians that do not take into account any other medicines a patient is taking
- Interactions between different drugs causing serious side effects
- Not filling prescriptions for some reason, including costs

For these reasons and more, management of the pharmacy benefit has grown beyond simply managing costs, and now includes some element of assisting medical managers in managing the care of individuals with chronic conditions through improving medication compliance.

Pharmacy Benefits Managers

Drug benefits are not only managed differently than other types of healthcare benefits, but are often managed by a different company or a different subsidiary of a large payer. In either case, the company or subsidiary managing the drug benefit is called, naturally enough, a pharmacy benefits manager (PBM). For insured coverage policies, the PBM contracts directly with the payer or is a separate subsidiary of a large health insurer, but rarely takes any financial risk for the cost of the drug benefit, although it may if the PBM is an MA-PDP. In many cases, PBM services are included in the overall administrative services for self-funded plans, but self-funded plans may instead contract directly with PBMs and do not combine PBM services with other administrative services. In all cases, UM, DM, and CM programs rely on claims data from PBMs to more effectively manage their programs.

Formulary

A formulary is a list of drugs covering typical medical needs, although it does not include all available drugs for each medical condition. In many cases, several drugs are equally useful for a particular condition but differ widely in price. In addition, the PBM, because of its size, may have negotiated volume discounts with the manufacturers of some drugs. The formulary, then, contains drugs that are effective and are the least costly among the alternatives. If one particular drug is clearly the most effective choice, however, it may be the agent listed on the formulary regardless of cost.

Each PBM has a pharmacy and therapeutics (P&T) committee that creates and manages its formulary, while simultaneously using clinical criteria and taking cost into account. A payer or self-funded employer group may accept the formulary as is, but many payers—especially large payers and HMOs—have their own P&T committees that adjust the formulary to meet the needs of the plan's network or community. A payer's P&T committee usually also reviews requests for patient-specific exceptions, such as for highly expensive and infrequently used drugs for which the indications for use are not always clear.

There are two basic types of formularies: open and closed. In an open formulary, all drugs legally prescribed by a physicians or other appropriate provider are covered at least to some degree, but a member will face significant cost sharing for any drugs not on the formulary. In a closed formulary, there is no coverage for any drug not on the formulary. The use of multiple tiers within a formulary is almost universal in health plans.

Benefits Design

Benefits design of prescription drug coverage has changed somewhat under the ACA. Specifically, such coverage is included as an essential benefit for qualified health plans, so it is no longer provided through a separate rider. However, the components of the benefits design for drug coverage are not required to mimic the medical/surgical benefits design, and remain similar to what was in place before the ACA.

Like benefits design overall, the drug benefit design must support the means used by a PBM and a payer to manage costs and access. Tiering stratifies drugs according to how much the member will share in their cost. For example, generic drugs may be classified as Tier 1, in which case the member has only a $20 copayment. Certain brand-name drugs that are effective and for which the MCO has favorable payment terms may be classified as Tier 2, in which case the member has a $30 copayment. Expensive brand-name drugs for which there is a good Tier 1 or 2 alternative may be classified as Tier 3, in which case the member has a $50 copayment. Some MCOs even designate a fourth tier for drugs for which cost sharing typically takes the form of coinsurance, not a copayment, such as 50%. Because of their high costs, specialty pharmacy medicines are often categorized separately and subject to their own benefits design, usually as coinsurance that varies between 20% and 50% cost sharing. Benefits may also be limited to a certain amount of a drug. For example, drugs for erectile dysfunction in men are often limited to 7–10 pills per month. Other drugs used strictly for cosmetic purposes, such as drugs for baldness in men, may not be covered at all.

Drug Utilization Review and Step Therapy

Drug utilization review (DUR) consists of activities and strategies for managing the volume and pattern of prescriptions. The most common DUR strategy is to create prescribing profiles and then provide this profile information to physicians so that they can compare their own prescribing patterns with those of their peers.

Another common strategy is to require precertification for new prescriptions of certain drugs. This requirement may apply to drugs that are normally prescribed only for specific diagnoses that do not match anything in the PBM's records for a patient—for example, prescribing human growth hormone for a 45-year-old man who has not previously taken it. In some cases, such as when an individual changes coverage, the new PBM will require precertification information showing that coverage was previously precertified and that the member has been taking the medication for some time.

Step therapy is a form of DUR in which precertification is used for costly drugs for which reasonable alternatives exist, especially specialty pharmacy. It is called step therapy because patients must demonstrate that they have side effects from, or an inadequate response to, treatment with less costly alternative drugs. In those cases, coverage for the more costly treatment is authorized.

Mail Order

All PBMs provide a mail order service. Members may be required to use this service for any chronic medications—that is, drugs that are always used by the member, such as blood pressure medicine. Mail order services typically dispense a three-month supply of the drug, but are never used for acute prescriptions that are limited as to how long the patient will take the drug. Such services lower the fill fee (i.e., the payment to a pharmacy to fill the prescription) and allow for greater discounts by purchasing drugs in bulk from their manufacturers.

Specialty Pharmacy and Compounding Pharmacy

Specialty pharmacy and compounding pharmacy are special categories. The definition of specialty pharmacy was once limited to biopharmaceuticals, meaning manufactured types of proteins requiring injection either by a provider or by the patient, as well as some agents that are taken by mouth. In the past decade or so, that definition has broadened to include the following types of medications:

- Biopharmaceuticals*
- Costly medicines used to treat rare conditions
- Costly drugs that require special handling or monitoring

---

* Specialty pharmacy does not include insulin, even though it is technically a biopharmaceutical.

- Costly drugs that are available only through very limited supply channels
- Any drug that exceeds some cost threshold—for example, $500 or $1000 per month to use

Examples of diseases and conditions for which specialty pharmacy medicines are commonly used include the following:

- Some common types of genetic diseases, such as the various forms of hemophilia (bleeding disease)
- Some hormone deficiencies, such as human growth hormone deficiency for short stature syndrome
- Certain uncommon genetic illnesses, such as Gaucher's disease, in which the body cannot make a critically important protein
- Certain types of cancers or forms of cancers, such as some lymphomas or certain forms of breast cancer
- Many types of inflammatory diseases, such as eczema, rheumatoid arthritis, or Crohn's disease
- Some other serious medical conditions, such as multiple sclerosis
- Some specific types of chronic infection, such as hepatitis C or human immunodeficiency virus infection and acquired immunodeficiency syndrome (HIV/AIDS)

Treatment ranges from expensive to enormously expensive; in some cases, drug costs can exceed $250,000 to $500,000 annually per treated patient. The overall cost of specialty pharmacy currently accounts for more than 20% of all drug costs, and it continues to rise rapidly. Many specialty pharmacy medicines are also riskier for a patient compared to less costly alternatives—a risk that can be worth taking if a patient is not responding well to less costly drugs but not for the sake of convenience or only a minor improvement. Management of the specialty pharmacy benefit is often managed by a division of a PBM or by a PBM that focuses only on specialty pharmacy.

Compounded pharmacy is another growing cost category for health plans. In compounding, medications are mixed together by a pharmacist before being given or administered to a patient. Examples include the following:

- A drug such as a steroid injected into a saline solution bag so the patient can self-administer an intravenous treatment
- A large dose of an injectable drug divided into small amounts, which are then mixed into a solution to be injected directly into an organ such as the eye

- Several drugs mixed together to create a lotion or ointment that a patient then applies to a body part

Pricing for compounded pharmacy comprises some combination of drug and labor costs, but there is little or no standardization and prices tend to be very high. There is also a higher potential risk involved when drugs are compounded. For these reasons, plans often use precertification and other DUR methods for these treatments, and they may restrict coverage to medications prepared by specific pharmacies. Reference pricing (as described in the *Provider Payment* chapter) may also be used to help manage costs.

QUALITY MANAGEMENT

All HMOs and POS plans based on HMOs are required to have QM programs under state laws and regulations, and some states require PPOs to have one as well. State requirements around QM apply only to insured plans, however. Private managed care plans of any type that serve Medicare or Medicaid beneficiaries must also have a QM program; QM requirements do not apply to MediGap coverage, which is indemnity insurance and not managed care.

Some large employers require plans to have a QM program, but not all do. Because self-funded benefits plans are not subject to state regulation, a self-funded benefits plan of any type is not required by law to have a QM program. Self-funded employer groups that contract with HMO, POS, or PPO plans that also have insured products may be included in the plan's QM program because it is already operational. Nevertheless, self-funded groups that contract with rental networks or use different companies for different administrative activities typically do not include QM requirements in their contracts, or only as a minor function.

Generally speaking, payers' QM programs are population based, meaning they look at quality elements applicable to a large portion of the plan's members. They also mostly use the types of data and information readily available to a payer, such as claims data. The QM programs typically look at specific conditions or medical care, such as prevention or treatment of diabetes.

Approaches to QM in Managed Care

QM has been an evolving activity for HMOs since passage of the HMO Act of 1973. The classic and most enduring model for QM is that developed by

Avedis Donabedian,* which classifies QM activities into three broad and interrelated categories:

- Structure
- Process
- Outcome

In 1999, the Institute of Medicine (IOM) issued two reports on quality, the second of which outlined six goals for providing high quality healthcare.[†] These goals call for health care to be:

- Safe
- Effective
- Patient centered
- Timely
- Efficient
- Equitable

Many HMOs have worked to incorporate the IOM goals into their QM programs. However, the IOM's six goals are provider oriented. In other words, the primary focus of both the IOM report and goals is how providers deliver health care—for example, reducing medication errors (particularly in the inpatient setting) or providing appropriate care more quickly to a patient having a heart attack. Except for group and staff model HMOs, however, payers are not providers and have little or no ability to directly measure and manage these six goals on a day-to-day basis. For that reason, payers that try to incorporate the IOM's six goals typically do so on a population basis, not a patient-by-patient basis.

Concepts of total quality management or total quality improvement that emphasize a cycle of measuring, analysis, planning changes, implementing changes, measuring the results, and then beginning the cycle again, are also incorporated into many QM programs.

Classic Quality Management

Avedis Donabedian's model of using structure, process, and outcome is the classic way of describing QM, so we will explore it a bit more.

---

* Donabedian A. *Exploration in quality assessment and monitoring: the definition of quality and approaches to its assessment, Vol. 1.* Ann Arbor, MI: Health Administration Press; 1980.

† Institute of Medicine. *Crossing the quality chasm.* Washington, DC: National Academy Press; 2001:5–6.

Structure

Structure focuses on the context in which care and services are provided, not *how* care is provided (process) or the *result* of that care (outcome). Examples of structure measures in a typical QM program include:

- Credentialing criteria
- Physical location and accessibility of a physician's office
- Cultural issues such as languages spoken by a physician
- Cleanliness of a physician's office

Chart reviews confined to medical records of its members may also be part of evaluating structure, often as a component of the recredentialing process for PCPs, OB/Gyns, and high-volume behavioral health providers. Structural medical chart reviews are typically confined to looking at whether the chart lists all the patient's diagnoses, current medications, drug allergies, and so forth. These reviews do not attempt to evaluate *how* a doctor practices medicine.

Structure is relatively easy to document, but structural measures are intended only to document that defined standards about the setting in which health care is provided are being met. Still, structure is a vital part of any QM program, and it is a regulatory requirement established by most states and CMS for HMOs and MA plans.

Process

Process focuses on the way in which certain medical services are provided—in other words, what is being done and how is it being done. Process cannot apply to everything a physician or facility does, but rather must be defined beforehand. QM programs select conditions or services to examine based on whether they occur commonly, whether there are variations in practice, and whether evidence-based medical practice guidelines are available. In this way, they are able to achieve statistical integrity, meaning the findings are more likely to be valid than if only a few events are observed. Such an approach also allows the QM program to affect a reasonably large proportion of the plan's membership and move providers closer to evidence-based practice.

Process studies are typically limited to data obtainable through the payer's claims data systems, including claims data from PBMs—for example, preventive services such as screening rates of mammograms and Pap smears for women, and immunization rates for children. The data are typically the same as those collected for the Healthcare Effectiveness Data Information Set (HEDIS).

Claims-based process studies typically look at common medical conditions such as heart disease, asthma, and diabetes. In this approach, claims data are analyzed to determine whether certain services and treatments are being provided—for example, prescribing beta blockers following a heart attack, prescribing inhaled steroids for patients with asthma, and patients with diabetes getting annual eye examinations.

Process studies may sometimes include chart reviews as well. When they are used, these reviews focus on selected common conditions (e.g., diabetes, heart disease). The typical approach is to review a set number of a PCP's charts for plan members, and to look for documentation of preventive or screening services, or services related to a specific condition (documentation of an annual foot exam in a patient with diabetes, for example). The review is confined to determining whether certain care was provided as documented in the provider's medical records, such as counseling a patient with congestive heart failure about lowering salt intake, for example, but not about how the doctor actually performs a physical exam, such as whether the physician uses her or his stethoscope or direct observation of patient care.

HMOs do not typically perform on-site QM studies in hospitals or ambulatory facilities. In recent years, some plans have developed target metrics for defined conditions, however, and have begun to require facilities to self-report those data. CMS does this as well, and both CMS and some payers may use those metrics in their pay-for-performance programs.

Outcome

Outcome focuses on the results of care that was or was not provided. Outcomes must be examined in context. For example, a good outcome for a patient who experiences a heart attack would be full recovery without complications, whereas a good outcome for a terminally ill patient would include pain control and the patient and family being fully informed. Because so many factors can influence outcome, it is sometimes difficult to tease out the relative importance of any one factor. Examples of outcomes in a payer QM program might include the following:

- Infection rates
- Improved blood pressure readings
- Fewer emergency department visits
- Hospital readmission
- Return to the intensive care unit
- Illness or injury
- Death

QM programs typically examine outcomes by looking for patterns based on claims data, similar to process studies. Also like process studies, they typically focus on specific conditions. Outcome studies are frequently associated with system-wide initiatives. For example, a plan may undertake a focused effort to increase medication compliance by members with congestive heart failure, and then analyze claims data to see if that program results in higher medication compliance and in fewer emergency room visits by those members.

Outcome may also be evaluated as a result of the inpatient utilization management process. In this case, if a UM nurse thought that she or he detected a pattern of less than desirable outcomes for a specific type of inpatient event—readmission to the intensive care unit, for example—a focused outcome review might be initiated. In addition, a focused outcome study could be initiated in response to specific member complaints.

Peer Review

Most HMOs and POS plans and many PPOs have established policies and procedures to evaluate potential service or quality issues related to specific providers. Those policies and procedures may apply to issues involving care provided to plan members by a network provider, or they may apply to the credentialing and recredentialing process, as discussed in the chapter titled *The Provider Network*. For that reason, peer review may be used by two different but related committees: one specific to QM and the other specific to the credentialing committee. Both of these efforts are still within the boundaries of QM, however.

Peer review policies and procedures consist of internal information gathering specific to a provider and relevant to the identified potential issue, review by a plan medical director, and peer review by a physician committee; all are considered part of the peer review process. The entire peer review process, including information gathering, internal evaluations, and deliberations by the peer review committee, is confidential and considered "protected information," meaning its confidentiality is protected by federal and state laws and the information is not typically shared outside of the peer review process.

Peer review is used in the credentialing process when a provider's credentials are found to be deficient—for example, when a physician is not board certified and the plan's credentialing policies requires it. It may also apply when information gathered during credentialing or recredentialing indicates a problem that

---

* The last two could also come up during credentialing or recredentialing.

might not cause the provider to be automatically excluded from the network—for example, several large malpractice awards or settlements in a short period of time. In those cases, the peer review process is similar to that used for other potential problems requiring review.

In addition to information obtained during credentialing or recredentialing, quality of care concerns about a specific provider or facility may be identified through member complaints or grievances, by a UM nurse during the course of regular inpatient concurrent review, by the actions of another organization (for example, a hospital restricting a physician's privileges), or by actions or sanctions by a state or federal agency.*

Potential problems, including complaints or grievances against a contracted provider by a member, are typically reviewed first by a plan medical director after plan personnel have collected any additional relevant information. In some cases, the medical director may determine that no further investigation is necessary. If the medical director concludes that the complaint may have substance, it is typically referred to the peer review committee at this point.

The peer review committee is made up of plan physicians and supported by nonphysician personnel. Physician members of the peer review committee are typically independent physicians who are in the network. Physicians who are plan employees may be members of the peer review committee, but often support it. Some physician members attend all peer review committee meetings, and the committee usually will bring in other professionals with similar training and education as the provider being reviewed to serve on the committee for that case.

The committee reviews relevant information provided by the plan and may request additional information from the plan, the member, and the physician. The process usually allows a physician to explain the deficiency and provide more information to the committee. After reviewing this information, the peer review committee may either close the case or recommend action and follow-up. Whatever the outcome, the plan typically does not communicate any conclusions or actions taken with members or with personnel outside of the peer review process so that the peer review confidentiality protections are not accidently violated.

If the quality of care concern is considered serious or an immediate threat to the health of members receiving care from that provider, the medical director and peer review committee may take immediate action—by suspending the provider's participation in the network, for example. Precipitous action by the medical director or the peer review committee that is unsupported exposes the payer to significant liabilities and is disruptive to patient care.

HEALTH PLAN ACCREDITATION

Health plan accreditation is a form of oversight in which an independent, private, nonprofit organization reviews an MCO and determines if it meets certain criteria or industry standards. If it meets these standards, the MCO is considered accredited, although accreditation levels vary.

In essence, accreditation is a "seal of approval" that is relied on by many employers and consumers. States also have required standards that the different types of payer plans must meet, as does CMS for MA plans. Accreditation is not important for all types of health plans, however. On one end of the continuum are health insurers or rental networks with few managed care features, for which accreditation may have little value. On the other end are HMOs, for which accreditation is often very valuable. State requirements follow similar lines.

The difference between accreditation and oversight by a government agency such as a state insurance department is that the accreditation is completely voluntary, whereas compliance with state and federal requirements is not. However, most states as well as CMS accept plan accreditation as meeting regulatory requirements for the functions that they review. Data reporting is also an element of some accreditation programs as well as a requirement by most states and CMS.

Under the ACA, plans participating in the health insurance exchanges must also meet standards for qualified health plans (QHPs). These standards are very similar to those for health plans generally, but include some additional measures specific to the ACA. The same organizations that accredit health plans for the marketplace and Medicare have established accreditation programs for QHPs.

This section includes a brief discussion of accreditation organizations in managed care, followed by a description of the two commonly reported data sets.

Accreditation Organizations

Three organizations are recognized as accreditation organizations for payers and MCOs, and each has additional programs as well:

- National Committee for Quality Assurance (NCQA)
- URAC (formerly called the Utilization Review Accreditation Commission, but now known only by the acronym)
- Accreditation Association for Ambulatory Health Care (AAAHC)

The accreditation process for all three begins with a "desk review" in which the accreditation organization reviews documentation and data sent by the plan. If the desk review is found to meet the standards, the next step is an on-site review to verify records, interview personnel, and otherwise assess a plan's compliance with the accreditation standards. All three accrediting organizations offer differing levels of accreditation, depending on how completely the plan meets or does not meet its accreditation standards.

The accreditation organizations also offer related accreditation, certification, or recognition programs for various types of managed care services, although those differ from one organization to another. Examples of such related programs include, but are not limited to, the following:

- DM programs
- CM programs
- Credentialing verification organizations (CVOs)
- Credentialing programs
- Utilization review or utilization management programs
- Patient-centered medical homes (PCMHs)
- ACOs
- Wellness and health promotion programs
- Health information websites

Because many health plans or payer companies have many different products, capabilities, and services, the same plan or company may have accreditation, certification, and recognition designations from more than one of these organizations.

NCQA

NCQA has been accrediting HMOs and other health plans since 1990. It was initially formed years earlier by members of the payer industry, but subsequently reorganized so that its governance was made up primarily of representatives from employers, consumers, providers, and regulators (payers are not excluded, but they hold few board seats).

Overall NCQA accreditation status is based on its performance in three areas:

- HEDIS measures
- Member satisfaction using the Consumer Assessment of Health Providers and Systems (CAHPS) survey
- A review of key structures and processes using NCQA standards and guidelines

HEDIS and CAHPS together account for approximately 45% of a health plan's accreditation results; the remaining 55% is based on compliance with NCQA's standards and guidelines, including the scope and function of key operations. NCQA evaluations include the following areas of review:

- Quality management and improvement (QM/QI)
- Utilization management (UM)
- Credentialing and recredentialing (CR)
- Members' rights and responsibilities (RR)
- Standards for member connections (MEM)
- Medicaid benefits and services (MED)
- HEDIS/CAHPS performance measures

URAC

URAC was formed in 1990 with the backing of a broad range of consumers, employers, regulators, providers, and industry representatives to provide an efficient and effective method for evaluating utilization review processes. Originally, URAC was incorporated under the name "Utilization Review Accreditation Commission." However, that name was shortened to just the acronym "URAC" in 1996, when URAC began accrediting other types of organizations such as health plans and preferred provider organizations.

The scope of URAC's accreditation program includes the following measures:

- Network adequacy
- Member access
- UM
- QM
- Provider credentialing
- Complaints and appeals
- Patient information programs
- Various other data and measures
- CAHPS

URAC does not require HEDIS data, but accepts it as part of its accreditation program.

AAAHC

AAAHC was formed in 1979 to assist ambulatory healthcare organizations in improving the quality of care provided to patients. The primary areas of focus for AAAHC accreditation are ambulatory healthcare organizations, including endoscopy centers, ambulatory surgery centers, office-based surgery centers, student health centers, and large medical and dental group practices.

AAAHC is included here, however, because it also surveys and accredits managed care organizations and independent physician associations (IPAs). Its managed care standards are developed with active industry input. Areas of focus include the following:

- Rights and responsibilities and protection of members
- Governance and administration
- Provider networks credentialing
- Case management and care coordination
- Quality improvement and management
- Clinical records and health information
- Environment care and safety
- Health education and wellness promotion

Standardized Reports

Three standardized reports are used in accreditation and, in some cases, regulation of managed care plans. HEDIS and CAHPS may be used in any type of plan. Another report, called the Health Outcomes Survey (HOS) or the Medicare Health Outcomes Survey (MHOS), is used primarily for MA plans. All of these standardized surveys and reports are used to report data and information about overall performance, but also focus on specific clinical conditions and outcomes. HEDIS includes a great deal of plan-generated data, while CAHPS and HOS/MHOS are consumer or member surveys.

HEDIS

HEDIS has become an industry standard for reporting data to employers and many government agencies. By specifying not only what to measure but also how to measure it, HEDIS allows true "apples-to-apples" comparisons between health plans. Every year, national news magazines, local newspapers, employers, and others use HEDIS data to generate health plan "report cards" during open enrollment. All HEDIS data are required to be independently audited and verified.

HEDIS, which was developed and is continually refined by NCQA, currently consists of approximately 80 measures, not including the CAHPS survey, across five broad categories. Many states require all HMOs to report HEDIS data annually, regardless of whether they use NCQA for accreditation. Different versions of HEDIS focus on commercial plans, MA plans, and Medicaid plans, although all three overlap to a considerable degree.

CAHPS

CAHPS is an initiative of the federal AHRQ that seeks to support the assessment of consumers' experiences with health care. The goals of the CAHPS program are twofold:

- Develop standardized patient questionnaires that can be used to compare results across sponsors and over time
- Generate tools and resources that sponsors can use to produce understandable and usable comparative information for both consumers and healthcare providers

The first CAHPS survey was developed in 1995 and focused exclusively on Medicare HMOs, and later on Medicaid HMOs. Primarily concerned with consumers' experiences, it examined numerous issues related to member satisfaction and access to care. Since then, the health plan version of CAHPS has continued to evolve and become more sophisticated, and is no longer confined to Medicare and Medicaid plans.

CAHPS for health plans asks questions about access to care, communications, and overall satisfaction; consumers' perceptions of how well a health plan carries out its administrative functions; and consumers' health status and chronic medical conditions. Specialized versions of CAHPS for health plans are used for behavioral health and for children with chronic conditions. NCQA requires that health plans seeking accreditation use a modified version of CAHPS.

The CAHPS Hospital Survey, sometimes known as Hospital CAHPS (H-CAHPS), is a standardized survey of adult inpatients who received hospital care and services. This consumer survey asks questions around communication between patients and their doctors, nurses, and hospital staff, as well as questions about communications about medications. Additional questions deal with pain management, general responsiveness and satisfaction, the hospital environment, and the patient's discharge experience.

The CAHPS Clinician and Group Surveys (CG-CAHPS) ask patients about their recent experiences with clinicians and their staff. Different versions focus on adults receiving primary or specialty care, children receiving primary care, and patents receiving surgical care. There is also a version specific to patient-centered medical homes.

HOS/MHOS

The HOS was developed through collaboration between CMS and NCQA, which now manages it. Its focus is on Medicare beneficiaries' experiences in the hospital. This instrument includes questions to gain information about the following topics:

- A general health survey
- Information to adjust case mix
- Questions specific to four HEDIS effectiveness of care measures
- Demographic information
- Additional health questions

CONCLUSION

Total medical costs are the product of price multiplied by volume, which equates to provider payment multiplied by medical utilization. Consequently, to manage costs effectively, efforts to obtain a better price for medical services, although necessary for controlling costs, must be combined with utilization management carried out through a variety of means. Managing costs is not the same as managing quality, so managed care plans use a variety of methods to address quality—but only within the boundaries of what they are capable of doing, because they are not healthcare providers. Accreditation serves to provide independent external assessments of how well a plan meets industry standards in network management, UM, QM, member services, and other functions.

Utilization management and quality management are constantly evolving. What worked well 10 to 15 years ago is now less valuable and in some cases has even been abandoned, replaced by new approaches and methods. As payers and providers become more sophisticated in dealing with issues of utilization and quality of care, managed care will continue to change to take advantage of these improvements.

Sales, Governance, and Administration

LEARNING OBJECTIVES

- Describe the basic structure of governance and management in payer organizations
- Identify the basic elements of the internal operations of payer organizations:
  - Information technology
  - Marketing and sales, including insurance exchanges
  - Underwriting and premium rate development
  - Eligibility, enrollment, and billing
  - Claims and benefits administration
  - Member services, including appeal rights
  - Statutory accounting and statutory net worth
  - Financial management

INTRODUCTION

Sales, governance, and administration (SG&A) is a term commonly applied to the various managerial and operational functions and processes performed by a payer organization. Sometimes referred to as "operations," it broadly encompasses the majority of the day-to-day activities within any insurer, managed care organization (MCO), or health maintenance organization (HMO). Although not topics covered in this chapter, strictly speaking administration also includes network and medical management activities, except for quality management (QM).

The Affordable Care Act (ACA) restricts the percentage of premiums collected by a plan that can be used for the combination of SG&A and profit or surplus (for a nonprofit plan). This medical loss ratio (MLR) limitation applies only to insured products; self-funded plans do not pay premiums and are not subject to this requirement. The only activities performed by an MCO that do not count against the MLR limitation are those of wellness and prevention, as well as QM.

Administrative services are often seen as a "middleman" and viewed as adding little value. Indeed, during the mid-1990s, the term "middleman" was wielded as an insult, with providers and consumers alike tending to believe that administrative services were largely a waste of money. Many providers at that time attempted to take over administrative functions themselves to "cut out the middleman"—and many, if not most, of those attempts ended in financial disaster. Any providers that succeeded found that they had to do all the same administrative functions as any payer did, and their administrative costs were also about the same. The exceptions were plans owned by medical groups, or health systems with many employed physicians or associated with a strong existing independent practice association (IPA), where all medical management was delegated to the medical group or IPA and not counted as administration; in other words, it still cost the same, but counted as a medical cost. The key point is that even if one considers administrative services to be a "waste of money," no health plan can succeed without them.

Not all administrative activities are discussed here; rather, only the key functions are included. Examples of important functions *not* addressed in this chapter include:

- Human resources
- Legal and regulatory support
- Facility management
- Mail room management
- Purchasing
- Internal distribution

For the topics we do cover, we will not strictly follow the lettering sequence of "SG&A." Instead, it makes more sense to follow a different order, beginning with the "G" as we explore the following major administrative functional areas:

- Governance and management
- Information technology (IT)
- Marketing, sales, and distribution
- Actuarial services
- Underwriting and premium rate development
- Eligibility, enrollment, and billing

- Claims and benefits administration
- Member services and appeals of coverage denials
- Financial management

Finally, this is the longest chapter in this text. The topics covered are essential to the operations of health insurers and MCOs, but there is no denying that most of us also find discussion of them to be painfully boring. For that reason, the reader may find it helpful to review the chapter in sections, not all at once.

GOVERNANCE AND MANAGEMENT

Governance and management are not the same thing, although they are related. Governance encompasses the overall policies, rules, goals or mission, and responsibilities for the organization as a whole, but not the day-to-day running of the organization, which is the role of management. The governance and management of a payer organization are influenced by its type, its structure (or that of its parent company), requirements under state or federal laws, and many other variables. This can affect the governance, and the functions and responsibilities of key officers and managers as well as some committees, but at a high level, the overall needs for governance and management are similar among plan types.

Board of Directors

Most, but not all, MCOs have a board of directors. Numerous factors influence the composition and function of the board, including various state and federal laws and regulations affecting board makeup in relation to ownership status, profit versus nonprofit status, and so forth.

Types of health plans that do not necessarily have their own boards include the following:

- Preferred provider organizations (PPOs) that do not need a state license
- PPOs or HMOs created solely for the purpose of serving a single company's employees
- PPOs that are set up by an insurer to provide a benefits plan and are not required to be licensed by the state
- An MCO that is a subsidiary of a larger company whose board of directors oversees the entire company, not just the subsidiary

Although most MCOs have boards of directors, not all those boards are fully independent. This is especially true for MCOs that are part of large national companies. For example, HMOs are typically required by law to have a board of directors, but it is not uncommon for a company to use the same corporate officers as the board for its subsidiary HMOs. Although this type of board meets the required legal function and obligation, control of the actual operation of the HMO is exerted by the management structure of the parent company, rather than through a direct relationship between the HMO executives and its local board. These types of boards are not the focus of this section, however.

Technically speaking, MCOs that only administer benefits plans on behalf of self-funded employer groups may not need a board because they are not the actual health plan. In a self-funded employer group benefits plan, it is the employer that is responsible; that is, the employer has "fiduciary responsibility" and is called "the fiduciary." The employer does not necessarily need to have a board for the benefits plan either, although many employers create one internally.

Board Composition

The composition of the board of directors varies depending on whether the plan is a for-profit entity, in which case the owners' or shareholders' representatives may hold the majority of seats, or a nonprofit organization, in which case community representation will be broader and the board cannot be dominated by any special interest. Some nonprofit health plans are organized as cooperatives (i.e., a legal entity in which the members, or enrollees, are as a group in control of the entity); in this arrangement, the board members are all members of the plan. The same is true for consumer-owned and -operated plans (CO-OPs) created under the ACA, which are also subject to some other unique requirements. Mutual insurers are similar, but their boards more closely resemble the boards of for-profit companies.

Board members generally should be truly independent and have no potential conflicts of interest. Depending on the situation, local events, company bylaws, and laws and regulations (for example, the tax code for nonprofit health plans) may dictate whether the board members come from outside the health plan and whether health plan executives hold any board seats.

Provider-sponsored nonprofit plans may restrict seats held by providers to no more than 20% of the board's membership. A provider-sponsored for-profit plan board of directors will usually be composed of participating providers, but they must take special precautions to avoid antitrust problems. For example, providers on the board of a provider-owned plan cannot set or influence how or how much providers are paid.

Board Responsibilities

The function of a payer board of directors is governance—that is, overseeing the payer's activities. Final approval of corporate bylaws rests with the board. These bylaws determine the basic structure of authority and responsibility, both that of the plan officers and of the board itself. As part of their legal responsibilities, members of the board typically review certain reports and sign particular documents. For example, a board officer may be required to sign the quarterly financial report submitted to a state regulatory agency, and the board chairperson may be required to sign any acquisition documents. Because significant liability issues surround the board of directors, each board member must undertake his or her duties with care and diligence. Plans also may buy a special type of insurance to financially protect board directors and officers from acts of commission and omission.

In freestanding plans, the board also has responsibility for hiring the chief executive officer (CEO) of the plan and for reviewing the CEO's performance. The board in such plans often sets the CEO's compensation package, and the CEO reports to the board. In addition, many boards oversee the compensation for all senior executives in the plan. The board of a publicly traded company has increased financial oversight requirements, created by the Sarbanes-Oxley Act of 2002 in the wake of a number of financial scandals.

Typical Board Committees

Most companies have certain board committees, which focus on nonmedical issues relevant to running a business. Most states also require HMO boards, and sometimes boards of PPOs, to assume final responsibility for the plan's QM program, even though the board does not actively participate in running it.

Typical board committees include the following:

- *Executive Committee*: Provided with board-level decision making authority for issues that must be addressed before the full board can meet.
- *Finance and/or Audit Committee*: Charged with direct oversight of issues relating to financial statements and relationships with the outside auditing firm. Reviews financial statistics, approves budgets, sets and approves spending authority, reviews the annual audit, and reviews and approves outside funding sources.
- *Compensation Committee*: Charged with determining the appropriate compensation and incentives to key executives. The board must also approve and issue stock options to plan officers, board members, and large institutional investors.

- *Quality Management Committee*: Charged with overall oversight of the quality management program of the plan through regular reports on findings and activities. This board committee, however, does not participate in the plan's internal credentialing, QM, or peer review committees.
- *Corporate Compliance Committee*: Charged with oversight of the corporate compliance requirements under the Health Insurance Portability and Accountability Act (HIPAA), the ACA, Medicare and/or Medicaid requirements for payers with those plans, and the Sarbanes-Oxley Act.

Management

Management refers to individuals with the authority and responsibility to operate the plan. The roles and titles of the key managers in any organization will vary depending on the type of organization, its legal status, its line of business, its complexity, and whether it is a freestanding entity or a satellite of another operation, among other factors. There is little specific consistency from health plan to health plan, but there is relative consistency in the overall duties described here.

Executive Director/Chief Executive Officer

Most plans have at least one key manager. Sometimes called an executive director, a CEO, a general manager, or a plan manager, this individual is usually responsible for the overrall operations of the plan. This is not always the case, however. Many large national or regional payer companies use vertical reporting, in which managers of the various functions such as marketing or network management report to regional managers, not to a plan's executive director.

In freestanding plans and traditional nonprofit HMOs, the CEO is responsible for all areas. The other officers and key managers report to the CEO, who in turn reports to the board of directors (or to a regional manager in the case of national companies). The executive director also has responsibility for general administrative operations and public relations.

Medical Director/Chief Medical Officer

Every health insurer and managed care plan will have a medical director, and often more than one. Larger plans typically designate a chief medical officer (CMO*) to whom the other medical directors report. The medical director usually has responsibility for QM, utilization management (UM), and medical

---

* Not to be confused with a chief marketing officer, who also may be referred to as a CMO.

policy. In some plans, a medical director is also responsible for provider management and provider recruiting, which may or may not include provider facilities such as hospitals. In addition, medical directors are involved in physician-specific activities such as provider credentialing, peer review, and benefits coverage denials. Under the ACA and in most states, a medical director, one who was not involved in the initial denial decision, must review appeals of denials of coverage as well.

Vice President of Network Management

In large health plans and insurance companies, it is common for provider relations and network management to be the responsibility of an officer other than the medical director. This officer may be a physician, but usually is not. Larger organizations also separate the management and recruiting of professionals from these responsibilities in facilities. Network management is responsible for the credentialing of those providers, as described in the chapter titled *The Provider Network*, but a medical director and a credentialing committee are typically responsible for any final deliberations or reviews of provider credentials for professionals.

Finance Director/Chief Financial Officer

In freestanding plans or large operations, it is common to have a finance director or chief financial officer (CFO). That individual is generally responsible for all financial and accounting operations, including fiscal reporting, and budget preparation.

Operations Director/Chief Operating Officer

In larger nonprofit plans as well as national plans, it is common to have an operations director or chief operating officer (COO). In very large companies, this position may carry the title of president. The person in this position usually oversees overall operations of the organization, but not finance, board and investor relations, and external relations. Strategy is usually the responsibility of the CEO, but a COO/president may assume this role as well.

Marketing Director/Chief Marketing Officer

The responsibility for sales and marketing the plan belongs to the marketing director or chief marketing officer (CMO*). These duties generally include oversight of marketing representatives, advertising, client relations, enrollment

---

* Not to be confused with a chief medical officer, who also may be referred to as a CMO.

forecasting, and public relations. In larger organizations, responsibility for marketing is typically separated from sales.

Director of Information Services/Chief Information Officer

Information services are so complex that all health plans have an officer dedicated to overseeing this function. Typical responsibilities of the director of information services or chief information officer (CIO) include oversight of the data center (the physical computing equipment itself), all software and system applications, personal computer networks, telecommunications, Internet portals, and outsourced services. In some cases, plans outsource this function to an independent company.

Chief Underwriting Officer

The chief underwriter is responsible for oversight of actuarial services, which may be provided by in-house actuaries or by external actuarial firms, and for generating premium rates.

Corporate Compliance Officer

Health plans have specific corporate compliance requirements under many different laws and regulations. Some of these requirements include appointment of a specific individual who is responsible for ensuring that the organization is in compliance. One corporate compliance officer may be able to fulfill all these responsibilities, but larger organizations may require multiple compliance officers; for example, there may be different compliance officers for financial matters and for oversight of privacy and security requirements.

Management Committees

The types of operational or corporate committees may vary from one organization to the next. Some may be standing committees that meet on a regular basis for specific purposes, whereas others are ad hoc committees that are created to meet a specific need and then dissolved. Each functional area of a payer organization is likely to have multiple committees, and cross-functional team committees are commonly encountered as well.

In contrast, some committees specifically related to medical management and to appeals of coverage denials are similar from plan to plan. The first four of the following medical management committees are found in most health plans, and the remaining two are found in many plans:

- Quality management committee
- Credentialing committee
- Peer review committee
- Pharmacy and therapeutics committee
- Medical advisory committee
- Utilization review/care management committee

INFORMATION TECHNOLOGY

A payer's IT system refers to the computer hardware, software, and telecommunications systems and support the organization uses to collect, store, transmit, operationally use, and analyze data and information, and communicate via voice and electronic data interchange. The IT system is the backbone of the payer's operations. All the activities performed by a payer depend on computer hardware and software. If this information system is not working efficiently and properly, neither is the payer.

The core of most payers' IT system is a mainframe system (sometimes more than one) used to handle high-volume day-to-day operations such as member enrollment and claims. Mainframe systems are usually licensed from a commercial vendor, and they typically contain multiple modules for performing different functions. Payers also often license different software modules that are able to perform specific functions yet are compatible with the mainframe system. Examples of such types of separate program modules include general ledger programs, medical management, and provider database management. Some large plans program their own mainframe systems, and even licensed modules are often heavily modified to suit a particular plan's requirements.

The IT system also includes an internal network that supports electronic communication within the organization, Internet and e-commerce capabilities for communication with the outside world, and telecommunications systems. In addition, it generally includes private communications systems for business-to-business electronic interchange, data storage, and analysis systems. Finally, IT supports all remaining work-related technology used by the organization, including personal computers and mobile devices, and all software licensed by the company.

While a payer's ability to conduct business and communicate with members, providers, and employers depends on IT, a surprising amount of paper is still used in the business of health care, although it continues to be replaced by electronic forms of information storage and transmission. The IT function often manages this stream of data as well through the use of imaging and storage.

HIPAA Requirements and Standards

One of HIPAA's biggest areas of impact is its requirements mandating that "covered entities," including payers, providers, and their business associates, comply with standards included in the section of HIPAA titled "Administrative Simplification." These standards, which apply primarily to electronic transactions, deal with the following issues:

- Code sets
- Electronic transactions
- Electronic funds transfers
- Identifiers
- Privacy
- Security

Code sets, electronic transactions, and electronic funds transfers are addressed in the *Provider Payment* chapter because most of them are related, directly or indirectly, to provider payment. The other three standards are discussed here.

Identifier Standards

The national provider identifier (NPI) is described in the chapter titled *The Provider Network*, so that discussion will not be repeated here. The existing employer identification number (EIN) that is used for tax purposes is also used to meet HIPAA's employer identifier requirement.

The health plan identifier (HPID) is to apply to health plans of all types with one exception: If a health plan is a controlled subsidiary health plan, meaning that it is fully controlled by another health plan, then it does not need to have its own HPID. The HPID requirement was to go into effect in late 2014, but shortly before the publication of this text, the government postponed its implementation indefinitely.

Privacy and Security Requirements Under HIPAA

The privacy and security provisions of HIPAA are complex. HIPAA allows states to establish stricter standards than those in HIPAA, but not less strict versions. These requirements are described here at a very high level, but additional information, including summary information provided by the U.S. Department of

Health and Human Services (DHHS), Office of Civil Rights (OCR), can be found on the following two websites (current at the time of publication):

- Privacy: http://www.hhs.gov/ocr/privacy/hipaa/understanding/summary /index.html
- Security: http://www.hhs.gov/ocr/privacy/hipaa/understanding /srsummary.html

Protected Health Information (Privacy)   Central to the privacy and security regulations is the concept of protected health information (PHI). PHI is individually identifiable health information that is transmitted or maintained in electronic media or in any other form or medium. In other words, all electronic, paper, and oral information is covered. PHI includes all past, present, or future information that is created or received by a covered entity about an individual and that individual's physical or mental health or condition or the health care he or she receives. PHI is "individually identifiable" because it includes the individual's name or some other information that can be used to identify the individual, such as an address or Social Security number. The definition of PHI is intended to be quite broad and includes most of the information used in managing health benefits plans.

Consumers' Control over Their Health Information (Privacy)   Patients have the right to understand and control how their health information is used. The regulations that apply to HIPAA privacy require covered entities to educate patients about their rights, provide patients with access to their own medical records and means to obtain copies of those records, and similar protections. Consumers do not have the right, however, to alter or delete health information created by a covered entity.

Limits on Medical Record Use and Release (Privacy)   With few exceptions, PHI can be used for healthcare purposes only, including health benefits management. Only the minimum necessary information should be disclosed, although that requirement does not apply to the transfer of medical records for the purpose of medical treatment. The main exceptions to the requirement that PHI be used only for healthcare purposes are some defined and limited marketing, fundraising, and outreach activities by provider organizations; an individual may also choose to "opt out" of any such use.

Examples of routine use of PHI that would apply to all covered entities are the use of this information for payment, treatment, and healthcare operations. For example, a hospital must use PHI to both provide care and bill a payer for that care, and a payer must have enough information to accurately process the claim.

PHI is used for nearly all major administrative processes, as well as for provider payment, UM, case management (CM), disease management (DM), and QM.

Administrative Requirements (Privacy) HIPAA's privacy provisions also have administrative requirements, including establishing policies and procedures to protect privacy, designating a privacy official to be responsible for maintaining privacy, workforce training, and having a way for patients or members to file complaints about potential HIPAA violations.

Physical and Electronic Data Protection Requirements (Security) Even though the HIPAA privacy provisions generally require covered entities to ensure the confidentiality of PHI by appropriately securing it, HIPAA has separate security requirements for electronic PHI, including e-mail. Fax, telephone, and paper records are generally not considered electronic PHI unless they are recorded and stored electronically, although these records are still subject to the privacy requirements. Eighteen different standards cover an even larger number of security rules and specifications related to PHI. These complex standards and rules are well beyond the scope of this text, however.

Analytics and Informatics

Most payers have a department dedicated to using data and information for analytic purposes. This function, often referred to as informatics, may have very specific areas of focus in particular areas, such as medical costs, or sales and marketing data. It may also be more generalized, such as creating useful operational reports for managers on an "as needed" basis. Regardless, informatics continues to be increasingly important for payers to succeed in today's market.

MARKETING AND SALES

Health plans must market to a wide variety of potential customers, from administrative services for large self-funded employer group plans to insured products for small groups and individuals. The approach to marketing and sales differs, at least somewhat, for each different type of customer. Many plans also participate in Medicare and Medicaid, which have their own stringent rules as discussed in the *Medicare and Medicaid* chapter.

The ACA has had a major impact on how payers market and sell their products. Many ACA requirements are confined to insured products, but some apply to all services.

Summary of Benefits and Coverage

The ACA requires all health plans, including self-funded plans, to provide existing and potential enrollees with access to a standardized summary of benefits and coverage (SBC), also called a summary of coverage (SOC). Similar but separate provisions apply to private Medicare and Medicaid health plans. The ACA further requires the SBC/SOC to adhere to a uniform and common format that defines the number of pages, the exact information that must be provided, and even the size of the font so consumers can compare plan benefits among and between carriers. The SBC does not replace the far more detailed evidence of coverage (EOC), sometimes called a certificate of coverage or certificate of insurance, that all health plans must make available to covered individuals.

SBCs must provide information in easy-to-understand language, including a description of coverage, cost sharing, exceptions, and limitations on coverage. In addition, they must provide examples to illustrate coverage for some common conditions, explain how to renew coverage, include a glossary of common terms, and explain where to go to find out more. A full description of the SOC, including some examples, can be found on the federal website: Access http://www.cms.gov /cciio and then click on the section titled "Consumer Support and Information."

Marketing

Although the two functions are closely related to each other, marketing differs from sales. Marketing generally refers to the various activities that support the sales effort and promote the plan in the marketplace, but it usually does not include actual sales. The marketing function in payer organizations typically includes responsibilities, such as:

- Brand management
- External communications and public relations
- Advertising
- Market research
- Lead generation
- Sales campaign support

Sales

Sales refer to the processes of actually selling the products and services that the health plan offers. It is the concrete means of adding or retaining employer group customers and their employees, and individual members. The sales process differs to some degree by market segments and distribution channels, and sales personnel employed by the plan usually specialize in one type of market segment or distribution channel.

Market Segments

The ACA defines distinct market segments that are similar to the way payers defined them before the law was passed:

- *Individual*: Health insurance purchased individually, not through a group.
- *Small employer group*: At least one (in those states that allow a business with a single owner/employee to be classified as a small group) or two employees, but not more than 100 employees on average. (Some states may cap this at 50 employees.)
- *Large employer group*: More than 100 employees on average.

Most payers actually use four levels and divide them a bit differently, adding a mid-sized group market segment applying to groups with more than 100 employees but fewer than 300 or so employees, and defining the large group market as applying to employer groups larger than that. They distinguish this additional type of market segment because the distribution channels usually differ for mid-sized and large groups. In the large employer group market segments, health plans typically apply some designation to reflect the risk arrangement, ranging from fully insured to self-funded administrative services only (ASO).

Distribution and Distribution Channels

The term "distribution" refers to how payers' products and services are sold, and the term "distribution channel" refers to the way the payer accesses the different types of market segments. Distribution channels may overlap, and sometimes more than one form of distribution may be used in the same market segment. Table 6–1 lists the most common types of distribution channels.

Health Insurance and SHOP Exchanges Under the ACA

The ACA created two similar but distinct distribution channels: health insurance exchanges for use by individuals and the Small Business Health Options Program (SHOP) health insurance exchanges for use by small businesses. It is worth exploring these new forms of distribution in a little more detail because of their importance.

Table 6-1   Distribution Channels by Market Segment

Distribution Channel	Individual Market	Small Employer Group Market	Large Employer Group Market
Individual health insurance exchange	Yes	No	No
Small Business Health Options Program (SHOP) exchange	No	Yes[1]	No[2]
Private health insurance exchange	No	Yes	Yes, but only for employee coverage options
Direct through web	Yes	Yes	No
Direct mail	Yes	Yes	No
Telesales	Yes	Yes	No
Retail stores	Yes, but Uncommon	Yes, but Uncommon	No
Plan sales personnel	Yes, but uncommon	Yes, sometimes with a broker	Yes, but usually with a consultant
Brokers and agents	Yes	Yes	Yes, but less common than in small group market
Benefits consultants	No	Rarely	Yes

[1] Not everywhere, however. SHOP exchanges have been delayed in many states until 2016.
[2] After 2017, states that operate their own exchanges will have the option of opening up the exchange to businesses larger than 100 employees.

Under the ACA, each state is to create its own health insurance exchanges, but if it either cannot or will not do so, then the federal government is responsible for doing so. The individual exchanges were originally supposed to be operational by late 2013 for coverage beginning in 2014, but states may build them at any point after that as well. The deadline for SHOP exchanges has been delayed twice, however, and at the time of publication it has been set as 2016 for some states, though a number of states already have operational SHOP exchanges, including states that are relying on a federally facilitated SHOP exchange.

Health insurance exchanges for the individual market and the small employer group market are separate, although a state that is operating its own exchanges may merge them. Only small employers with 100 or fewer employees (or 50 or fewer employees in some states) may use the SHOP exchange if one is available. Except for individuals who qualify for a premium subsidy and small employers that qualify for a tax subsidy, no individual or small business is required to use this exchange.

Some states have chosen to create and run their own exchanges, some have chosen to create and operate exchanges in partnership with the federal government, a few states initially ran their own exchanges but have since defaulted back to the federally run exchanges, and some states elected to not create or operate any exchanges and defaulted to the federal government's exchanges. As of 2014, health insurance exchanges for individuals are available in all states in one way or another, while SHOP exchanges are available in many, but not all, states.

The federal government is also operating a website that provides similar information at www.HealthCare.gov. Consumers can directly access an exchange through www.healthcare.gov/marketplace.

The ACA does not require an insurer or HMO to offer its plans through the exchange, but a state may prohibit one from participating in an exchange based on several criteria. Any insurer offering coverage through an exchange must offer at least one Gold-level and one Silver-level benefits plan for each product it offers. It is not required to offer Platinum or Bronze plans, although many offer those options as well. Insurers may offer different products through the exchange than they do outside of it, the biggest difference being the size of the provider network, with exchange-based products using narrower networks. They are not required to offer an exchange-based product outside of the exchange, but if they do, they must charge the same premium rates for a product that is offered both inside and outside of an exchange.

The insurance exchanges have many functions and requirements under the ACA:

- Certifying, recertifying, and decertifying qualified health plans (QHPs) offering coverage through the exchange
- Assigning ratings to each plan offered through the exchange on the basis of relative quality and price
- Providing consumer information through the SBC for each QHP's offerings
- Operating an Internet site and toll-free telephone hotline offering comparative information on qualified health plans and allowing consumers and small businesses to apply for and purchase coverage if eligible
- Determining eligibility for the coverage through the exchange
- Determining eligibility for premium subsidies or tax credits
- Facilitating enrollment in those programs, by directing consumers to a health plan's website for enrollment or by enabling enrollment on the exchange

Exchanges for individual coverage have additional functions and requirements:

- Determining exemptions from requirements that individuals carry health insurance, and granting approvals of these exemptions to individuals related to hardship or other criteria
- Determining eligibility for coverage outside of the normal enrollment period
- Determining income-based eligibility for coverage through Medicaid or for premium subsidies
- Creating an electronic calculator to allow consumers to assess the cost of coverage after application of any advance premium tax credits and cost-sharing reductions
- Managing a navigator program to assist consumers in making choices about their healthcare insurance options and accessing their new healthcare coverage

To meet many of the ACA's requirements, an insurance exchange must also have two-way information exchanges with the following entities:

- The U.S. Department of Homeland Security, for validation of citizenship
- The U.S. Department of the Treasury, for reporting of coverage and verification of eligibility for premium subsidies
- State Medicaid agencies, for determination of eligibility for Medicaid coverage, including facilitating enrollment
- Health insurers and HMOs participating in the exchanges for a wide variety of transactions

Private Health Insurance Exchanges

Private health insurance exchanges are not the same as the exchanges under the ACA. Private exchanges are private commercial web-based marketplaces operated by payers or by benefits consulting firms. They focus primarily on small to mid-sized employer groups, though some large employers are using them too. The products offered in a private exchange may be the same as those offered in a public exchange, but they do not need to be.

Private health exchanges are both a new form of digital distribution channel as well as a means of providing more services to employers and their employees. As a distribution channel, a private exchange replaces the more traditional sales approaches and, therefore, can lower sales costs by eliminating or reducing commission payments to outside brokers and agents, eliminating or reducing costs for printing traditional hard copies of sales materials and enrollment forms, and even increasing revenues through the use of captive agents and brokers (i.e., brokers and agents employed by the payer or the benefits management consulting firm).

Private exchanges can also provide benefits administration services to smaller employers, reducing their costs as well. Insurers that offer private exchanges often use private exchanges to allow the employees of a group customer to choose from various coverage options offered by the payer rather than imposing a single type of benefit plan—something most large employers have been doing for many years.

Web Sales

A plan may have its own web-based portal for direct purchase of coverage for eligible individuals or small businesses, although many require going through an exchange first to determine eligibility for coverage and subsidies. Online brokers may also run web-based sales portals, and plans often provide web-based sales tools to brokers to be used in selling to consumers. What sets this portal apart from a private exchange is who may use it and what it does, although the distinction is not necessarily clear cut. Web sales are more like customer self-service for purchasing whatever the insurer chooses to offer to that market segment, which may include options it does not offer in the public exchange. It is usually not used for mid-sized or large group sales.

Direct Mail

Direct mail to consumers and/or small businesses is a common sales tool, although it is slowly giving way to use of electronic media. A mailing may be informational only, directing the individual or business owner to another channel, or it may provide an application form that can be mailed or faxed in.

Telesales

Telesales are more common in the individual than in the small business markets. This distribution channel is similar to direct mail, with the caller using a specific script intended to promote the sale of a product or service.

Retail Stores

Sometimes health plans set up stores that enable walk-in, in-person purchasing of health insurance. Sales associates in the retail store consultatively engage the consumers and guide them through the purchase process. This avenue is not a commonly used distribution channel, but when it is used, other channels (e.g., web, mail) are leveraged to stimulate traffic to the retail store.

Brokers and Agents

Brokers and agents are major distribution channels in the individual, and the small and mid-sized employer group markets. Brokers must be licensed by the state in which they work, and may offer products and services both within an exchange and outside of it. Brokers also help service accounts. They usually must be appointed or certified by a plan before being able to sell any of the plan's products.

Brokers and agents are paid a commission by the health plan. In the past, this meant a percentage of the premiums paid by the employer or individual that bought coverage through the broker. Plans could not or did not vary premiums depending on whether a broker was involved. As a consequence, when healthcare cost inflation drove premiums up, the amount paid to brokers rose at the same rate. In response to the MLR limits created by the ACA, some plans now pay brokers through a flat commission payment, meaning a fixed dollar amount. Percentage of premium commissions are still used, however, and where the individual and small group markets have become more competitive, commissions have once again begun to grow.

Benefits Consultants

Benefits consultants focus on larger, self-funded employers. Consultants are paid by the employer, not the payer, and their payments usually take the form of fixed fees and are not directly related to the amount of premium. The consultants help negotiate administrative agreements with payers, obtain reinsurance, and often manage nonmedical benefits. In many cases, a benefits consulting firm may manage all aspects of all employee benefits programs for a large employer other than payroll.

Sales Personnel Employed by the Payer

Payers employ sales personnel who work in a variety of capacities. They often specialize or focus on specific types of sales, such as direct sales to small and mid-sized employer groups, sales to individuals (no longer as common as it once was), working mostly with brokers, or working with benefits consultants. Many states require employed sales personnel to be licensed to sell insured products.

One unique form of sale that occurs in the large group market is a type of "second sale." The first sale is to the employer group. Large employers, however, typically contract with more than one payer to provide their employees with choices in benefits plans and costs. The second sale refers to selling to each individual employee—that is, persuading the employee to choose one payer over another. Some large companies restrict how a payer handles this contact with employees during the employer's open enrollment period—for example, by controlling the types of information a payer can make available to employees, or by limiting the locations and allowed time for sales presentations to employees and dependents.

ACTUARIAL SERVICES, UNDERWRITING, AND PREMIUM RATE DEVELOPMENT

A fundamental requirement for any payer is to know what to charge in premiums for its insured products. Because of the MLR limits, overcharging results in having to pay rebates to customers, and undercharging means having to deal with premium payments that are insufficient to cover costs for a full year, without ever being able to recover the losses. It is the responsibility of the related but distinct actuarial and underwriting functions to calculate what the premium needs to be each year.

Actuarial Services

The most important things that actuaries do are to estimate current medical claim liabilities and future medical expenses by building on past and current experiences. The estimates of future medical expenses are influenced by the design of the benefits plan, changes in laws such as benefits mandates, provider payment rates, assumptions about utilization patterns, and so forth. The end result is a model in which these factors are used to estimate the average amount of money required to cover medical costs on a per-member per-month (PMPM) basis. Projections developed by actuaries are used as a basis for developing premium rates, but the actual premiums will differ from those base numbers.

Actuaries also perform ongoing estimates of how much money a plan needs to reserve to cover expected costs (more on this later in the chapter). Small and mid-sized payers typically contract with external actuarial firms rather than hire staff actuaries. Even when a payer does have staff actuaries, it is standard practice for outside actuaries to examine reserve calculations as part of the payer's annual audit. Many states require actuarial certification as well.

Underwriting and Premium Rate Development

To calculate the premiums that will be charged, underwriters must combine what the actuaries' calculations with a determination of the levels of risk for groups and products. Under the ACA, some new requirements will have a very large impact on premium rate development for the individual and group markets:

- Guaranteed issue and renewability
- MLR limitations
- Restrictions on rate variations (individual and small group markets only)
- State review of rates and a requirement for plans to justify increases (individual and small group markets only)

Guaranteed Issue and Renewability

All insurers and HMOs are required under the ACA to provide guaranteed issue and renewability, meaning that no group or individual may be denied coverage as long as they apply during an open enrollment period (which usually takes place once per year) or based on a "life event" (also called a "special event"), and have not failed to pay their premiums or committed fraud. This results in a higher level of financial risk to insurers and HMOs because sicker people are more likely to want and need coverage than are healthier people—a consideration that must be taken into account during the underwriting process.*

Medical Loss Ratio Limitations

The ACA created limitations on the MLR, meaning the proportion of premium dollars spent on clinical services and quality improvement, and provided rebates to consumers if the percentage of premium spent on clinical services and quality that is less than 85% for plans in the large group market and less than 80% for plans in the individual and small group markets. This requirement does not apply to self-funded groups because they pay only administrative fees, not premiums.

Premium payments in excess of the MLR limitations must be paid back as rebates. In the individual and small group markets, the rebates are paid out evenly to each covered individual or small employer group, in proportion to how much they actually paid in premiums. In the large group market, rebates are paid on a company-specific basis, meaning they are paid only to companies for which the MLR was less than 85%.

The MLR limitation operates in one direction only; if a plan experiences a higher than expected MLR, meaning it spends more on benefits than it

---

* This is the reason for the "individual mandate" discussed in the chapter titled *Health Benefits Coverage and Types of Health Plans*, so healthier people will still buy coverage.

anticipated, it cannot recover the difference. The MLR requirement also does not allow a payer to use a group's *overall* medical costs if it is providing coverage for that employer in more than one state; instead, the MLRs are calculated exclusively on a state-by-state basis. In other words, if a single large group employer has an MLR of 75% in one state but an MLR of 92% in an adjoining state, the insurer must rebate 10% of the premiums for the first state and is not allowed to apply that rebate to losses experienced in the second state. The MLR cannot be averaged over time, either; separate calculations are made for each year.

Underwriters must take these requirements into account. However, because only rebates apply and plans cannot recover any losses, underwriters are particularly careful to not calculate rates that are too low because low rates will incur unrecoverable losses for an entire year.

General Approach to Premium Rate Determinations

A few concepts must be considered in terms of how premium rates (or premium-equivalent rates that will be discussed shortly) are calculated. There are some significant differences in how rates are calculated for the individual and small group markets versus for the mid-sized and large employer group market, but the following descriptions generally apply.

Underwriters calculate the actual premiums based on a combination of the actuarial projections, risk level assessments, various product design elements (such as the amount of cost sharing) or the type of product (such as a PPO, HMO, or POS plan), and the mix of adults and children in the group overall. The individual market is treated like a single group, as is the small group market, whereas each larger employer group is treated separately.

The calculation begins with the projected PMPM base cost developed by the actuaries to cover all benefits costs, before taking any other information into account. Benefits design and cost sharing for each product in each market segment or large group is now included, and the more required cost sharing, the lower the premium rates. This approach is applied for two reasons. The first and most obvious reason is that any amount paid by individuals in cost sharing is not paid by the plan. The second reason is that as the amount of cost sharing rises, people tend to use fewer medical services or are more willing to choose less costly alternatives as discussed in the *Utilization Management, Quality Management, and Accreditation* chapter.

The next element to be applied is the mix of adults and children. The monthly rate charged to a single individual is always higher than the PMPM base cost, and monthly family rates are lower than what they would be if each person were charged the same base amount. The reason for this difference is that the average medical costs for children are far lower than they are for adults. Premium rates are often calculated for different mixes of adults and children. For example, there may be different rates for single coverage versus family coverage, or different rates for different combinations of subscribers and dependents such as the following:

- Single coverage only
- Two adults only
- One adult plus one or more children
- Two adults plus one or more children

Premium Rating in the Individual and Small Group Markets

The ACA is very specific about the type of rates that may be charged in the individual and small group markets, requiring plans to use what is known as "community rating." Unless a state that is running its own health insurance exchange chooses to combine the individual and small group markets, those two segments have their own sets of community rates.

Community rating means that premium rates cannot be different for people or small groups that are sicker or healthier than average. Instead, the overall average forms the basis of the rates. The ACA allows for some exceptions to the requirement for using strict community rating, however. Plans may charge individuals premiums that are up to 1½ times higher than the community rate if they smoke. The ACA also allows rates to vary by age (or average age for small groups), but the highest age-based rates can be no more than 3 times higher than the lowest age-based rates.

Experience Rating in the Mid-sized and Large Group Markets

Experience rating may be used for fully insured employer groups with more than 100 employees. With this approach, the rates reflect the actual medical experience of an employer group. If the group has had high medical expenses in the past, it will be charged a higher premium than a group whose medical costs have been low. Underwriters calculating experience rates also try to differentiate between trends and just plain bad luck. For example, a group may have high expenses one year because of a single terrible auto accident (such cases are sometimes referred to as "shock claims"). Conversely, another group's high expenses may be due to factors that are not one-time events—for example, such might be the case with a group such as the National Association of Asbestos Smoking Snack Food Enthusiasts.* The first group's prior year's high expenses was owing to bad luck and does not indicate that its expenses will remain high, whereas the high expenses of the second group are likely to continue, at least for the few years they remain alive.

Determination of Premium Equivalent or Imputed Premium Rates for Self-Funded Employer Groups

Self-funded employer groups are not insured by a health plan, although they typically do purchase reinsurance. Nevertheless, even a self-insured employer needs to have "rates" calculated so that the employer knows the likely future cost of employee health benefits and can determine how much the employees must contribute through payroll deductions. These are not true premium rates, but rather are typically referred to as a "premium equivalent" or "imputed premiums." The calculations are often done by a payer contracted to administer the benefits plan, or they may be performed by an actuarial firm or the employer's benefits consultants. In either case, the methods used are similar to those described for experience-rated large groups.

ELIGIBILITY, ENROLLMENT, AND BILLING

Nothing can happen in any payer until it has members enrolled. The first step in that process is determining whether an individual is even eligible for coverage in the first place. The enrollment process itself simply means creating a record in the transactional processing system that an individual is eligible for benefits coverage, and linking that record to a specific benefits schedule and a specific network of contracted providers. It is the basis for many of the other transactions that take place in a payer organization, including claims processing, member services, and medical management. Enrollment is a dynamic process, with changes being made every day and seasonal surges in enrollment being associated with open enrollment periods in all markets. Even benefits plan changes for existing members require changes in the enrollment system.

Billing is how the payer itself is paid. For insured or at-risk commercial businesses, bills are generated for premiums. For self-funded accounts, bills are sent for administrative fees only. This is also a dynamic process, with billing, payment,

---

* Thankfully this is not a real group.

reconciliations, and changes occurring daily as well as significant changes during open enrollment periods.

Eligibility, enrollment, and billing differ for commercial group coverage, commercial individual coverage, Medicare Advantage, and managed Medicaid plans. The ACA also created a new avenue for enrollment and billing through the health insurance exchanges for individuals and small employer groups, although at the time of this text's publication this capability was not yet functional.

Eligibility for Coverage in the Commercial Market

Eligibility in the commercial market may be thought of as comprising three categories:

- Eligibility for coverage through an employer-sponsored group benefits plan
- Eligibility for individual coverage
- Eligibility for coverage based on "life events" or "qualified life events" that can affect both individual and employer group eligibility

Eligibility for Coverage Through an Employer-Sponsored Group Benefits Plan

Employers are not compelled to offer group health benefits, so employment by itself does not necessarily mean an employee will have health insurance. However, the ACA created penalties for employers with more than 25 employees if they do not offer coverage, although these penalty costs are generally lower than are coverage costs. The ACA also created tax incentives for employers with fewer than 25 employees if they offer coverage. In any case, most large employers offer health benefits coverage to their employees, and many smaller employers offer coverage as well. If an employer does offer this benefit, coverage cannot discriminate between people based on such factors as income, position in the company, or health status.

Nothing compels an employee to take up the employer-offered coverage, although the ACA does provide for individual penalties, as discussed earlier in the text. Sometimes employees may not accept coverage through their employer because they are covered under a working spouse's health plan.

In the large group market, employers typically have an annual open enrollment period if they offer more than one plan, which large employer groups almost always do. The annual open enrollment period is the only time when employees can change plans except in the case of life events (sometimes called qualified life events). New employees must enroll within a specific time period after coming on board, typically 30 days. In some cases, a waiting period applies before a new employee is eligible to join the employer's plan, but the ACA limits any waiting period to no more than 90 days.

In the small group market, small groups are eligible to purchase coverage through the SHOP exchange or through guaranteed issue benefits plans during the same open enrollment period in the fall of each year that applies to the individual market.

Eligibility for Individual Coverage

Eligibility for individual coverage applies to coverage for single individuals as well as coverage for single families, not including coverage through Medicare or Medicaid. Individuals who do not have access to coverage from other sources may obtain coverage through the health insurance exchanges operating in their states. They must apply for this coverage during the annual open enrollment period, which takes place in the fall of the year before that coverage goes into effect. States may opt to have longer or more open enrollment periods, but cannot have a shorter enrollment period. Individuals must also pay their premiums before coverage goes into effect.

Eligibility for Coverage Based on Life Events or Qualified Events

Eligibility may be affected by changes that occur in an individual's life, which is why they are referred to as "life events"; because they qualify an individual for coverage, they also may be called "qualified events" or "qualified life events." Life events are directly affected by several federal laws including the Consolidated Omnibus Budget Reconciliation Act (COBRA), the federal Employee Retirement Income Security Act (ERISA), HIPAA, and the ACA. State laws and regulations can also affect eligibility and may provide greater protections than federal laws, but not less.

When a life event occurs, an individual or that individual's dependents qualify for coverage as long as they act within a defined time period, usually 60 days from the event. If they fail to do so, then they lose eligibility for coverage outside of the normal open enrollment period. These events allow for periods of eligibility involving employer-based coverage as well as coverage extensions. Table 6–2 provides examples of life events and their associated coverage eligibility options.

Table 6–2   Life Events and Eligibility Options

Life Event	Coverage Eligibility Options
The following apply in any situation.	
• Marriage • Birth or adoption of a child	• Extension of existing coverage to new dependent • Typically must apply within 30 days of the event
• Job change	• Eligible for coverage through new employer • Typically must apply within 30 days of employment • May obtain coverage through the health insurance exchange if the new employer does not offer coverage
• Coverage loss due to job loss • Coverage loss due to reduction in	• Eligible for coverage extension under COBRA • Must pay full cost and apply within 60 days of the event • Eligibility for COBRA extension lasts for only 18 months • May obtain coverage through the health insurance exchange immediately, or else upon loss of COBRA coverage
• of a	• Eligible for coverage extension under COBRA on the basis of the spouse's coverage • Must pay full cost and apply within 60 days of the event • COBRA coverage extension lasts up to 36 months

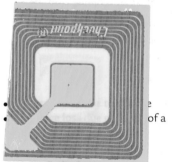

The following only apply to coverage obtained through a health insurance exchange. In all cases, an individual must apply for new coverage or coverage change within 60 days of the event.

• Change geographic location	• Obtain new coverage through the health insurance exchange at the new location
• Change in citizenship status	• New citizens may apply for coverage • May be eligible for a premium subsidy
• Change in income level	• May be eligible for higher, lower, or loss of premium subsidy • May be eligible for Medicaid coverage, or changing from Medicaid to subsidized commercial coverage
• Experience government error	• May reapply for coverage

Extension of Coverage or Special Enrollment Eligibility

In addition to allowing employees to change their coverage in their group plan, life events change eligibility for coverage through two other means: an extension of existing coverage or the ability to obtain coverage through an insurance exchange or through Medicaid.

Under COBRA, people who lose their employer-based group coverage due to a life event are usually able to extend that coverage for up to 18 months (or 36 months in some cases). The specific rights and requirements are see in Table 6–2. The individual must pay the full premium plus 2%, and any failure to pay results in loss of coverage and loss of eligibility for COBRA continuation. Once eligibility for coverage under COBRA runs out, coverage may be extended under HIPAA—although there is no longer any need for that option.

Eligibility for coverage through the health insurance exchange is normally limited to the open enrollment period. Coverage lost as the result of a life event, however, qualifies an individual for coverage through the exchange under a special enrollment period that has much the same requirements as other life event changes listed in Table 6–2. In most cases, an extension of employer-based coverage under COBRA is less costly than similar benefits obtained through the exchange, but lower-cost plans with greater cost sharing or subsidized coverage offered through the exchange may be preferable for some individuals. For those who elect the COBRA extension, the expiration of that coverage extension is itself a life event that qualifies an individual for coverage through the exchange.

Lastly, loss of coverage based on a life event may qualify an individual for coverage under Medicaid or a subsidized premium for commercial coverage through an exchange, based on the individual's expected income level.

Enrollment

Enrollment is the process of entering or changing enrollment data and information for each subscriber or member in the plan's processing system. One way or another, most of the payer's core processes and systems depend on accurate enrollment data.

Provider Verification of Patient's Eligibility for Coverage

Before discussing enrollment further, it is appropriate to point out that the payer is not the only organization that depends on accurate enrollment data. Providers depend on such data as well—not just for one payer, but for all the payers covering any patients who receive care from the provider. The same may be said for other companies or organizations that are involved in managing benefits; for example, pharmacy benefits managers rely on accurate enrollment data for managing the drug benefit.

HMOs that pay any or all providers through capitation use enrollment data to calculate capitation payments as well as to inform capitated providers which members are attributed to them. The most common use of enrollment and eligibility data by providers is simply verifying that a patient is covered at the time of service. For instance, a hospital will want to confirm that a patient is covered under a health plan so that it can properly bill for its services. If it is not possible for the hospital to verify eligibility (or if the patient is using an ID card for coverage that has lapsed), the facility will make other payment arrangements with the patient.

Provider eligibility verification is increasingly handled through automated self-service means. Examples of these types of self-service include secure lookup functions via the Internet, secure direct communications between the payer's and provider's respective IT systems, interactive voice response via the telephone, and use of swipe-card or radio frequency identification (RFID) technology (working with established credit card issuers) at the time of service.

Sources of Enrollment Data

Enrollment in employer-based plans begins with the employer. In most cases, the employer is responsible for providing the payer with accurate and timely data on the employees and dependents covered under its plan as well as identifying those individuals who are no longer covered. This includes new employees as well as those employees who gain, extend, or lose coverage through life events. The enrollment information may be transmitted through paper forms, computer tape cassettes or optical media, or batched electronic transmissions, or input directly by the employer into the payer's system. In some cases, employees apply or make changes through a dedicated web portal.

The public insurance exchanges are supposed to be able to handle enrollment for individuals who buy health insurance through the exchanges. This is particularly important for individuals receiving premium subsidies because they can qualify for those only by going through an exchange. At the time of publication, they were able to handle enrollment but were not yet able to provide disenrollment information (to change plans, an individual must not only enroll in one plan but must also disenroll from his or her prior plan). The same process is to apply to coverage obtained by small employers through the SHOP exchange, but as of this text's publication, both the availability of coverage through the SHOP exchange and the transmission of enrollment data have been inconsistent.

Enrollment in individual coverage may also occur through direct interaction with an insurer or an HMO, in which case the data and information come through the plan's website or through data entered on a paper form.

Enrollment Errors

Enrollment problems and errors can affect operations elsewhere in the payer organization. Enrollment errors can be caused by both internal and external factors. Errors add to administrative costs because resolving them often takes manual work. Errors in enrollment can result in payment of claims for someone who is no longer covered or denial of payment for someone who is covered, incorrect capitation payments, more calls to member services from angry members, and so forth.

Internal errors in enrollment are often the result of enrollment backlogs that occur during heavy enrollment periods, particularly from the fall through the end of January, when the largest number of open enrollment periods take place. In addition, they result from paper enrollment forms being incorrectly read by the optical recognition system and not corrected manually. A related error can occur when new members enroll through self-service portals and enter incorrect information.

Errors in enrollment can occur for a variety of external reasons as well. The insurance exchanges are one source of potential errors, as occurred in their initial rollout in late 2013. While their performance has steadily improved, they are still building and refining their capabilities, which also means the need to continue to reduce errors.

In the group market, an employer may transmit inaccurate or late data about who has been hired or is no longer employed, or which employees changed from one plan option to another. Larger employer groups may also use more than one database for human resources, and those database do not always match up accurately.

In both the group and individual markets, employees or individual members may wait until the last moment to add or change coverage based on a "life event." Also, both employers and individuals typically have a "grace period," meaning that if their payments are past due but are ultimately paid in full within a defined period of time, coverage will be reinstated.

Billing

For both insured and self-funded accounts, payment is made before the coverage period begins. Coverage ends if payments are not received, although "grace periods" for reinstatement are typically required. Chronic late payment may be a cause for termination, however. It is a central concept in any type of insurance that you cannot purchase coverage for something that has already occurred, although the ACA now allows it under its guaranteed issue provision, which prohibits insurers from refusing to issue coverage based on preexisting conditions. Nevertheless, the concept of prepayment still applies for continued coverage.

Payers bill employers for premiums or administrative fees based on enrolled members. For individual coverage, they send bills directly to the individual policy holders, and they may require individuals to allow for direct billing of a checking or credit card account. The health insurance exchanges are also supposed to facilitate billing, but that task currently remains the responsibility of the payers participating in the exchanges. As would be expected, billing errors often mirror enrollment errors.

CLAIMS AND BENEFITS ADMINISTRATION

The claims department is responsible for ensuring that the network providers are paid directly for the medical goods and services they provide to members, and that members who have paid providers out-of-pocket receive the reimbursement to which they are entitled. Even when providers are capitated, the claims department typically still processes encounters, usually through claims submitted by capitated providers that are counted for purposes of data capture only (these are often called "null" claims). The complexity of medical claims and benefits administration is almost universally underestimated by those not thoroughly familiar with health plan operations. Moreover, it is affected by almost every other function in a payer organization. In this section we will take a very high-level look at some of the basic elements or functions of the claims and benefits administration process.

Claims Capture

The first function performed by the claims department is to capture the claim, which means entering a received claim into the claims processing system. All claims are accounted for, either manually or electronically and regardless of how they are received, and assigned unique identifiers. Without logging and entry, claims would be impossible to track.

Claims may come in from a variety of sources, but most commonly arrive through HIPAA-standardized electronic submissions. Claims may also arrive through the U.S. mail, fax, secure e-mail, electronic imaging, and self-entry via the web. They usually come directly from the providers, but when a member receives care from a nonparticipating provider and pays for that care at the time of service, the subscriber (the member who has the coverage, regardless of whether the patient was the member or one of the member's dependents) typically will submit the claim.

Claims Screening

Captured claims are first screened to ensure that they contain the necessary data and information. If they do not, they are rejected and returned to the submitter. Claims that contain all required data are called "clean claims" and are usually processed quickly. Claims that are missing some required data elements or that have obviously incorrect data—for example, not enough digits in the NPI—are not considered clean and are rejected.

Conversion into a Standardized Electronic Record

Claims are converted into electronic records within the payer's processing system. HIPAA-compliant electronic claims are converted almost immediately. Paper or other nonelectronic types of claims are scanned into an image file, then converted by using optical recognition software. Images of any claims that cannot be quickly and easily converted are marked for manual entry. Even a sample of those that are successfully converted may be manually reviewed for quality management purposes.

Basic Benefits Administration

After capturing and converting the claim, the claims system must then go through a series of steps before it either goes through final adjudication (basic benefits administration), or it proceeds on to additional steps before being adjudicated. For clean claims, basic benefits administration is almost always auto-adjudicated, meaning the processing is fully automated with no human intervention.

Approximately 80% of all claims are auto-adjudicated on their first pass through the claims system. The rate is somewhat higher for claims originally received electronically, and somewhat lower for paper claims. The reason for this difference is that even after they pass initial screening and are converted to an electronic format, paper claims are more likely to contain other types of errors that do not show up until they are actually processed.

Determining Coverage

One of the first steps in the process is to check the enrollment system to see if the member was even covered at the time he or she received medical care. If the member is or was eligible, the claim proceeds to the next step. If the member is not or was not eligible for coverage on the date of service, the claim is denied at that point and the member and provider are so notified.

If the member is or was covered at the time of service, the claims system is then responsible for determining which level of benefits to apply. For example, the coverage levels typically differ in POS plans and PPOs for elective in-network care versus out-of-network care. Benefit plan designs also change over time and members may change the type of plan in which they are enrolled, so the system must determine exactly which coverage was in effect on the date of service. For example, the copayment for a visit to a specialist may have been $30 in December but increased to $40 in January.

The claims system must also determine whether the member has fully or partially met his or her deductible. If not, the claims system applies the appropriate amount against the deductible. The same concept applies to the maximum out-of-pocket costs that an individual or family must pay each year, which the claims system must track because cost sharing stops once that maximum is reached.

The system must then determine if a medical good or service requires authorization or precertification. If so, it looks for a record that such preapproval was obtained. If there is no such record, the claims system must determine if the service was elective or an emergency: Emergency services are covered at the in-network level, whereas there is less coverage, or no coverage in some cases, for non-authorized elective services; this can be a difficult determination to program into a claims system, some of these claims may instead be pended to obtain additional information.

Pricing Claims Payments

Once a claim is determined to be covered to any extent, the claims system must determine the correct amount to pay (or apply against cost sharing) for each submitted claim, based on its diagnostic and procedure codes. Payment terms and amounts often vary between different types of products (e.g., HMO and PPO products offered by the same payer), and payment amounts may change each year for the same type of product. Thus, in addition to coverage levels, payment amounts must account for terms and payment schedules that were in place for the appropriate network and the appropriate product at the time the covered service was provided.

Many providers of all types "unbundle" their claims, meaning they include separate charges under separate billing codes for services that are supposed to be paid through one payment. For example, an outpatient facility will often include separate charges for gauze dressings, sutures, and other supplies, and a hospital with employed physicians may tack on a "facility fee" for routine office visits, something that the basic office visit fee is supposed to include. The system must determine when unbundled charges are inappropriate and not payable, and when they must be covered. This is sometimes a difficult exercise, especially in the case of noncontracted providers who can and do charge what they want.

Application of Routine Medical Payment Policies

Routine medical payment policies are rules for using clinical information to make commonplace claims payment determinations. For example, one common medical policy is to pay an assistant surgeon no more than 50% of the fee that the primary surgeon receives. Another common policy is to pay for only one abdominal surgical procedure even if a surgeon bills for multiple procedures. Most routine medical policies are fully integrated into the basic claims adjudication system and are applied on an automated basis at the time that the claim is actually adjudicated.

Management of Pended Claims and Adjustments

A claim may be pended by the claims system, which means that it is neither paid nor denied, but rather put on hold so further information can be obtained. When a claim is pended, the claims department must have a system in place to make sure that the claim does not wind up in limbo. The department needs to track each pended claim and make sure that action ultimately is taken on those claims, usually within a defined time period.

A claim might be pended for any number of reasons. For example, there may be a diagnosis–procedure mismatch, which means just what it sounds like. In such a discrepancy, claims systems typically automatically generate a notice to a contracted provider about the problem and request the claim be resubmitted with the correct codes or additional information. The system may do the same for claims from noncontracted providers, or it may not pend the claim, but deny it and notify the member why it was denied. Claims that require manual review and determination based on medical necessity are also first pended before being forwarded to the appropriate clinical personnel in the plan.

Paid claims may sometimes be reopened for adjustments. This occurs when a claim is processed but then an error is corrected or additional information is provided, resulting in a change to the coverage and/or payment amount. Adjustments may also occur after a member successfully appeals a benefits coverage denial.

Finally, a claim may be pended or even reopened to determine whether another party is responsible for paying all or part of the claim, which is the next thing we will look at.

Coordination of Benefits, Other Party Liability, and Subrogation

There are three common situations in which another party has primary responsibility for payment of all or part of a medical claim. It is the responsibility of the claims department to identify and handle these situations so that the plan does not pay when another organization is obligated to pay first.

Coordination of Benefits

The most common situation in which another party has responsibility for payment of a claim is called coordination of benefits (COB). This happens when an individual is covered by two or more health plans, such as when two working parents each and have employment-related health benefits. If both parents elected family coverage, then their children are covered by both benefits plans. COB is the process for determining which parent's plan pays first. There are many other situations in which COB is involved, and payers follow a complex set of rules in determining which health plan has primary payment responsibility and which one is secondary. Benefits from both policies may also be available under certain circumstances.

Other Party Liability

Other party liability (OPL) means that some other type of insurance may be liable for all or part of the healthcare costs incurred, such as automobile insurance or worker's compensation. When the other coverage has benefit maximums or limitations, the health benefits plan may then become responsible once the other insurance no longer covers costs.*

Subrogation

Subrogation refers to the right of the payer to recover any legal settlement or award dollars associated with healthcare costs if a member was harmed by a third party. For example, if a legal settlement or award is calculated based on a combination of lost income, medical costs, and pain and suffering, the payer can sue to recover that portion of the award that was based on medical costs that the plan has already paid. Subrogation is required in some states, but is illegal in others.

---

* Technically this is a form of COB; indeed, some sources refer to both COB and OPL as one or the other. But the more common usage, however, separates the two.

Management of Claims Inventory

Claims inventory refers to the number of claims that have been received but not yet processed. Claims are rarely processed immediately upon delivery, and a typical inventory level is somewhere between 7 and 14 days' worth of claims, though that can vary quite a bit. Plans typically establish a policy regarding inventory levels: If the length of time it takes for routine processing exceeds that level, a claims backlog is said to exist. Claims that have been pended do not count as part of the backlog. Many states, as well as large employers, also have standards for how quickly a clean claim must be paid, generally referred to as "timely payment."

A backlog can arise if claims productivity drops or if too many errors occur at any of the various places where the claims system depends on accurate data. Backlogs can generate problems throughout the plan. For example, providers and members will become unhappy, leading to more work for the member services and network management departments. Claims backlogs are associated with an increase in processing errors as the claims department tries to dig its way out, and managing errors in coverage and payment requires costly manual interventions. In addition, such backlogs may result in providers submitting duplicate claims in the belief that the original claims were lost, adding to the volume of claims and worsening the backlog, and increasing the number of payment errors.

Finally, a claims backlog reduces the accuracy of calculating reserves, or the amount of money that must be available to pay the claims that will eventually be processed. This is can lead to a very dangerous condition, as we will see later in the chapter.

Payment and Explanation of Benefits Statements

Final adjudication usually does not mean instant payments. Once a claim has been approved and finalized, it is routed to the accounts payable function in the system, which has its processes that take a certain amount of time to complete. How the claim is paid depends on who is receiving the money and which, if any, agreements are in place. Most payments to network providers are through EFT or by mail. The provider is also sent a notification of payment or remittance advice, providing relevant information about how the claim was processed and the amount(s) paid.

When a member receives elective care from a noncontracted provider, the member is sent a paper check for the amount covered, and he or she is responsible for paying the provider. Some noncontracted providers send in the claim to the payer after asking the patient to sign an "assignment of benefits" form, in which the provider and the patient ask the payer to send the check directly to the provider rather than to the subscriber. Most payers refuse to assign benefits to a nonparticipating provider, because direct payment is one of the benefits of participation for a provider. Some states, however, require plans to direct payments to nonparticipating providers if the member signed the form.

Payers also send an explanation of benefits (EOB) statement to the subscriber (even if a dependent received the care) that describes what was covered (or not), which adjustments were made and why, how much the plan paid, and how much the subscriber may need to pay. The EOB also informs the subscriber of the right to appeal coverage denials and explains how to do so.

Archiving

The final step in the claims management process entails storing all the information about each claim, from its initial submission up through final adjudication and any postprocessing adjustments. These records are important in cases of appeals and grievances for reconciling self-funded accounts, for audits, for analysis, or in the event of a lawsuit. The data and information are stored electronically, including electronic images of paper documents (the actual paper documents are stored separately). How long records are stored is usually dictated by any applicable laws or regulations limiting the length of time that they may be audited or the subject of a lawsuit. This span can vary but typically ranges from 7 to 10 years.

MEMBER SERVICES

Member services acts as the interface between members and a payer. In other words, when an individual member has a problem or needs assistance, the member services department helps the member handle it. Interactions between members and member services may occur on the telephone; via secure e-mail; through secure, live web-enabled chat; by correspondence sent via U.S. mail (or any other document delivery service); or face to face in a customer service center. The member services department has the following responsibilities, among others:

- Providing information to members
- Assisting members with problems or complaints
- Undertaking proactive member outreach
- Monitoring member satisfaction and conducting member surveys
- Managing the appeals and grievances process

Providing Information

A health plan must regularly communicate with its members. Such communication begins before enrollment, when the plan provides information through the SBC and other marketing materials, and it continues for as long as the member is covered (and often beyond that, too). Examples of routine types of communications include keeping members informed about any significant changes in the network, ways to obtain assistance, help with understanding benefits, and so forth. Member services may also help coordinate or conduct informational sessions about particular topics.

Some types of communications are required by law or regulation. Examples include the SBC and providing or making the EOC available upon request, extension of coverage rights, privacy and confidentiality rights, and denial of coverage appeal and grievance rights (which are also communicated to members in the SBC, the EOC, and the EOB).

Assisting Members with Problems or Complaints

Member problems can range from something as simple as an incorrect identification card to something as complex as a mishandled claim for medical expenses. HMOs and POS plans have a special interest in helping members select physicians and straightening out problems with authorization and other unique aspects of managed care.

Complaints can vary widely as well, but share one thing in common: They are informal. Formal complaints take the form of grievances or appeals of coverage denials. A complaint can progress to a formal grievance or appeal, but most do not. Complaints often focus on coverage or payment policies and deal with issues such as an error in enrollment or claims processing, misspelled names, and so forth. Many are resolved quickly, but some take more time. This aspect of member services can be one of the most stressful roles in a payer organization, so member services representatives undergo specific training to help them manage this role in a professional manner. Also, more complex complaints or particularly upset members are often referred to the more experienced member services representatives.

Proactive Member Outreach

Proactively reaching out to members can have a positive impact on member satisfaction and on the operations of the payer. For instance, a welcoming call to new members can help them understand how the payer operates, help with physician selection in an HMO, answer any questions they have, and take care of any issues that may have already arisen. Contacting members who have not extensively used the payer's services is one way to make sure that they are satisfied with their membership. Outreach by member services representatives is costly, however. Recently, under the pressure of the ACA's MLR limits, many plans have adopted automated electronic systems that encourage members to use the plan's self-service resources rather than contact the member services representatives.

Monitoring Member Satisfaction and Conducting Member Surveys

A payer must continually gauge the level of member satisfaction. Periodic surveys can allow the payer to discover how members view their health plans and pick up on trends at an early stage. A survey may contain general questions intended to expose the overall level of satisfaction with the payer, or it may contain narrow questions targeted at specific issues, such as the adequacy of the provider network. In some cases, formal member satisfaction surveys are required, such as the Consumer Assessment of Healthcare Providers and Systems (CAHPS) for Medicare or Medicaid managed care plans. Further, states and some accreditation programs require payers to conduct broad member satisfaction surveys, including CAHPS, and act on the results.

Managing the Appeals and Grievances Process

Appeals and grievances are two different types of formal notifications by members that require formal responses from health plans. An appeal is a formal request for another review of a denial of coverage. A grievance is a formal complaint about anything other than a coverage denial, such as a formal complaint about a quality of care issue or about an interaction between the member and the plan. In both cases, a written response is required in a timely manner, but the process for handling each type of complaint differs.

Members are informed of their appeal rights on the SBC, on the EOC, and on all EOB statements. In addition to specifying what those rights are, those documents provide the information necessary for members to begin the appeals process and point members to resources where they can find more information. Note that appeals and grievances apply only to members, not to providers, although providers frequently become involved in the process on behalf of their patients.

Managing the appeals and grievances process is typically the responsibility of the member services department. The volume of formal appeals and grievances is very low compared to all interactions between plans and members, but its importance is very high. Managing this process is a support function that requires timely correspondence between involved parties, obtaining information, maintaining records, and keeping the process on track.

Appeals of Denials of Coverage

Denials of coverage that are appealed are often a result of denial determinations based on medical necessity, although consumers have the right to appeal other types of coverage denials, too. A denial of benefits coverage can apply to any point where coverage determinations are made, ranging from precertification denials for care not yet provided, to denials of coverage after the care has been provided. An appeal of a coverage denial may begin with an informal review request. If the dispute is resolved at that point, it does not become a formal appeal. If an informal review does not resolve the issue, then the member has the right to proceed to a formal process. An appeal can also begin with the formal process.

Formal appeal rights include an internal review of the coverage denial by health plan professionals not involved in the initial decision, and the right to request an external review by impartial professionals. Appeal rights are governed by the ACA as well as ERISA for self-funded benefits plans. Most states also have laws providing appeal rights to individuals covered through insured plans. State laws and regulations can be more stringent than what is required under the ACA, but not less; if a state does have less stringent laws, then the federal government will handle the process as needed.

During the appeal process, the plan's documented coverage policies and evidence of coverage document, as well as its definition(s) of medical necessity in the EOC document, are very important for all reviewers to understand. Additional documentation that is sent in by either the member or the member's physician(s), notes by UM nurses or member services representatives, or other relevant information must be available as well. Only the relevant portions of any records, including a member's medical records, are required, however.

The main elements of the appeals processes are summarized in Table 6–3 for internal reviews, and in Table 6–4 for external reviews.

Table 6–3 Main Elements of the Internal Review Process for Appeals of Coverage Denials

- A member must file the appeal within 180 days of being notified of the denial.
- If the member requests it, the plan must provide the member with copies of documents that are relevant to the claim, and identify any medical experts involved in the review.
- The member and/or the member's physician or other provider may submit additional information if they wish.
- The appeal must be reviewed by someone new who looks at all of the information submitted and consults with qualified medical professionals if a medical judgment is involved.
  - This reviewer cannot have been involved with the initial decision or be a subordinate of the person who made the initial decision.
  - The reviewer must give no consideration to the initial decision.

- After an appeal request is received, it must be reviewed within defined time periods:
  - If the appeal is urgent (based on the medical needs of the member), it must be reviewed within 72 hours.
  - Preauthorization appeals must be reviewed within 30 days.
  - Appeals for coverage after a service has already been provided must be reviewed within 60 days.
- If the reviewer overturns the denial, the decision is binding on the plan, but the member can still request an external review.
- An individual may obtain an independent external review of a denied appeal, and must be allowed to file for it no less than 4 months following notification of the upheld denial.

Summarized by author based on 26 CFR Parts 54 and 602, 29 CFR Part 2590, and 45 CFR Part 147 in the Federal Register, Vol. 75, No. 141.

Grievances

A grievance is a formal complaint, demanding resolution or a formal response. It may come directly to the payer, but more often is submitted through a regulatory agency such as a state insurance department or CMS. If the member belongs to a self-funded benefits plan, the grievance will usually come from or through the employer. Examples of grievances include a formal letter to the insurance commissioner charging an insurer with deceptive sales and marketing practices, or a Medicare beneficiary's letter to CMS complaining about poor service. In each case, the agency requires a response from the plan and, if it deems this step to be necessary, may investigate further. A pattern of grievances or particularly egregious acts may lead to fines, restrictions on operations or sales, revocation of licensure, or even disbarment from the program.

Table 6–4 Main Elements of the External Review Process for Appeals of Coverage Denials

- An individual must request an external review within 120 days of being notified that the denial was upheld by the internal reviewer(s).
- The cost to the member for an external review request cannot exceed $25.
- External reviews must be conducted by an accredited independent review organization (IRO) selected on a random basis by the state or the federal government.
- Reviews will be conducted by clinical personnel with the appropriate training and education relevant to the type of coverage denial.
- The plan must provide relevant documentation to the reviewer within 5 days of notifying the IRO. It must include material related to any internal review, but only as information, and the reviewer must give no consideration to the initial decision.

- The member may provide additional information and/or the reviewer may request additional information.
- If the reviewer concludes that the request is not eligible for external review, the reviewer will notify the parties; otherwise, the review will proceed.
- After an external review request is received, the IRO review must be completed within defined time periods:
  - An expedited external review for an urgent case must be decided within 72 hours.
  - A standard external review must be completed within 45 days.
- The decision by the IRO is binding on both the plan and on the member.

Summarized by author based on 26 CFR Parts 54 and 602, 29 CFR Part 2590, and 45 CFR Part 147 in the Federal Register, Vol. 75, No. 141.

FINANCIAL MANAGEMENT

The finance department is responsible for managing the payer's money. It has four main areas of responsibility:

- Operational finance
- Budgeting
- The treasury function
- Reporting

Three Important Accounting Concepts

Accounting is well beyond the scope of this text, but three important accounting concepts should be addressed before briefly describing the areas of responsibility.

Accrual Accounting

There are two ways to approach financial accounting: cash accounting and accrual accounting. This distinction is not unique to the insurance industry, and most companies other than very small ones use accrual accounting. Cash accounting means that all of the financial numbers are based on the actual movement of cash, as currency, deposits, bill payments, and so forth. This method is what most of us use to manage our personal finances. It is not suitable for financial management of a large company, however, and is especially unsuitable for a payer.

Accrual accounting means accounting not only for cash, but also for money that will be received and will be paid.* It includes known amounts, such as the payroll or payments that will be received, as well as estimates of amounts not yet known. For a health insurer or HMO, the most important of these estimates is how much will be needed to pay claims on its insured business, even if the payer does not actually know what those claims will be. Those estimates are used to accrue money (meaning, in this case, put money aside) as a reserve to be used to pay the claims as they come in. We will revisit this topic shortly when we look at calculating claims and reserves for incurred but not reported claims.

Statutory Accounting and Statutory Net Worth /Reserves/Surplus

Almost all companies use Generally Accepted Accounting Principles (GAAP)—a set of rules and definitions that provide for uniform financial reporting—in their accounting practices. Payers use GAAP as well, but they must also use another form of accounting, albeit only for their insured business: Statutory Accounting Principles (SAP). SAP is used by regulators as part of their financial oversight responsibilities, which accounts for the "S" in SAP. GAAP and SAP differ most importantly in how they define what counts as an asset. Specifically, many assets under GAAP have limited (or no) value under SAP.

A company's net worth is made up of its assets minus its liabilities. SAP accounting rules directly affect how *statutory* net worth is calculated by reducing the amount that can be considered an asset (in comparison to GAAP), without reducing the liabilities. Said another way, assets under SAP rules are the only

---

* Technically it means measuring the performance and position of a company by recognizing economic events regardless of when cash transactions take place, in order to better understand the company's financial state.

assets a payer may use to calculate its statutory net worth for purposes of meeting state laws and regulations regarding net worth requirements.

Statutory net worth, sometimes called statutory reserves or statutory surplus, is an asset. It is defined by state insurance laws and regulations, and it comprises the amount of cash or readily available money, meaning cash or liquid investments that are considered "cash-equivalent," that a plan is required to have on hand at all times to continue paying claims for a defined period of time even if all revenue stops. In other words, if the payer stopped doing business and stopped collecting premiums, how much cash is on hand and how much cash could be raised *immediately* by disposing of the payer's assets in order to continue to pay claims.

Under SAP, only cash and assets that are easily and quickly convertible to cash, such as short-term notes or liquid investments, may be considered assets. Unlike GAAP, SAP places a limit on how much value may be placed on nonliquid assets such as computers, buildings, nonconvertible long-term investments, and so forth, limiting this value to no more than 5% of total assets.*

Statutory net worth is recorded as an asset (or assets) on the payer's books, but a payer cannot use it, or at least a portion of it, for anything because the payer must be able to meet the statutory net worth requirements at all times. The amount of cash or cash-equivalent money that a plan must have on hand to meet its minimum statutory net worth requirement is established by the state, but the minimum is usually enough to continue to pay claims for at least 3 months. States typically expect payers to have much more than that amount available, though, and regulators will usually take action if the amount begins to approach the minimum.

The minimum statutory net worth requirement is based on the amount of financial risk the plan has, meaning its insured business, based how much the plan pays out each month in medical claims on its insured business as well as some other liabilities. It ignores self-funded business because the payer is not at risk for payment of those claims. This also applies when an HMO has transferred some risk to the providers through capitation, although capitation only reduces but does not eliminate the HMO's financial risk for capitated medical services. How much the statutory net worth is affected by self-funded business and provider risk sharing is known as "risk-based capital" (RBC) and it is determined by specific accounting rules and definitions.

---

*Technically, a binding guarantee agreement with a bank that says the bank will provide a certain amount of cash if the payer needs it can also be counted as an asset.

Claims Reserves and Incurred But Not Reported Claims Reserves

Claims reserves, unlike statutory reserves (if a plan uses that term), are a liability, not an asset. That is because the claims reserves are what the payer estimates will actually be used in the normal course of business to pay claims for any given period of time. Claims reserves are made up of two parts: (1) the amount of money in known claims and (2) the amount of money the plan estimates will be needed to pay claims that have been incurred but not reported (IBNR). This is a critical concept: If a plan determines its total claims liabilities by counting only claims that it has paid or that are in its system, then it will not set aside enough money to pay all of the claims that have yet to come in. While premium payments come in right away, claims arrive much later. Failing to appreciate and account for this difference in timing has been the demise of many smaller health plans in the past as well as some plans that had rapid growth.

Each month's claims reserves are calculated, reserved for, and tracked separately. As claims for medical care provided in that same month come in and are paid, the reserves for that month are reduced by the amount paid out. Claims can take a long time to straggle in, so most payers calculated reserve estimates that last for 18 to 24 months, with anticipated claims payments steadily dropping off over that time. Timely filing terms in provider contracts help in this regard, but have no effect on claims from noncontracted providers.

The estimated part of the claims reserve—the IBNR—is more than an educated guess. It is calculated on a monthly basis using a combination of data, including enrollment data for insured business, benefits levels and cost-sharing data, actual versus expected volume of claims received that month, actual versus expected claims inventory, seasonal and regional utilization trends, pricing trends, historical trends, and more. By tracking each month separately, these data are more effectively used and the plan can monitor how accurate its IBNR calculations are and make adjustments to its reserves as needed.

Operational Finance

Operational finance refers to the day-to-day functions of the finance department. The most important of these functions is tracking all money that comes in and goes out. Broadly speaking, the following categories are tracked:

- Revenues, including premiums for insured business, administrative fees for self-funded business, and other revenues (e.g., from subsidiaries)
- Costs, including medical costs (both paid and estimated) for its insured business, administrative costs, and other fees and costs

- Surplus and reserves
- The bottom line, before and after taxes

Treasury

The treasury function refers to managing cash and short-term investments. It may also include managing long-term investments, but not always. Payers generally have a lot of cash on hand, mostly for both operational claims reserves and for statutory reserves, but also because premiums and fees are paid before the fact, whereas claims and services occur after those payments have been received. Managing such a large amount of cash to keep it safe and, when possible, earn some investment income is an important element in managing finances overall.

Budgeting

All organizations require a budget to properly manage their operations, and payer organizations are no different. What makes budgeting for a payer unique is the need to create one budget for medical expenses and a separate budget for operational expenses. Further, different financial tools and techniques are used to create the two budgets. Budgeting is essential, for it is only through this process that the payer can test assumptions about how much to charge in premiums, how much it can or cannot spend on administration, and how much it can afford to invest in administrative improvements.

Reporting

Reporting is discussed separately from budgeting because the finance department must do several types of reporting, though some payers have a separate department for report filing. Specifically, the finance department is usually responsible for creating reports for each employer, state insurance departments, state health departments (in some states), the U.S. Department of Health and Human Services, the U.S. Department of the Treasury and the Internal Revenue Service, the U.S. Securities and Exchange Commission (if it is publicly traded), the U.S. Department of Labor, CMS (if it has a Medicare plan), and a state's Medicaid agency (if the plan participates in that program). An independent form of reporting known as internal auditing frequently resides in the finance department as well; it is responsible for ensuring that all areas of the payer are both reporting accurate numbers and operating according to the company's policies and guidelines.

All of these reports use special types of forms, though state financial filings use forms called "blanks." In some cases, if the payer is based in a different state, a state insurance department may accept the results that have been reported to the insurance department in the payer's home state. Most financial reports are submitted quarterly as well as annually, and some (though not all) reports use both SAP and GAAP.

Finally, the finance department is responsible for maintaining the organization's financial records in such a manner as to be considered acceptable to an independent external auditor. For-profit plans must have their annual statements certified by an accredited auditing firm, and the chief executive officer must attest to the accuracy of the financial statements.

CONCLUSION

Administrative activities make up most of what an MCO does from day to day, even though it represents only 15% to 20% of the total amount of dollars paid out in medical claims. Typical administrative functions include enrolling members; checking and verifying eligibility for coverage; billing groups and individuals for premiums or administrative fees; managing authorizations and other aspects of medical management; managing benefits and claims; helping members resolve problems; managing the complaints, appeals, and grievances processes; managing operational finances and maintaining adequate reserves; filing a variety of state and federal reports; and continually developing and managing the IT systems necessary to perform all of these tasks and more.

CHAPTER 7

Medicare and Medicaid

LEARNING OBJECTIVES

- Understand the basic issues involved with Medicare Advantage and managed Medicaid plans
- Explain the difference between plans serving the typical Medicare and/or Medicaid population and those serving beneficiaries who have special needs and/or who are dual eligibles
- Understand key legal and regulatory issues in the government entitlement programs that affect health plans
- Identify the different types of organizational models to manage benefits in the public sector programs
- Explain the Medicare benefit structure and how private health plans may provide and manage those benefits
- Explain in general how the Medicare Quality Bonus Payment Program, or "Stars" works

INTRODUCTION

Most commercial payers offer Medicare and/or Medicaid managed care plans that are different from their commercial health plans. Medicare and Medicaid share their origins in laws passed in 1965 and represent two of the most significant healthcare marketplace reforms ever passed in the United States. Both are entitlement programs, meaning eligible individuals are entitled to coverage (see the *Health Benefits Coverage and Types of Health Plans* chapter); in some cases, individuals may be eligible for both, in which case they are referred to as dual eligibles. There are some shared elements in how private managed care organizations (MCOs) operate within the Medicare and Medicaid markets, but more than not, they differ in their approaches to these markets.

MEDICARE

Medicare provides healthcare benefits for the elderly, for persons with end-stage renal disease (kidney failure), and for some disabled persons. The Medicare program is administered by the federal Centers for Medicare & Medicaid Services (CMS), which is part of the U.S. Department of Health and Human Services (DHHS). CMS administers the program from a policy and regulatory standpoint, but all of the day-to-day operational administration, such as handling claims and benefits administration, is actually done by private companies called "intermediaries." Another DHHS agency with which the intermediaries must work is the Social Security Administration (SSA), which manages eligibility and enrollment for both Social Security and Medicare benefits.

Medicare benefits coverage is divided up into separate parts. Much like the earliest Blue Cross and Blue Shield plans, the traditional benefits consist of Part A (benefits for hospital services) and Part B (benefits for medical services), both of which have always been covered under Medicare. Part A is mandatory for all individuals eligible for Medicare coverage, but Part B is voluntary and requires monthly premium payments taken as deductions from Social Security payments. Few seniors do not take up Part B. In the traditional Medicare program, providers are paid through fee-for-service (FFS), which is why traditional Medicare is sometimes referred to as "FFS Medicare."

Parts A and B include cost sharing but no limits on total out-of-pocket spending, although there are limits on some types of benefits. Neither Part A nor Part B provides benefits for coverage of prescription drugs or for preventive services. For many years, the only way seniors could obtain coverage for costs that Medicare did not cover was through a type of supplemental insurance policy referred to as "MediGap" coverage.

In the mid-1980s, another option became available when a pilot program was authorized that allowed private plans that met various criteria—federally qualified health maintenance organizations (HMOs), for example— to market and sell private Medicare plans. The private plans could cover more than what traditional Medicare covered, but not less. That created a new option for seniors in some markets, because many private HMO plans included coverage for prescription drugs and prevention, although they were not required to do so.

In 1997, Medicare Part C was passed as part of the Balanced Budget Act (BBA; see the discussion in the chapter titled *A History of Managed Health*

Care and Health Insurance in the United States). Part C is not a benefit, but rather a provision that made permanent the option for beneficiaries to receive their Medicare benefits through an approved private plan if one was available to them. When it was originally implemented, the Part C option was called "Medicare+Choice." The BBA also expanded the different types of private plans that could be approved under Part C, including preferred provider organizations (PPOs), point-of-service (POS) plans, a new type of Medicare plan called private fee-for-service (PFFS), and a demonstration program for medical savings accounts (MSAs). Finally, the BBA created an ill-fated Medicare pilot program for provider-sponsored organizations (PSOs).

To be eligible to join a Part C plan, beneficiaries had to already have Medicare Parts A and B. Also, they could not have both a Part C plan and a MediGap policy—they had to select one or the other.* Those requirements remain in place today.

The Medicare Prescription Drug Improvement and Modernization Act, better known as the Medicare Modernization Act (MMA), was passed in 2003. This act created a new benefit, Medicare Part D, which added an optional drug coverage benefit for all Medicare beneficiaries. The MMA also changed the name of the Part C Medicare+Choice program to Medicare Advantage (MA). More importantly, it changed how MA plans are classified, how they are paid, and how performance is measured, among other things.

The Patient Protection and Affordable Care Act (ACA) contains many provisions that apply to Medicare. Many apply primarily to the traditional FFS program, such as accountable care organizations (ACOs; discussed in the chapter titled *The Provider Network*) and the Medicare Shared Savings Program (MSSP) payment methodology (discussed in the *Provider Payment* chapter). Some provisions are specific to Parts C and D, however. For example, ACA required reductions in payments to Part C plans, although the levels of these reductions varied by type and location of plan. It also created a new bonus payment program for plans based on quality ratings, and as of 2014 it required MA plans to maintain a medical loss ratio (MLR) of at least 85%, which mirrors the ACA's MLR limitations for insured large groups in the commercial market (discussed in the *Sales, Governance, and Administration* chapter).

The Medicare Part D Drug Benefit

The MMA added drug coverage as a benefit to be administered entirely by private entities—either "stand-alone" prescription drug plans (PDPs) or Medicare

---

* MediGap is not discussed beyond this point in the text.

Advantage Prescription Drug plans (MA-PD or MA-PDPs) in which the Part D drug benefits plan is combined with the Part C medical benefits plan. Unlike PDPs, MA-PD plans can use savings from their Part C plan to make their Part D benefit more attractive to beneficiaries; for example, by offering better drug coverage or lower cost sharing.

Part D is voluntary for regular Medicare beneficiaries, but dual eligibles are automatically enrolled in the program. This benefit is primarily paid for by federal subsidies, with a portion of the voluntary benefit being paid by beneficiaries in the form of premiums and cost sharing, and a portion being financed by plans that are partly at risk for the provision of the benefit. Access standards apply to ensure that beneficiaries have convenient access to pharmacies.

Part D Benefit Design

The Part D benefit is complicated and is characterized by a coverage gap sometimes called a "doughnut hole." In 2011, before the ACA provisions began to go into effect, the benefit design was as follows:

1. A small deductible of approximately $300 must be met before any coverage applied.
2. An enrollee paid 25% coinsurance after the deductible was met, up until total costs reached approximately $2900.
3. A coverage gap existed between total drug benefit costs of $2900 and approximately $6500 in which the Part D enrollee paid 100% out-of-pocket for medications, although many PDPs and MA-PDPs continued to provide some coverage for generic drugs.
4. Enrollees paid only 5% coinsurance after total costs rose to more than $6500.

The ACA contains provisions to plug this coverage gap over time. Between 2014 and 2020, the coinsurance amounts in the coverage gap will decline until they reach 25%, although there are some differences between brand-name and generic drugs in terms of how much their coinsurance amounts decline each year. As before, once total costs reach a certain level, cost sharing drops to 5% coinsurance. The exact dollar figures for when the coverage gap begins and ends may be adjusted annually.

Formularies and Drug Utilization Review

Part D plans are allowed to develop formularies that limit which drugs are covered under the plan. These formularies must include drug categories and classes that cover all disease states. Each category or class must include at least two drugs unless only one drug is available for a particular category or class, or only two drugs are available but one drug is clinically superior to the other. The formularies are submitted to CMS in April of each year and are reviewed to assure that they are "adequate," that they include a range of drugs in a broad distribution of therapeutic categories and classes, and that they are not designed to discourage enrollment by individuals with significant illnesses. PDPs and MA-PD plans may also use drug utilization review (DUR) strategies, including prior authorizations, step therapies, quantity limitations, generic substitutions, and other approaches described in the *Utilization Management, Quality Management, and Accreditation* chapter.

Medication Therapy Management Programs

Part D plan sponsors are required to offer a medication therapy management (MTM) program that targets beneficiaries who have multiple chronic diseases and high drug costs. For example, MTM programs must target chronic conditions such as hypertension, heart failure, and diabetes. In addition, these programs must target beneficiaries who incur annual drug costs of $3000 or more. MTM programs include a comprehensive medication review, ongoing monitoring, and beneficiary or prescriber interventions if necessary. Such programs are also built into the requirements for ACOs.

Types of Medicare Advantage Plans

In addition to PDPs, the MMA defines three categories of MA plans that private payers can offer to Medicare beneficiaries:

- Coordinated care plans, which are required to offer at least one plan with Part D benefits throughout their service area (they are free to also offer plans without Part D)
- Private fee-for-service (PFFS) plans, which are allowed, but not required, to include Part D coverage
- Medical savings account (MSA) plans, which are not allowed to include Part D at all
- Group retiree plans that are restricted to only employer or organized labor groups that include coverage for healthcare in their defined benefits plans for retirees

CMS refers to these plans broadly as Medicare Advantage organizations (MAOs). CMS must approve any plan offered, and other than retiree plans, most are also regulated by the states as risk-bearing insurers or HMOs. As discussed elsewhere in this text, the PSO pilot program under the BBA was a failure and its authorization expired, so PSOs are no longer part of the Medicare landscape.* At the time of this text's publication, approximately 30% of all Medicare beneficiaries were enrolled in an MA plan, and that number has been steadily growing since the MMA was passed.

Coordinated Care Plans

Coordinated care plan (CCP) is the broad term used by CMS to describe the different types of health plans that use a network of providers to deliver the benefits package approved by Medicare. CCPs include HMOs, POS plans, and PPOs, as well as a new type of MA plan called the special needs plan (SNP).

CCPs may enroll beneficiaries only within their defined service areas (see the discussion in the *Health Benefits Coverage and Types of Health Plans* chapter). CMS must approve the provider network to assure that the enrolled Medicare beneficiaries will have sufficient access to covered services, and plans must routinely monitor and report on network adequacy. Coordinated care plans may use financial incentives or utilization review to control the use of services and must meet quality requirements. For each type of plan (e.g., HMO, POS or PPO), requirements for utilization management and use of network providers are the same for Medicare products and commercial products.

Coordinated care plans may also be used for dual eligibles. In some cases, that plan will be an SNP; in other cases, it is a standard type of MA plan, albeit one that focuses on the unique aspects of dual eligibility such as different coverage benefits and the unique challenges of medical management in this population.

HMOs and POS Plans   Medicare HMOs and POS plans are similar to HMOs and POS plans in the commercial market, but are subject to additional Medicare-related requirements as described elsewhere in this section. Medicare HMOs, including POS plans based on HMOs, are the oldest coordinated care plan type and have the highest enrollment among all types of MA plans.

Preferred Provider Organizations   Like HMOs, Medicare PPOs are similar to PPOs in the private sector, in that they do not use primary care physician "gatekeepers," typically have larger networks, and usually provide some coverage for services provided by noncontracting providers (with some exceptions). Unlike many purely commercial PPOs, MA-PPOs must meet MA quality

---

* The acronym "PSO" lives on in Medicare, however. CMS recycled it so that it now stands for "patient safety organization."

requirements, albeit only for services provided on an in-network basis, and must meet network adequacy service area requirements that they are not necessarily subject to in all states. PPOs must establish a maximum out-of-pocket limit for in-network services and a catastrophic limit on in-network and out-of-network services.

Medicare offers two types of PPOs: local PPOs and regional PPOs (RPPOs). Local PPOs have the flexibility to choose the service area where they will operate (e.g., one or multiple counties). RPPOs were added to Medicare by the MMA to provide increased access to private plans, particularly in rural counties. RPPOs must serve all counties in one or more of 26 statewide or multiple-state regions designated by CMS. To encourage the growth of regional PPOs, CMS did not allow any new local plans to start up for two years in the designated regions, but that restriction was lifted in 2008.

Special Needs Plans   SNPs (often referred to informally as "snips") are coordinated care plans, usually HMOs, that limit enrollment to individuals with special needs. These beneficiaries include those with significant chronic medical conditions, such as persons with multiple chronic conditions—for example, individuals with diabetes who also have advanced-stage conditions such as kidney failure and heart disease. While not as widespread as other types of MA plans, SNPs have been steadily growing.

Three types of SNPs are distinguished:

- D-SNPs: Dual-eligible SNPs for beneficiaries who are eligible for both Medicare and Medicaid (i.e., "dual eligibles" or "duals," or less commonly, "Medi-Medis"*)
- I-SNPs: Institutional SNPs for beneficiaries who are institutionalized in a skilled or intermediate nursing facility, or in an assisted living facility
- C-SNPs: Chronic care SNPs for beneficiaries with one or more severe or disabling chronic conditions

The ACA created a new requirement that all SNPs meet a scored set of standards in an SNP Model of Care (MOC), which is based on standards created by the National Committee for Quality Assurance (NCQA), the major accreditation organization for healthcare plans. MOCs are scored, and SNPs must achieve a minimum score of 70% to pass, and at least 75% to be able to contract with CMS for more than one year.

---

* Pronounced "Med Eee Med Eees"

Private Fee-for-Service Plans

PFFS plans were authorized in 1997 and are a model unique to Medicare. Enrollees are permitted to self-refer to any Medicare provider willing to accept the individual as a patient consistent with the rules of the plan regarding coverage. The PFFS plans pay providers on a FFS basis at Medicare fee schedule rates, do not place the provider at financial risk, and do not vary their payment rates based on utilization data. A PFFS plan, however, is permitted to vary its payment rates based on the provider's specialty, location, or other factors not related to utilization. For example, such plans may increase payment rates to a provider based on increased utilization of specified preventive or screening services.

PFFS plans and enrollment grew very rapidly beginning in 2006 when MMA payment rates, which were relatively high, went into effect. Because there was no cost associated with establishing provider networks, there was little barrier to entry. Consequently, by 2008, PFFS plans were available to almost all Medicare beneficiaries in the United States. In 2011, PFFS plans were required to establish networks and the amount they were paid was reduced, leading the majority of PFFS plans to drop out of the market.

Medical Savings Account Plans

MSAs authorized under the BBA were intended as a demonstration only and, in fact, few were ever sold. The MMA continued to authorize MSAs, however, including a new Medicare MSA demonstration program. An MSA plan is similar to a consumer-directed health plan (CDHP; discussed in the *Health Benefits Coverage and Types of Health Plans* chapter). Like CDHPs, Medicare MSA plans have a special type of high-deductible Medicare Advantage plan (Part C), a high-deductible health plan, and a medical savings account.

MSAs have not had much success in the Medicare market (or the commercial market, for that matter). The plans are confusing to beneficiaries, and the plan design does not allow beneficiaries to contribute to their tax-free accounts. Furthermore, Medicare MSA plans do not provide Part D coverage of drugs, so this coverage must be purchased separately.

Group Retiree Plans

CMS has historically offered MA plans wide latitude to negotiate with employers and unions for retiree coverage under MA. The MMA went even further by including a very broad waiver provision to encourage employer- or union-sponsored plans to offer retiree coverage through MA plans and PDPs, and it added a new option whereby employers or unions could directly contract with CMS as MA, PDP, or MA-PDP plans. As part of that revision, retiree MA plans do not need to meet many of the requirements that commercial MA plans do, such as minimum enrollment levels or service area restrictions, and they follow the employer's or union's eligibility rules for enrolling retirees.

Payment of Medicare Advantage Plans

CMS's method of paying MA plans is complicated and can be described here only in very broad terms. It has two components. The largest component is the basic method used to pay MA plans, and a smaller but still substantial component is the Quality Bonus Payment (QBP) program.

Basic Payment of Medicare Advantage Plans

Payments to MA plans and cost sharing by MA plan members are determined through a competitive bidding system. Prior to the MMA, Medicare+Choice plans were paid based only on average FFS Medicare costs in the same area in which the plan operated. Under the MMA, however, payment to MA plans changed significantly, as is described below. The ACA also reduced payment rate increases to MA plans overall, but it also readjusted payment averages into four categories so that plans in high-cost areas received lower payment percentage increases, while plans in low-cost areas received higher payment increases.

Bids for Part D benefits are calculated separately from bids for medical benefits. No plan can provide benefits that are lower than Medicare, but it may provide more benefits if approved to do so by CMS. If an MA plan has claims history data, it uses those data to predict its costs for the coming year to cover Part A and Part B benefits. If it has no history, then it must estimate costs. The amount that it submits to CMS is called a "bid." CMS compares the bids of local MA plans to a benchmark that it calculates each year based on county-specific payment rates used for MA plans prior to 2006, adjusted for cost trends. If a plan's bid is higher than the benchmark, then enrollees must pay a premium. If the bid is lower than the benchmark, then CMS keeps a percentage of the difference, and the MA plan can use the remaining percentage to fund additional benefits for enrollees. The percentages used are affected by a plan's QBP star rating as discussed in the next section.

The actual payments to each MA Plan are based on multiple factors that account for specific characteristics of the MA plan's enrollees. These factors include the age, gender, place of residence, and prior health condition of each individual beneficiary enrolled in the MA plan (CMS does not use data on non-Medicare members). Payments are also affected by a risk-adjustment model using CMS-Hierarchical Condition Categories (CMS-HCCs) that projects the expected relative risk for each enrollee. MA plans submit data on an ongoing basis, and CMS periodically conducts audits to test the validity of submitted claims and other data.

Quality Bonus Payment Program

A QBP program was put in place as a demonstration under the MMA, and under the ACA it is now a substantial factor in payment. The QBP is also referred to as the Medicare "Stars" program because a plan's rating is summarized by the number of stars it receives, with five stars being the highest rating. The QBP program is designed to be modified from time to time, so its description here reflects only what was in place at the time of this text's publication. Updates and changes to the QBP program can be found on the CMS website.

Only plans that receive four or more stars are eligible to receive any bonus payment, which is added to the plan's overall payment rate from CMS. A bonus can add as much as 5% to the amount paid to a plan—a sum that can mean the difference between profit and loss. The amount of savings from a bid that is lower than the benchmark is also affected, such that plans with higher star ratings may keep a higher percentage of the savings for use in funding additional benefits for MA enrollees. MA plans with five stars are also allowed to market and sell to beneficiaries all year long, not just during annual open enrollment periods.

The QBP rating program includes five broad categories that carry different weights (Table 7-1). The measures used are described in the next section about requirements for quality and performance. Medicare beneficiaries can obtain not only the overall star ratings for each MA plan, and also more detailed information about individual measures.

Table 7-1   Weighted Measurement Categories in the QBP Program

Measure	Weighting Factor
Health outcomes	3.0
Intermediate outcomes	3.0
Patient experience	1.5
Access	1.5
Process	1.0

As important as the bonus payment is for plans with four or more stars, the star rating program also contains penalties for plans that have fewer than three stars—plans that are dubbed "poor-performing" plans by CMS. If a Medicare beneficiary or an individual who will soon become eligible for Medicare coverage uses CMS's www.Medicare.gov website to find a plan, the site only provides links to plans with three or more stars. For plans with fewer than three stars for three years, the website provides no links and it advises beneficiaries to not enroll in such plans. To enroll in a poor-performing plan, an individual must contact that plan directly. CMS also can remove a poor-performing plan that has had fewer than three stars for three years in a row from participating in the MA program altogether.

MA Quality and Plan Performance Requirements

In addition to the QBP program, each MA plan (other than PFFS and MSA plans) must meet several other requirements related to quality and plan performance programs. Data and information for these programs are used not only by the QBP program, but for other evaluations by CMS as well. A brief description of these requirements follows.

Overall MA Quality Program Requirements

Quality program requirements for MA plans, which are at least partly similar to NCQA's accreditation requirements (discussed in the *Utilization Management, Quality Management, and Accreditation* chapter), include the following:

- Quality improvement projects (QIPs), which are more or less the same as quality management (QM) programs
- Chronic care improvement programs (CCIPs), which are similar to disease management (DM) programs
- A health information system (HIS) that collects, analyzes, and reports data
- Written policies and procedures that reflect current standards of medical practice and mechanisms to detect both underutilization and overutilization of services
- Formal annual evaluations measuring the impact and effectiveness of the program; problems that were revealed through internal surveillance, complaints, or other mechanisms; and resolution of those problems

CMS requires the annual submission of the QIP and the CCIP in July of each year. Projects are reviewed at the contract level to identify those that show improvement or deterioration. CMS also determines an MA plan's overall compliance with the requirements.

MA External Review and Reporting Requirements

Coordinated care plans are subject to external review by quality improvement organizations (QIOs) under contract to CMS to also review hospital quality of care in the FFS Medicare program. QIOs review complaints by MA enrollees about the quality of care in an MA plan and process beneficiary requests for review of hospital discharge decisions. QIOs also play a significant role in member appeals of benefits denials.

Plan reporting requirements are similar to the requirements that NCQA places on health plans for purposes of accreditation. The first four of these data sets are described briefly in the *Utilization Management, Quality Management, and Accreditation* chapter. MA plans report the following specific data sets to CMS, based on measures that are specifically modified for Medicare:

- The Healthcare Effectiveness Data and Information Set (HEDIS), which provides information about service and quality
- The annual Consumer Assessment of Healthcare Providers and Systems (CAHPS) survey
- The quarterly CAHPS Disenrollment Reasons Survey
- The Health Outcomes Survey (HOS), also called the Medicare Hospital Outcomes Survey (MHOS)
- Plan information: Contract performance measures such as call center performance and appeal and grievance rates

Deemed Compliance with Quality Requirements

Deemed compliance means that plans accredited by NCQA, URAC, or Accreditation Association for Ambulatory Health Care (AAAHC) meet or exceed MA requirements for plan participation in six categories:

- Quality assessment and improvement
- Access to services
- Provider participation
- Advance directives
- Information about antidiscrimination
- Confidentiality and accuracy of enrollee records

Member Appeals

Member appeals for Medicare resemble the processes discussed in the *Utilization Management, Quality Management, and Accreditation* chapter, but there are some specific differences. In particular, the QIOs are involved in reviewing appeals of coverage denials. If the QIO upholds the denial, an MA member can have another review performed by an administrative law judge depending on the size of the claim(s).

Eligibility and Enrollment

Newly eligible Medicare beneficiaries may enroll in an MA plan as soon as they become eligible, as long as they also sign up for Medicare Part A and Part B benefits. The initial enrollment period begins three months before an individual is first entitled to Medicare Part A and B benefits, and ends on the later of the last day of the month before entitlement to Parts A and B, or the last day of the individual's Part B initial enrollment period. An additional initial coverage election period applies to Part D that allows individuals newly eligible for such benefits to join a Part D plan. Most newly eligible Medicare beneficiaries who are Medicaid recipients may also enroll. Newly eligible beneficiaries who do not choose an MA plan are deemed to have chosen the traditional FFS Medicare option. If they choose not to enroll for Part D when it is first available to them, they must pay higher premiums later should they decide they want Part D during a subsequent open enrollment period.

The only Medicare beneficiaries who are not entitled to enroll (and to whom a plan must refuse enrollment under the law) are those who have end-stage renal disease (ESRD), whether aged, disabled, or entitled to Medicare solely because of their disease. However, enrollees who acquire ESRD after enrollment in the plan may not be disenrolled because they have ESRD, and individuals who were enrolled as non-Medicare members of a plan who have ESRD may be retained as Medicare enrollees upon becoming eligible for Medicare. The one exception to this rule is that special needs plans may be offered to individuals with ESRD who would not otherwise be entitled to enroll in an MA plan.

All MA plans, unless they are at capacity and unable to accept new members, hold an annual open enrollment that takes place from October 15 through December 7 of each year.* During this "annual election period," beneficiaries receive comparative information on all their healthcare options, including traditional Medicare and MediGap supplemental coverage as well as available MA plans. During this period, beneficiaries may change MA plans, elect new coverage, or switch back and forth between MA and traditional Medicare, effective the following January.

---

* Open enrollment dates are subject to change, so these dates are only a guideline and the reader should check the CMS website for the most current open enrollment periods.

The annual open enrollment period is followed by a disenrollment period that goes from January 1 to February 15, at which time a beneficiary can disenroll from an MA plan and return to Medicare FFS. After that, beneficiaries are "locked in" to whatever option they chose for the remainder of the year, with some exceptions. Note that this election period does not allow for enrollment in a new MA plan. Individuals who switch to Medicare FFS during this time period have the option to join a PDP to add drug coverage.

Special election periods also apply to enrollment in MA plans. As with most private health insurance election periods, special election periods are related to certain events such as changing residence, losing employer/union health coverage, membership in an MA plan that loses its contract with CMS, or new eligibility for Medicaid.

Finally, the MA plan must provide an evidence of coverage (EOC) document that is similar to the document for non-Medicare plans described in the *Sales, Governance, and Administration* chapter. It includes information on benefits and exclusions; the number, mix, and distribution of plan providers; out-of-network and out-of-area coverage; emergency coverage (i.e., how it is defined and how to gain access to emergency care, including use of 911 services); prior authorization or other review requirements; grievances and appeals; and a description of the plan's quality assurance program. On request, the organization must provide information on utilization control practices, the number and disposition of appeals and grievances, and a summary description of physician compensation.

Sales and Marketing

Except for employer- or union-sponsored retiree MA plans, MA plans market and sell their products to individual Medicare beneficiaries, and a beneficiary's decision to join an MA plan is a personal one. Whereas marketing and sales of insured products in the commercial markets are regulated only by the states, marketing and sales of MA plans must not only meet state requirements, but also federal requirements. These requirements are extensive and complex. At a high level, they align with requirements included in the ACA such as the following:

- The MCO must market throughout the entire service area in a nondiscriminatory manner.
- All marketing materials, including membership and enrollment materials, must be approved by CMS before use (although there is a time limit on CMS's review process, and model language exists as well).

- Prospective enrollees must be given sufficient descriptive materials to allow them to make an informed decision regarding enrollment.
- Prospective enrollees must be given a summary of benefits form that uses standard definitions of benefits and a standardized format.

Many sales and marketing activities are explicitly prohibited, and an MA plan that engages in these activities is subject to fines, suspension of its ability to sell to or enroll new members, and other sanctions. These strict prohibitions were established because of abusive marketing and sales practices in the past. The list of prohibited marketing and sales activities is quite extensive, so only some examples can be provided here:

- Using a purchased list of e-mail addresses or other types of lists to contact nonmembers
- Door-to-door solicitation or leaflet distribution
- Referring to a plan as "the best" or anything similar to that
- Comparing one MA plan to another, unless using only CMS's star ratings
- Discriminatory marketing (e.g., avoiding low-income areas or people with medical problems)
- Misleading marketing or misrepresentation in the marketplace
- Requesting any beneficiary identification numbers such as a Social Security number or personal contact information
- Providing gifts worth more than $15 to attend a meeting
- Offering monetary incentives as an inducement to enroll
- Completing any portion of the enrollment application for a prospective enrollee
- Any sales by any means by a person who is not trained and certified to sell MA plans
- Any marketing or selling by providers, other than having some type of signage in the provider's office or facility that lists the plans in which the provider participates

Even prior to the MLR restrictions imposed by the ACA, CMS had created limitations on the amount of commissions that brokers could be paid for enrolling members into an MA plan. These restrictions vary by location and are periodically updated. CMS also requires any brokers, agents, or plan sales personnel to obtain MA-specific training from an organization approved by CMS. In addition, CMS has established requirements for websites and call centers that facilitate sales, marketing, and/or enrollment.

Corporate Compliance

Corporate compliance activities are directed toward (1) ensuring that the organization conforms to legal and regulatory requirements and (2) preventing and detecting illegal behavior. Corporate compliance applies to all MCOs under a variety of laws and regulations, including Medicare. Because there is considerable overlap, it is permissible and practical to combine the corporate compliance activities for most or all of the different laws and regulations into one overall compliance function.

For MA plans specifically, CMS, through the Office of the Inspector General (OIG), has created corporate compliance guidelines that an MA plan must follow. The full set of corporate compliance requirements is, as you would expect, complex, but in general an effective MA corporate compliance program must include the following requirements:

- Creation of a special compliance committee
- Designation of a corporate compliance officer
- Creation of standards of conduct for employees
- Creation of policies and procedures specifically designed to ensure compliance with MA rules
- Special training for employees
- Employee surveys that focus on compliance issues
- A "hotline" for employees to report violations of MA rules
- Exit interviews of employees in which they are asked about possible rule violations
- Audits of compliance
- Screening for individuals or entities barred from participation in federal programs (applies to employees, providers, and vendors)
- Creation of an internal investigation program that focuses on MA rule violations

MEDICAID

Medicaid is an entitlement program that provides benefits coverage to low-income individuals and families as well as the aged, blind, and disabled. It has been expanded over the years to increase coverage for children through the State Children's Health Insurance Program (SCHIP or simply CHIP) and to provide assistance to certain individuals with dual eligibility. All of the Medicaid programs combined cover more people than Medicare does.

Unlike Medicare, Medicaid is administered by the states, although approximately half of its funding comes from the federal government. Policies, rules, and regulations pertaining to eligibility, coverage, payment, and services vary from state to state, although the ACA addressed some of those differences, and federal regulations define certain baseline standards for eligibility and covered services that states cannot go below. In addition to the original act passed in 1965 and the SCHIP program, other legislation directly affects Medicaid, including the Americans with Disabilities Act (ADA), welfare reform legislation, the BBA, the MMA, and the ACA.

Many Medicaid beneficiaries are, by default, covered through their state's traditional FFS Medicaid program—for example, individuals in nursing homes and individuals living in an area that does not have a managed Medicaid plan. The states, however, have become reliant on private managed Medicaid plans, which now cover the majority of Medicaid beneficiaries in each state.

Eligibility for Coverage

Eligibility for coverage under Medicaid follows two sets of rules. One set applies to traditional Medicaid programs in all states. The other set applies to coverage expansion under the ACA, which not all states have undertaken.

Eligibility for Coverage Under Traditional Medicaid

Broadly speaking, Medicaid provides coverage primarily for three groups:

- Low-income individuals, mostly healthy women and children, who make up approximately 70% of Medicaid enrollees, through Temporary Aid to Needy Families (TANF) and SCHIP programs.
- Aged and younger persons who have a chronic illness or condition and are disabled, who make up the second largest group.
- Institutionalized individuals, who make up the third group, which is really a subset of the second group. This population includes aged persons needing nursing home care who are either impoverished at the time of their admission or become so during their stay, and persons in specialized facilities for the developmentally disabled or mentally retarded.

Not including the provisions in the ACA (discussed shortly), states must cover a core group of people with incomes below specified minimum thresholds based on a percentage of the federal poverty level (FPL), including the following subpopulations:

- Pregnant women
- Children
- Parents, but not to the same degree as children
- Elderly individuals
- Individuals with disabilities

Eligibility for coverage of children is broader than for their parents because the SCHIP program provides coverage to children in families with incomes that are low, but not necessarily low enough to qualify for Medicaid. Not all low-income people must be covered, either. Non-elderly adults without dependent children, referred to as childless adults, have not been considered eligible for traditional Medicaid coverage, though they may qualify in states that expanded Medicaid coverage under the ACA.

Only American citizens and specific categories of lawfully present immigrants can qualify for Medicaid, and most lawfully present immigrants cannot qualify for coverage for the first five years they reside in the United States. The states can eliminate that waiting period for lawfully present children and/or pregnant women, but not for other adult immigrants.

Medicaid Expansion Under the ACA

In addition to expanding coverage through reforms in the commercial market, the ACA sought to broaden the number of people who would be eligible for coverage under Medicaid by overriding each state's differing rules for who is or is not eligible for coverage. It set a standard of eligibility at or below 133% of the FPL,* above which individuals and families would be eligible for subsidized premium credits for coverage through private plans sold through the health insurance exchanges. The amount subsidized decreases on a sliding scale until income reaches 400% of the FPL, above which they no longer apply. The ACA also greatly simplified the process for determining and maintaining eligibility.

The cost for the expansion is 100% paid for by the federal government until the year 2017, when the federal government's share begins to slowly decline; it continues to decrease until 2020, after which the federal government pays 90% of the cost associated with the coverage expansion. The amount of the subsidy is based on a relatively low level of eligibility prior to expansion, not necessarily

---

* This percentage is actually 138% because the first 5% of income is automatically ignored in the calculation.

pre-ACA eligibility requirements in a state; in this way, the ACA does not "short-change" states that had already established more generous eligibility standards.

Medicaid expansion under the ACA was significantly affected when the 2012 ruling by the U.S. Supreme Court that determined the ACA was constitutional also ruled that states were not required to accept the Medicaid expansion, and that not expanding Medicaid would not change how much federal money the states received under their existing programs. Not expanding Medicaid also meant that a state would not receive any funding related to expansion.

At the time of this text's publication, 28 states plus the District of Columbia had expanded or were in the process of expanding Medicaid eligibility under the ACA, and several more states were actively considering it. There is no deadline for states to adopt expansion, so more states may expand their coverage over time. In states that have not expanded coverage, anyone who has an income that is greater than that state's cutoff for Medicaid eligibility but less than 133% of the FPL is also not eligible for a premium subsidy for private coverage under the ACA, leaving those people without any affordable means to obtain coverage.

Benefits Coverage Under Medicaid

Medicaid benefits include more services than do most MA and commercial health plans, including the following:

- Oral and dental care
- Vision care
- Transportation
- Nursing home and community-based long-term care

In addition to the preventive benefits available under the ACA, Medicaid requires coverage of early and periodic screening, diagnostic, and treatment (EPSDT) services for individuals younger than age 21. Prescriptions drugs are typically covered as well. States can require some beneficiaries to pay a premium as well as some level of cost sharing, but the amount of cost sharing is limited.

Managed Medicaid Plans

The traditional Medicaid program is a FFS program, but CMS can grant states a waiver, referred to as a Section 1115 waiver,* that allows them to use different

---

* An example of industry jargon referencing Section 1115 of the Social Security Act that gives the Secretary of Health and Human Services authority to approve experimental, pilot, or demonstration projects that promote the objectives of the Medicaid and CHIP programs.

types of plans including managed care plans. Indeed, the majority of Medicaid beneficiaries are currently enrolled in managed Medicaid plans. There are three main types of plans, two of which apply to beneficiaries who are covered only under Medicaid: the primary care case manager (PCCM) model and the managed care organization (MCO) model. SNPs, the third type of plan, can include individuals with dual eligibility and were discussed earlier in the chapter.

In a PCCM plan, primary care physicians (PCPs) are paid a monthly fee to manage the care of their Medicaid patients. Beneficiaries are not "locked in" to seeing only the PCP, however. Providers, including PCPs, are paid through traditional FFS and there is no provider risk sharing. The service area for PCCMs typically covers the entire state, and this type of coverage may be the default plan for those covered under the TANF and SCHIP programs when an MCO is not available. PCCM plans are often run by the state, although the state may contract with a private company to administer it. PCCMs may also be privately run and share some level of financial risk with the state. In recent years, states have been moving away from PCCM models because they do not provide the same value as MCOs do.

Although it varies by state, most Medicaid MCO plans are risk based, meaning the MCO is at risk for costs, and does not refer to how MCO providers are paid. The state capitates the plan, which refers to a type of premium payment, and once again not how the providers are paid. How that capitation amount is calculated varies. In some states, only age and sex of beneficiaries (and often urban versus rural residence as well) are used to adjust payments. Other states are now experimenting with adjusting payments based on how ill a Medicaid member is; that is, they provide higher capitation payments if the plan has sicker-than-average members and lower payments if members are healthier on average. This approach is similar to the one used to pay MA plans. At the time of publication, Medicaid MCOs are not subject to MLR restrictions, but in reality most states negotiate "give back" provisions under which the MCO can retain only a relatively modest percentage of any leftover funds or profits. Whether MLR restrictions will be placed on Medicaid MCOs in the future cannot be predicted at the time of publication.

State Medicaid agencies employ multiple approaches to select which MCOs they will contract with. Some states establish participation qualifications for interested plans—including payment rates—and select all plans that meet them. Others require periodic bidding and may award a limited number of contracts.

States have become more detailed and demanding in their contracting with health plans, including key requirements like provider network access standards, customer service standards and obligations, performance data submission, external reviews, and many other criteria that must be met to merit a contract. In some states, arrangements are in place for certain services to be carved out and provided separately from the basic health plan—pharmacy benefits, for example, which may then administered by a separate pharmacy benefits management program. Specialized models have also been developed in some states for behavioral health and special needs populations (e.g., children in foster care, developmentally delayed children).

Medicaid MCOs pay providers in ways similar to those described in the *Provider Payment* chapter, and provider capitation is common. Most providers who already participate with a state's Medicaid program also participate with private MCOs as well, and Medicaid MCOs frequently contract with providers who do not participate with traditional Medicaid.

Similar to MA plans, Medicaid MCOs can enroll only members who live within the MCO's service area. In some states, commercial HMOs enroll Medicaid members as well as commercial members. Most states also have privately operated Medicaid-only plans that look much like traditional HMOs or PPOs that specialize in having capabilities specific to meeting the needs of Medicaid beneficiaries. Such private Medicaid-only MCOs may be part of a traditional multi-line payer, part of a national for-profit company that specializes in Medicaid, or locally owned and operated. Locally owned and operated plans may be for-profit or not-for-profit entities and, in some cases, are owned or sponsored by provider organizations.

Sales, Marketing, and Enrollment

All of the regulations created by CMS for MA plans that were discussed earlier in the "Medicare" section apply equally to managed Medicaid plans, but states are free to apply additional requirements as long as they do not violate the federal regulations. Most states currently require low-income women and children to be enrolled in a Medicaid MCO or PCCM plan. Often beneficiaries are allowed to choose the plan in which they will enroll; if they do not choose a plan, they may be automatically enrolled in the PCCM plan. Other states assign beneficiaries to a plan. The ACA also created a requirement for the health insurance exchanges for the individual market (exchanges are discussed in the *Sales, Governance, and Administration* chapter) to provide a seamless entry point or transition for individuals eligible for Medicaid as well as commercial health insurance.

Cultural diversity is highly important in Medicaid plans, including the need to accommodate non-English-speaking individuals. Because of the low educational levels prevalent in some Medicaid populations, materials that explain the program must be written in easy-to-understand language. Transportation services, proactive outreach, attentiveness to physical and social environmental factors, and increasing cultural competency are all areas in which plans must develop proficiency to have positive, sustained impacts on their members.

One of the most frustrating administrative concerns for Medicaid managed care plans is member turnover due to changes in eligibility, commonly referred to as "churning." This occurs most often because a person's income increases enough for that individual to lose eligibility. Under the ACA, the health insurance exchange is supposed to help such persons make a seamless transition to subsidized commercial coverage, but this is not an option for some low-income people in those states that did not expand Medicaid eligibility. Churning can also occur when a member forgets to reapply or for coverage or simply stops contacting the Medicaid agency. Even prior to the ACA, laws and regulations for the SCHIP program provided for longer periods of eligibility to smooth out this problem, and the ACA does the same for other Medicaid beneficiaries in those states that agreed to the expansion.

Management of Utilization and Quality in Medicaid MCOs

Medicaid managed care is a demanding line of business, requiring plans to serve populations with complex medical and social needs and forcing them to develop provider networks of considerable diversity—in terms of both service capabilities and cultural competencies. UM, case management (CM), DM, and QM in Medicaid MCOs are similar to the programs used in MA plans, but must accommodate the differences in this population. They must also meet prevention program standards that apply only to Medicaid and SCHIP such as the Early Periodic Screening, Diagnosis, and Treatment (EPSDT) program.

Medicaid MCOs must be able to address a number of special challenges, of which only a few examples follow. As a group, adult Medicaid beneficiaries are more likely to smoke cigarettes and abuse alcohol and/or other drugs, so treatment and prevention programs must be more proactive and must incorporate the socioeconomic pressures many of these beneficiaries face. There is also a high concentrations of high-risk pregnancies in this population, as well as higher than average rates of chronic conditions like asthma, diabetes, depression, and behavioral health problems, requiring well-planned interventions to promote member well-being and to achieve cost-effective outcomes. Finally, lack of transportation is often a major factor in the ability of beneficiaries to even see a provider.

External Review and Reporting Requirements for Medicaid MCOs

States monitor the activities of Medicaid MCOs in much the same way that the federal government monitors the activities of MA plans. External review and required reporting are similar to the processes described for MA, except that both the review and the reports contain measures and metrics that are specific to Medicaid.

CONCLUSION

Medicare and Medicaid, as entitlement healthcare programs managed at the federal and state levels, together represent enormous expenditures of U.S. tax dollars. Medicare, by implementing managed care, has been able to better measure and manage certain aspects of quality of care, improve its healthcare benefits, and better realize the value of the money it spends. The creation of the Part D drug benefit provided greater benefits to those persons who enroll in that program, and managing this benefit has become a major area of focus for managed care.

State Medicaid programs have also successfully used managed care to manage costs, improve access, and enhance the coordination of care, which explains why most states have incorporated managed care into their Medicaid programs. The ACA contains provisions for the expansion of Medicaid eligibility as part of its overall goal of increasing coverage, but because of a ruling by the U.S. Supreme Court, states can choose to not expand Medicaid coverage. Because Medicare and Medicaid are government programs and have widely different characteristics, MCOs that undertake to serve Medicare and Medicaid populations must be prepared to focus or modify their operations to meet the programs' special requirements.

CHAPTER 8

Laws and Regulations in Managed Care

Tom Wilder, JD

LEARNING OBJECTIVES

- Describe the basic structure of state and federal oversight of managed care organizations (MCOs)
- Identify key state and federal laws and regulations governing managed care
- Explain the interaction of state and federal laws affecting managed care, what happens when there is a conflict between state and federal requirements, and the role of the courts
- Discuss the role of nongovernmental organizations in the regulation of MCOs

---

INTRODUCTION

Note to the Reader

Many of the topics covered in this chapter are discussed in greater or lesser detail in other chapters as well, but usually only as they apply to some aspect of operations. This chapter brings them all together to provide the overall framework for the regulation of MCOs. The Medicare Modernization Act (MMA) of 2003 also has a significant impact on private Medicare Advantage (MA) MCOs, but since that topic occupies more than half of the Medicare and Medicaid chapter, it has been omitted from this chapter.

Traditionally, states have regulated health insurers and health maintenance organizations (HMOs), referred to collectively as MCOs. State oversight traces its origins to the enactment of the McCarran-Ferguson Act by the U.S. Congress in 1945; this act gave states the authority to oversee insurance products, including health coverage. As more individuals and employers purchased health insurance, states began passing laws regulating managed care. The laws covered issues such as the following:

- Establishing solvency requirements, also referred to as statutory net worth
- Requiring coverage for certain medical conditions, also referred to as mandated benefits
- Establishing requirements for healthcare provider networks, also referred to as access requirements
- Setting standards for medical review of claims, including appeals of benefits coverage denials
- Standards for licensing MCOs and insurance agents
- Other consumer protections

Increasingly, MCOs and managed care are subject to federal laws and regulations in addition to state oversight. Starting with the passage of the Health Maintenance Organization (HMO) Act in 1973, Congress and the federal regulatory agencies have played a significant role in how managed care is provided. Laws such as the Employee Retirement Income Security Act (ERISA), Health Insurance Portability and Accountability Act (HIPAA), and the recently enacted Patient Protection and Affordable Care Act (ACA) have vastly expanded federal regulation of MCOs.

There is a great degree of interaction between state and federal laws and regulations. For example, the insurance market reform provisions of HIPAA were based in large part on existing state laws regulating insurance. Similarly, many of the requirements in the ACA enacted in 2010 modified state laws and regulations affecting MCOs and managed care.

This chapter provides an overview of the state and federal agencies regulating MCOs, discusses the key state and federal laws and regulations on managed care, and explains what happens when state and federal laws governing MCOs and managed care conflict. It also discusses the key role played by the courts and by certain types of nongovernmental organizations—such as the National Association of Insurance Commissioners (NAIC)—in setting standards for MCOs.

It should be understood, however, that state and federal laws on managed care are evolving. While this chapter provides a general understanding of how MCOs are regulated at the time of publication, up-to-date resources should be consulted for legal or compliance guidance.

MCO STRUCTURE AND ORGANIZATION

All health insurers use managed care techniques to one degree or another in providing health coverage. While this chapter discusses state and federal regulation of MCOs, the same laws and regulations apply equally to other types of health insurers. MCOs are typically divided into several broad types of structures:

- HMOs, which provide coverage of physician services either directly as a closed panel plan (group or staff model) or through a network of contracted physicians as an open panel plan (independent practice association [IPA] or direct contract model). Enrollees must receive care from one of the physicians or hospitals participating in the HMO network. In the HMO structure, members usually must select a primary care physician (PCP), who is then responsible for the individual's care, and who must approve any referral of a patient for services provided by a specialist provider.
- Point-of-service (POS) plans, which have the structure of an HMO but also cover some level of out-of-network care. The enrollee is responsible for the cost that is not paid by the POS plan.
- Preferred provider organizations (PPOs), which provide coverage through a contracted network, but also cover services obtained on an out-of-network basis. Medical services outside the PPO network will be paid at a lower rate by the MCO, with the enrollee being responsible for any cost difference.
- High-deductible health plans (HDHPs) and HDHPs with optional pretax savings accounts such consumer-directed health plans (CDHPs)

using either a health savings account (HSA), a healthcare reimbursement account (HRA), or the somewhat related medical savings account (MSA).

MCOs and other health insurers provide coverage in three distinct markets: (1) insurance coverage purchased by individuals, (2) group coverage provided by employers and/or labor unions and paid for by employer and employee premiums, and (3) government programs such as Medicaid and Medicare.* This chapter discusses state and federal regulation of the individual insurance market and coverage provided to groups; Medicare and Medicaid are discussed in their own chapter.

STATE REGULATION

State oversight of MCOs generally focuses on two aspects of health care: how managed care is provided to individuals and what MCOs can and cannot do in carrying out their business operations. Most of state regulation is carried out through the Department of Insurance. In some states, the Department of Health or Department of Managed Health Care may be responsible for regulating HMOs. For example, the California Department of Managed Health Care oversees HMOs, and in Pennsylvania the Department of Health has primary responsibility for HMO oversight.

At a basic level, state laws and regulations are intended to make sure individuals get the health coverage they pay for. These laws establish a wide range of managed care standards and requirements for MCOs, although they apply only to "insured" benefits coverage, meaning the MCO is at risk for costs.

Licensing MCOs

States typically require MCOs to conform to licensing requirements geared toward ensuring the MCO has sufficient management expertise, financial support, and adequate healthcare provider networks to do business. MCOs must obtain state approval to engage in operations and provide health coverage. For health insurers and any types of MCOs operated by a health insurer, state approval comes through an insurance license; for HMOs and any HMO-based MCOs (e.g., most POS plans), state approval comes through a certificate of authority (COA). States also regulate any holding company that owns or controls the MCO and any subsidiaries of the MCO.

---

* Benefits plans for governmental employees and elected officials are considered to be forms of employer-based group coverage.

In addition, the state licenses insurance agents and brokers who sell insurance coverage on behalf of the MCO to individuals and employers. The agent and broker licensing requirements address compensation paid to the agent or broker, education and training, and consumer protections. States may also require agents and brokers to post a bond or other evidence of financial responsibility as a condition of doing business.

Informing Consumers

States have established extensive requirements for information given to individuals when they enroll in coverage provided by an MCO. MCOs must provide enrollees with an evidence of coverage (EOC) document that contains information about what is and is not covered, any requirements for preapproval of medical services, the doctors and hospitals that are in the MCO's provider network, procedures for filing grievances, and conditions under which the individual will be expected to pay part of the cost for medical care. States also control the language included in the application for coverage submitted by the individual or employer. Almost all states require the MCO to submit insurance forms and applications for preapproval prior to use.

In addition, states have laws and regulations requiring MCOs to provide an explanation of benefits (EOB) form to individuals after a claim is submitted. The EOB describes the name of the doctor or hospital, the medical services that were provided, the cost for the services, and the portions of that cost that are the responsibility of the MCO and the individual. The EOB must also disclose information on any denied claims and the individual's rights to appeal if the claim is not paid in full or in part by the MCO (for example, if the claim is denied because the MCO does not believe the service was medically necessary).

Protecting Health Information Privacy

State laws require MCOs to protect the privacy of any health information that is collected, used, or shared by the MCO. These laws typically give the MCO the right to use the individual's health information without consent for purposes of providing medical care or for carrying out business operations such as paying claims. Many state laws provide specific protection for certain types of "sensitive" information such as mental health conditions, substance abuse disorders, and sexually transmitted diseases. In addition, laws and regulations require MCOs to provide data security protections and to inform individuals if their information is compromised.

Requiring Coverage for Doctors and Medical Conditions

Almost all states have laws requiring MCOs to cover specified medical conditions (e.g., breast cancer, substance abuse disorders, mental health conditions), certain categories of medical providers (e.g., chiropractors, midwives, physician assistants), and medical services (e.g., bone marrow transplants, maternity care, hearing aids). These "mandated benefits" vary from state to state. The laws are intended to make sure patients have access to a full range of healthcare benefits from the MCO. MCOs are permitted, however, to determine whether a mandated benefit or service is medically necessary before providing coverage.

Overseeing Utilization Review and Quality Assurance

Utilization review (UR), also called utilization management (UM), is the process used by MCOs to determine if a covered medical service is medically necessary and, as a result, is a covered benefit. Typically, the MCO will use nationally recognized medical guidelines and input from healthcare provider specialists to develop medical necessity review standards for various types of services. In some cases, the MCO will require a patient to get prior authorization before an elective service is provided; in other situations, retrospective review may be applied. Almost all states have laws and regulations governing the situations in which UR may be used by the MCO and the qualifications of any healthcare providers used by the MCO to determine if the service is medically necessary.

Most states also require MCOs to have a quality assurance (QA) program, also referred to as a quality management (QM) program. The most common types of MCO that are required to have a QA/QM program are HMOs and HMO-based POS plans. Some states also require PPOs to have one. The definition of an acceptable QA/QM program varies from state to state, and many states default to the standards set by a health plan accreditation organization.

Contracting with Healthcare Providers

MCOs contract with physicians and hospitals to provide services to enrollees. State laws and regulations govern healthcare provider networks and contracts between the MCO and the providers. These laws address how disputes between the provider and the MCO must be handled, how quickly claims from the provider must be paid (and penalties for late payment), and when an MCO is allowed to drop a provider from the network. In addition, a number of states have passed "any willing provider" laws that require the MCO to accept any healthcare provider who is willing to accept the terms and conditions of the network.

Assuring Adequate Provider Networks

Most states have network adequacy laws requiring MCOs to have sufficient healthcare providers available for enrollees. Network adequacy, also called network access, is typically measured based on the ratio of healthcare providers to enrollees, the location of a physician's office or inpatient facility in relation to the enrollee, and waiting times for appointments. In addition, a number of states have laws mandating that HMOs that require an enrollee to designate a primary care physician must allow the individual to designate any healthcare provider or specialist as his or her primary care physician.

Protection Against Balance Billing

Most MCOs use a contracted provider network to deliver care to the plan's enrollees. In turn, states typically have laws requiring MCOs' provider contracts to include language prohibiting the provider from requiring patients to pay any amount of the cost for medical services not paid by the MCO except for any copayments or coinsurance specified in the EOC document. If an enrollee goes outside the network for care, he or she will end up paying more of the cost for those services because the provider has no contract with the plan.

Assuring a Fair Insurance Market

State insurance market rules govern how much the MCO can charge in insurance premiums for coverage offered to individuals and employers. The laws generally divide the market into three segments: (1) coverage sold to individuals, (2) coverage offered to small employers (generally, businesses with 1 to 50 employees), and (3) coverage offered to large employers (businesses with more than 50 employees). The ACA, however, changed the definitions so that starting in 2016 a small group will mean a business with up to 100 employees and a large group means a business with more than 100 employees.

The insurance market rules typically apply the following standards to MCOs when establishing insurance premium rates and offering coverage to individuals and employers:

- Guaranteed availability: The health coverage must be provided to all individuals and employers that want to purchase coverage, although this ability may be limited to designated open enrollment periods.
- Guaranteed renewability: The MCO is required to renew health coverage provided to individuals and employers for another year unless the individual or employer fails to pay premiums or has engaged in fraud.

- No preexisting condition exclusions: The MCO cannot exclude or limit coverage for any conditions (e.g., diabetes or cancer) that the individual had when he or she enrolled in coverage.
- Rating factors: MCOs are prohibited from varying the cost of coverage except for factors based on the age of the individual, family composition (e.g., self-only versus family coverage), and the individual's participation in a wellness program (e.g., some MCOs may provide a premium credit if the enrollee successfully completes a tobacco cessation program).
- Limits on rating: States set limits on the premiums that can be charged by an MCO in the individual and small group markets. States typically take one of three approaches to the insurance market: (1) a pure community rating, in which all individuals or groups are charged the same rate; (2) an adjusted community rating, in which rates may vary based on demographic or other factors; and (3) rating bands, where rates may vary for individuals or groups based on a percentage factor. With the last approach, for example, rates charged to small businesses might be allowed to vary no more than 20% between the lowest premium and the highest premium charged by the MCO for coverage in the market. The ACA includes limits as well.
- Nondiscrimination: MCOs may not charge individuals more for coverage based on a health status factor such as their health condition, disability, and prior medical history.
- Preapproval of premium rates: Most states require MCOs to submit rates in advance to the state Insurance Department, Department of Health, or Department of Managed Care for approval prior to use.
- Continuation of coverage: Most states require MCOs to offer individuals who lose coverage through an employer the opportunity to purchase coverage in the individual insurance market (these requirements may be limited to businesses with fewer than 20 employees because of federal ERISA continuation coverage requirements applicable to employers with 20 or more employees).

Assuring MCO Solvency

States typically require MCOs to meet solvency standards, thereby assuring that the MCO has sufficient financial resources available to pay medical claims for members for which the plan, not the employer, is at risk. This requirement is also called statutory net worth or sometimes statutory reserves. The state laws establish rules that require MCOs to submit quarterly and annual financial reports, including the amount of surplus financial capital the MCO must have available at all times, as determined under statutory accounting principles (SAP), based on risk-based capital (RBC) levels.

States have the authority to examine the accounting and financial records of MCOs and to take action if an MCO's statutory surplus levels fall too low. Many states have a guarantee fund that is available to assist MCOs in financial trouble; the guarantee funds are subsidized by MCOs and other health insurers doing business in the state. When the statutory surplus falls to a certain level but is still higher than the statutory minimum, a state has the right to intervene and place specific demands on the MCO for improving its surplus within a set period of time. If an MCO's surplus levels fall too low, the state has the authority to take over the MCO. At that point, it may attempt to rehabilitate the MCO, but it is far more likely that the state will seek to sell the troubled MCO to another, healthier plan. Failing that, the state may be left with the prospect of dissolving the MCO and distributing its members to other plans in the same service area.

Assessing Market Conduct

Market conduct involves the state's regulation of MCO practices that directly affect consumers—for example, marketing, advertising, sales practices, and language used in documents provided by the MCO to prospective purchasers and enrollees. Many states have enacted laws prohibiting unfair or deceptive trade practices such as not promptly handling a claim for benefits or engaging in misleading advertising. State insurance regulatory agencies will periodically carry out market conduct examinations at MCOs to review how complaints are handled, how products are marketed and sold, and other processes affecting consumers.

Resolving Enrollee Grievances and Appeals

State laws dictate how MCOs must resolve grievances with an enrollee as well as enrollee appeals of benefits denials. Grievances are formal complaints by enrollees that do not include a denial of benefits coverage. MCOs typically must respond to formal grievances in writing, although other laws such as medical peer review confidentiality protection laws may limit the amount of detail in the response.

Laws about appeals of benefits denials typically provide for additional review of the claim, establish the time limits for review, and permit the individual or his or her physician to present additional documentation on why the medical service should be covered. This process is called an internal review. If the appeal involves a denial of a medical benefit based on medical necessity, the MCO reviewer must have specific training and expertise in the service that is being appealed—for example, a cancer specialist must review appeals involving benefits denials related to services for cancer.

If the MCO and the enrollee are not able to resolve the appeal of a medical claim where the denial is based on a determination by the MCO that the service was not medically necessary, the dispute may be submitted to an independent review organization (IRO)* that will determine whether the individual is entitled to coverage. This process is called an external review. The IRO cannot be affiliated with the MCO and must have a panel of medical experts qualified to review medical claims. Most states require that more than one IRO be available, and the state, not the MCO, determines which cases go to which IROs.

Premium Taxes

All states assess a surcharge on every premium dollar paid to MCOs. These taxes are used to fund the operations of the state regulatory agencies as well as other state general fund expenditures. In many states, premium taxes are the second largest source of state revenue after revenues from individual and business income taxes.

FEDERAL REGULATION

Starting with the HMO Act in 1973 and ERISA in 1974, the federal government has assumed increasing oversight of managed care and MCOs in the United States. These laws typically work in coordination with, and sometimes take the place of, state laws and regulations. Conflicts between state and federal laws pose challenges for MCOs as well as for their individual and employer customers.

Federal regulation and oversight of MCOs is carried out by a number of agencies:

- The U.S. Department of Health and Human Services (DHHS) has primary responsibility for establishing managed care rules and providing oversight of MCOs. DHHS also sets the regulatory standards for health information privacy, data security, and electronic healthcare transactions and code sets.

---

* IROs are also used by Medicare and state Medicaid programs in very specific ways. The same term—IRO—is often also used in the commercial sector for external reviews, though not always. Medicare and Medicaid typically contract with only one IRO in a region, while most states require at least two IROs for external reviews in the commercial sector. A Medicare/Medicaid IRO may also participate in external reviews in the commercial market, but not always.

- The U.S. Department of Labor (DOL) sets rules governing health coverage benefits provided by employers and unions. These rules are enforced under the federal ERISA law.
- The U.S. Department of the Treasury has authority to enforce tax laws governing health coverage. The federal tax code has an important role in determining how individuals and employers purchase health coverage offered by MCOs.
- The U.S. Department of Justice (DOJ) has responsibility for enforcing criminal laws and penalties against MCOs for violations of federal standards such as the health information privacy laws and laws on fraud and abuse involving government programs such as Medicare.

Although Congress has enacted an extensive set of laws and regulations governing managed care, five laws have the most significant impact on MCOs:

- The HMO Act, which provided the first federal recognition of health maintenance organizations and set standards for managed care
- ERISA, which established uniform national rules for employer- and union-sponsored health coverage
- HIPAA, which includes health insurance market rules, health information privacy and data security protections, and standards for electronic healthcare transactions and code sets
- The ACA, which built on the standards in ERISA and HIPAA and enacted additional requirements applicable to health insurance markets
- The federal tax code, which provides tax preferences to encourage individuals and employers to purchase health coverage

Legislation does not operate in a vacuum, and new laws frequently involve issues addressed in other laws that existed prior to a new law's passage. In almost all cases, it is neither practical nor desirable to repeal an older law, so new legislation typically must amend each relevant existing law accordingly. Because of that, the HMO Act, HIPAA, and the ACA also amend the Public Health Service Act (PHSA), which was passed in 1941.

Health Maintenance Organization Act (1973)

The HMO Act established the first federal requirements for "federally qualified" HMOs and provided loans and other financial guarantees for HMO start-up costs. Prior to the HMO Act, managed care organizations were found in only a handful of states such as California and the Pacific Northwest. Federally qualified

HMOs were required to provide a specified package of "basic" and "supplemental" health services to enrollees including inpatient and outpatient care, home health services, preventive care, laboratory services, and emergency care. The HMO Act also required HMOs to meet solvency standards, provide procedures for handling member grievances and appeals, and establish programs for quality assurance.

Employee Retirement Income Security Act (1974)

ERISA was enacted by Congress to provide a uniform legal framework for health and pension benefits offered by employers and unions. Congress passed this law in response to the varied and sometimes conflicting standards for health and pension benefits that raised operational challenges for businesses with workforces in multiple states. ERISA generally preempts state laws affecting health benefits provided by employers and unions.

Employers and unions have two options for providing health coverage: They can "fully insure" the benefits by purchasing insurance from an MCO or other health insurer, or they can "self-fund" by assuming the risk for the benefits' cost by setting aside sufficient financial resources to pay claims. In the latter case, the employer or union may contract with an existing MCO or a free-standing third-party administrator (TPA) to handle the various administrative functions of the health plan.

ERISA sets out a number of requirements for employer and union health plans that frequently mirror state rules governing MCOs and managed care. The ERISA standards include the following considerations:

- Consumer information disclosures: The health plan must provide enrollees with a summary plan description (SPD) describing the coverage available under the plan and any limits or restrictions, the doctors and hospitals in the plan's network, procedures for grievances and appeals, and information on the financial structure of the plan (i.e., are the benefits insured or self-funded by the employer or union).
- Fiduciary standards: Health plans are required to appoint a fiduciary that is responsible for operating the health plan and maintaining solvency. The fiduciary must operate in the interest of plan enrollees and in accordance with the plan documents such as the insurance coverage provided by the MCO. Fiduciaries are also prohibited from engaging in any self-dealing or other prohibited transactions. If the fiduciary breaches its duties to the health plan or enrollees, it may be subject to legal action by plan enrollees or the Department of Labor.

- Claims and appeals: ERISA requires health plans to establish procedures for enrollees to appeal denials of health coverage and places limits on how quickly reviews must be conducted by the MCO. Enrollees must be permitted to present evidence to the plan challenging the denial and to have their appeal reviewed by a plan representative with healthcare expertise. Denials of health coverage based on medical necessity may be submitted to an IRO if the enrollee is dissatisfied with the result of the appeal to the health plan. If the claim dispute is not resolved by the health plan or after submission to the IRO, the enrollee may file a lawsuit against the plan in federal court to recover the amount of the healthcare benefit.
- Reporting: Health plans are required to file annual reports with the Departments of Labor and the Treasury describing the type of coverage provided, the means by which coverage is financed, and the number of enrollees in the plan.
- Continuation of coverage: A later amendment to ERISA requires employer and union health plans to allow enrollees to continue coverage for a period of time after they leave employment. Spouses and dependent children may also be entitled to continuation coverage in certain instances. Premiums charged for continuation coverage may not exceed 102% of the cost originally paid by the individual and his or her employer under the employer or union health plan. The continuation coverage requirements apply to group plans sponsored by employers with 20 or more employees (as discussed elsewhere in this chapter, states typically establish continuation of coverage requirements for businesses with fewer than 20 employees). This provision is intended to help individuals preserve their health coverage options after they lose their employer- or union-sponsored health coverage.

Health Insurance Portability and Accountability Act (1996)

Congress enacted HIPAA to provide a standard set of insurance market requirements for health insurers, including MCOs. HIPAA set out the first significant set of federal standards for managed care for individuals and coverage provided to employer and union health plans. Many of these standards had previously been enacted by states, but the specific state requirements varied. The federal law also established the first national requirements for health information privacy, data security, and electronic healthcare transactions and code sets. Key provisions of HIPAA include the following:

- Definition of group size: HIPAA defined a small employer as a business with up to 50 employees and a large employer as a business with more than 50 employees. As discussed elsewhere in this chapter, the ACA subsequently modified these definitions: Starting in 2016, small employers will be businesses with up to 100 employees.
- Guaranteed availability of coverage: HIPAA required MCOs to provide health coverage to any small employer (or an employee of the small employer) that wants to purchase coverage, but only if certain conditions were met, such as only a small time lapse having passed between when prior coverage ended and when new coverage was applied for. The ACA subsequently extended this right to all employers regardless of group size and to all enrollees in the individual market.
- Guaranteed renewability of coverage: MCOs are required to renew coverage for any employer (or any employee of the employer) that wants to continue its health plan for another year unless the employer or employee fails to pay premiums or engages in fraud or the MCO is leaving the market in a state or discontinuing a particular type of coverage. The ACA extended this right to enrollees in the individual insurance market.
- Preexisting condition limits: Under HIPAA, MCOs were not permitted to impose preexisting condition limits on enrollees for coverage sold to employers and unions, except in very limited situations. The ACA eliminated all preexisting condition limits or exclusions.
- Discrimination based on health status: HIPAA prohibits employers and MCOs from denying coverage or charging more for coverage based on the health status of the individual. Health status includes the individual's medical condition, claims experience, medical history, disability, or genetic information. This requirement was extended by the ACA to enrollees in the individual insurance market.
- Special enrollment periods: Employer- and union-sponsored health plans typically enroll individuals once each year during an open enrollment period. HIPAA gives individuals the right to enroll in group coverage outside of the open enrollment period due to certain "life events," such as the birth or adoption of a child, marriage, divorce, or a spouse losing coverage.
- Health information privacy and data security: HIPAA established standards for the protection of personally identifiable health information, including

protections for the collection, use, and disclosure of such information by the MCO. MCOs are restricted from using an individual's health information without the person's consent unless the use is for purposes of payment, provision of health care, or certain types of healthcare operations. MCOs are also prohibited from using health information for marketing purposes, such as selling the addresses of their enrollees to other businesses. These requirements extend to the business associates of the MCO that may be collecting, disclosing, or using health information on behalf of the MCO.

- Electronic healthcare transactions and code sets: HIPAA developed requirements for the electronic sharing of information between doctors and hospitals and MCOs, such as the transmittal of claims and information concerning the individual's eligibility for coverage.
- Mental Health Parity Act and Mental Health Parity and Addiction Equity Act: These two amendments to HIPAA set out requirements to provide coverage for the treatment of mental health conditions and substance abuse disorders on the same basis as coverage provided for medical and surgical benefits. For example, MCOs cannot impose limits on the number of days of treatment for a mental health condition if they do not impose similar treatment limits for medical conditions. The parity requirements also extend to "nonquantitative" treatment limits such as utilization review—for example, the process used by the MCO to determine the medical necessity of mental health treatments must not be more restrictive than the process used for reviewing medical and surgical benefits.
- Genetic Information Nondiscrimination Act: This amendment to HIPAA placed limits on the collection and sharing of genetic information, including family history, and prohibits use of genetic information in setting premium rates.
- Newborns and Mothers' Health Protection Act: This amendment to HIPAA requires MCOs to provide coverage for hospital stays of up to 48 hours after a vaginal delivery and 96 hours after a delivery by cesarean section.
- Women's Health and Cancer Rights Act: This amendment to HIPAA requires MCOs to provide coverage for reconstructive breast surgery after a mastectomy.

Patient Protection and Affordable Care Act

The ACA significantly amended the standards set out in ERISA and HIPAA and imposed changes on how coverage is offered by MCOs. The provisions of the ACA also affect, and in many cases supersede, state laws governing managed care and MCOs. Many of the ACA provisions discussed in this section became effective upon the law's enactment in 2010, while others—such as the creation of the health insurance exchanges and the individual and employer coverage mandates—did not start until 2013 and 2014.

Key provisions of the ACA include the following:

- Definition of markets by size: The ACA defines a small employer as a business with 1 to 100 employees, while a large employer is any business with more than 100 employees. States are, however, permitted to retain the old definitions of a small employer (up to 50 employees) and a large employer (more than 50 employees) until 2016.
- Guaranteed availability and renewability of coverage, and limits on preexisting conditions: The ACA extended and broadened HIPAA's requirements for MCOs to make coverage available to nearly all individuals and companies. HIPAA's guaranteed renewability requirements were extended to enrollees in the individual market. Additionally, MCOs are prohibited from imposing any preexisting condition limits or exclusions for coverage in the individual or group markets.
- Nondiscrimination: MCOs are prohibited from varying the premiums paid by individuals—whether purchasing coverage in the individual market or provided through their employer—based on their health status (e.g., an individual's health condition, disability, or medical history). This provision expanded on the earlier HIPAA requirements applicable to coverage provided to employees.
- Rating restrictions: The ACA limits the variability in premiums that may be charged by an MCO for health coverage. Rates may vary only based on family composition, geographic region, age (but only within restricted limits), and whether the individual uses tobacco (however, to assess a tobacco use surcharge, the MCO must waive the extra cost if the individual participates in a tobacco cessation program).
- Consumer information: MCOs are required to provide any prospective purchasers and enrollees with a summary of benefits and coverage (SBC) document that describes what is covered or excluded, any cost-sharing requirements such as deductibles and coinsurance, and the amounts the individual may be expected to pay for certain types of medical services.
- Coverage for preventive benefits: MCOs must provide coverage for a specified list of preventive benefits such as routine physical examinations,

laboratory tests, immunizations, and contraceptive services for women. The enrollee cannot be charged for the preventive services—for example, routine physician office visit copayments are no longer permitted. The list of preventive benefits is maintained and periodically updated by the U.S. Preventive Services Task Force, the Advisory Committee on Immunization Practices of the Centers for Disease Control, and the Health Resources and Services Administration.

- Coverage for children up to age 26: MCOs that offer family coverage must agree to continue coverage for children up to age 26.

- Coverage for emergency services: MCOs must provide coverage for emergency services for all enrollees and cannot require the individual to pay a higher level of cost sharing for emergency care provided by non-network providers than the individual would pay if it has been provided by network providers. The MCO is also prohibited from imposing any precertification or authorization requirements for emergency care.

- Access to primary care: Individuals enrolled in MCOs that require enrollees to designate a primary care physician cannot limit the individual's choice of providers. For example, women are permitted to designate their OB/GYN as their primary care physician.

- Essential health benefits: MCOs are required to provide an essential health benefits (EHB) package to all enrollees in individual and small employer group market coverage, including prescription drugs, inpatient and outpatient services, mental health and substance use disorder coverage, and habilitative services. In addition, coverage offered to families must include pediatric dental and vision benefits. The EHB coverage must provide an actuarial value of at least 60% (i.e., the value of the health benefits provided to an average enrollee is at least 60% of the total allowed benefits cost).

- No annual or lifetime benefit limits: MCOs are prohibited from imposing any annual or lifetime coverage limits on EHBs.

- Health insurance exchanges: The ACA established insurance exchanges (called "marketplaces") in each state as a mechanism for individuals and small businesses to purchase coverage. The state may choose to run the exchange or may partner with the federal government in running the exchange; the federal government is responsible for the exchange if the state fails to do so. Coverage in the exchange is divided into "metal levels": Copper plans (at least 60% actuarial value); Silver plans (at least 70% actuarial value); Gold plans (at least 80% actuarial value); and Platinum plans (at least 90% actuarial value). In addition, MCOs may offer individuals younger than age 30 the option to purchase "catastrophic" coverage with a higher deductible (and therefore lower premiums and actuarial value).

- Premium tax credits: Individuals with lower family incomes are eligible for a tax credit to assist with the purchase of health coverage through an exchange. Additionally, certain small businesses may qualify for tax credits for exchange health coverage offered to their employees.

- Medical loss ratios: MCOs offering insurance coverage are required to meet annual medical loss ratio (MLR) standards. In general, the MLR is defined as the amount of the premium dollar that spent by the MCO on healthcare claims and on activities to improve health care (for example, wellness programs). In each state, coverage sold to individuals and small employers must have an MLR of 80% or higher, and coverage sold to large employers (and to individuals in MA plans) must have an MLR of 85% or higher. If the MCO does not meet the MLR target in a particular state, the MCO must refund any excess to enrollees. For example, if an MCO has an MLR of 75% for coverage sold in the individual market in a state, the MCO must refund 5% of the premiums collected back to individuals.

- Individual coverage mandate: As of 2014, almost all individuals are required to have minimum essential coverage (MEC) such as insurance coverage purchased in the individual market or an exchange, coverage from their employer, or coverage from Medicaid or Medicare. Individuals who do not maintain MEC for themselves and any family members will be assessed a penalty. There are exceptions for low-income individuals and those with religious objections to maintaining insurance coverage.

- Employer coverage mandate: Starting in 2015 all employers with 100 or more full-time employees (50 or more in 2016) must provide coverage or pay a penalty (this requirement was originally scheduled to go into effect in 2014, but was delayed one year). The employer-sponsored health coverage must be affordable (i.e., the cost cannot exceed 9.5% of the employee's household income) and provide minimum value (i.e., the coverage must provide an actuarial value of at least 60%). The employer penalty applies only if the employer has one or more full-time employees who receive a tax credit for purchasing coverage through an exchange.

- Health insurance fees: Starting in 2014, a new federal annual fee is assessed on MCOs and other health insurers. The total industry fee in 2014 was $8 billion, increasing to $11.3 billion in 2015 and 2016, $13.9 billion in 2017, and $14.3 billion in 2018. The total industry fee is indexed for inflation thereafter. Each health insurer's share of the total industry fee is based on its respective share of the insurance market for insurance sold to individuals and employers and government programs (e.g., Medicare and Medicaid). For nonprofit insurers, only 50% of premiums are taken into account for purposes of assessing the fee, and nonprofit plans that receive 80% or more of their income based on covering low-income, elderly, and/ or disable individuals are exempt from the fee.

- Drug and medical device manufacturer fees: Starting in 2012, fees are assessed on manufacturers of drugs and medical devices. The total fees for 2013–2014 were $2.8 billion. They increase to $4.1 billion by 2018, but then fall back down to $2.8 billion in 2019 and thereafter.
- High-value plan tax: Starting in 2018, employers that provide high-value coverage (or their insurer or MCO) will be assessed an excise tax of 40% of the cost of the plan that is above a benchmark set by statute ($10,200 for self-only coverage and $27,500 for family coverage). These cost benchmarks will be adjusted upward for inflation in later years. In addition, individuals in certain types of "high-risk" professions, such as public safety employees, are subject to higher benchmarks in determining if their health coverage is subject to the excise tax.

The ACA provisions are still being implemented by the federal regulatory agencies, and the overall impact on MCOs and managed care will not be fully realized for many years. In addition, the ACA has been subject to several legal challenges and litigation involving the law will continue.

Federal Tax Code

The federal tax code provides incentives for individuals and employers to purchase health coverage. For example, the cost of health coverage is fully tax deductible to employers and to their employees. Enrollees purchasing coverage in the individual insurance market may deduct the cost of health insurance premiums and other medical costs to the extent these expenses exceed 10% of the individual's adjusted gross income. In addition, the ACA allows certain individuals purchasing coverage through an exchange to qualify for a tax subsidy.

The tax code also recognizes a number of tax-advantaged spending accounts—namely, health reimbursement arrangements (HRAs), health savings accounts (HSAs), and health flexible spending arrangements (FSAs). HRAs and health FSAs may be offered only in conjunction with employer- or union-sponsored health coverage. HSAs may be used by individuals or by enrollees in employer- and union-sponsored health plans. With all of these accounts, the individual (and in some cases the employer) contributes money into the account on a fully tax-deductible basis; this money may then be used for qualified medical expenses.

CONFLICTS, PREEMPTION, AND THE ROLE OF THE COURTS

State and federal laws and regulations frequently address the same issues involving managed care and MCOs. For example, the states had long-standing insurance market rules that were duplicated—and in some cases addressed differently—by HIPAA and the ACA. While ERISA governs self-funded employer- and union-sponsored health benefits plans and is regulated at the federal level by the DOL, states are responsible for oversight of the MCOs that provide insured health benefits plans, meaning health insurance coverage, to the employer's health plan. Determining whether state or federal laws should prevail and resolving conflicts poses challenges for MCOs and for state and federal regulatory agencies.

Two general legal principles govern whether a state law is preempted by the federal requirements. First, state laws may be preempted only if they directly conflict with a specific federal requirement. HIPAA and the ACA are generally enforced by the Department of Health and Human Services through its authority under the PHSA. The PHSA preempts state laws that "prevent the application" of the federal law. More plainly stated, if the MCO is unable to follow both the state law and the federal law, the federal requirements prevail.

For example, states typically provide that MCOs count only the number of full-time employees when determining whether the business is a small employer or a large employer. However, HIPAA and the ACA are structured such that the employer counts all employees—both full-time and part-time—in determining whether the business is a small employer or a large employer. Because it is not possible for the MCO providing coverage to employers to follow both the state counting method and the federal requirements, the federal standards take precedence and the state standards are preempted. In another example, the HIPAA electronic transaction and code sets standards preempt any state laws that are intended to regulate the electronic exchange of information between healthcare providers and MCOs.

In another example, states typically require MCOs to cover certain medical conditions and/or healthcare providers. Because federal law generally does not include similar coverage mandates (other than the ACA requirements to cover preventive services and emergency care), MCOs must comply with the state coverage mandates.

There are, however, situations in which a federal law is structured such that states are never permitted to regulate the same set of issues. One of the most significant of these areas involves ERISA, which generally preempts any state attempt to regulate a self-funded employer- or union-sponsored health benefits plan. For example, states are not permitted to tell the employer that self-funds its benefits how quickly claims must be paid, because ERISA leaves such regulation to the Department of Labor. However, a state can—and frequently does—regulate an MCO that is insuring the employer plan. In other words, the state can tell an MCO that is the insurer of an employee benefits plan—but not an MCO that is administering a self-funded benefits plan—how quickly claims must be paid.

Resolution of these conflicts is frequently handled by the judicial system. State and federal courts are often asked by an MCO, or by enrollees, employers, or healthcare providers, to determine whether state law is preempted by the federal requirements. One of the primary areas of conflict and federal lawsuits involves questions of whether ERISA or state law should prevail.

Courts are also frequently asked to interpret other state and federal laws governing MCOs and managed care. Significant litigation has arisen over implementing the ACA, with the federal courts ruling on the validity of various provisions of the law. The U.S. Supreme Court has determined that the ACA is a valid law. However, it also found that two provisions of the ACA—one requiring states to expand Medicaid coverage and another telling certain types of closely held corporations that have religious objections that they must provide contraceptive coverage—are void. Additional legal challenges to the ACA are ongoing, and the Supreme Court is expected to handle more ACA-related appeals over the next few years.

ROLE OF NONGOVERNMENTAL ORGANIZATIONS

MCOs are impacted by a number of nongovernmental organizations,* including the following:

- Two different types of standards setting entities
- Independent review organizations
- National Association of Insurance Commissioners (NAIC)

---

* Nongovernmental organizations are often referred to by the acronym "NGO," but its use is inconsistent. For example, NGO is used more often for organizations working in other countries than for organizations working within the United States. This practice explains why a chapter—and an entire text—that are otherwise stuffed with acronyms does not use the acronym "NGO."

Standards-Settings Entities

Two types of standards-setting entities influence MCO operations. The first are organizations that establish the electronic healthcare transactions and code sets used by MCOs and healthcare providers to exchange information; the second are health plan accreditation organizations.

Designated Standards Maintenance Organizations

Under HIPAA, the Department of Health and Human Services (DHHS) is responsible for the development, maintenance, and modification of relevant electronic data interchange standards that must be used by covered entities. DHHS does so by delegating these tasks to designated standards maintenance organizations (DMSOs). Six of the DSMOs are public organizations. For example, the National Council for Prescription Drug Programs (NCPDP) develops the format requirements for electronic healthcare transactions related to drug benefits, and the Accredited Standards Committee X12 (ANSI ASC X12) develops the format requirements for electronic healthcare transactions related to the business interactions be
tween healthcare providers and MCOs.

An additional three DSMOs are nonpublic—for example, the American Medical Association, which maintains the Current Procedural Technology, Fourth Revisions (CPT-4) procedure codes, and the Centers for Disease Control and Prevention (CDC), which maintains the versions of the International Classification of Disease (ICD) codes.

Accreditation Organizations

Health plan accreditation organizations also set standards that most plans follow, although unlike HIPAA transaction and code sets, being accredited by virtue of following accreditation standards is not mandatory. Accreditation standards apply to a wide variety of managed care operations, such as UR/UM, QA/QM, provider network credentialing, and policies and procedures for making medical necessity determinations.

There are three recognized accreditation organizations in the United States. While they differ in their approach to accreditation, their standards are similar. Of these three accreditation organizations, the first two account for nearly all health plan accreditations, while the third focuses more on ambulatory healthcare facilities and providers:

- National Committee on Quality Assurance (NCQA)
- URAC (only the acronym is used)
- Accreditation Association for Ambulatory Health Care (AAAHC)

Accreditation may be voluntary, but most states accept accreditation as meeting the state's standards in the functional areas addressed by accreditation. CMS accepts accreditation as well for MCOs in the MA program.

Independent Review Organizations

State law and the ACA require claim disputes involving medically necessity determinations to be submitted for review by an independent review organization if an individual covered under a healthcare benefits plan wishes to appeal a coverage denial, including a denial following an internal re-review by the plan. The IRO provides a panel of medical experts who review claims. Both enrollees (or their healthcare providers) and the MCO have the opportunity to present additional information that may be needed to determine if the MCO must provide the coverage.

National Association of Insurance Commissioners

As the name indicates, the National Association of Insurance Commissioners is an association of chief state insurance and managed care regulators in the 50 states, District of Columbia, and U.S. territories. The NAIC provides the insurance regulatory agencies and their staffs with the opportunity to share information on developments involving MCOs and to discuss legal and regulatory challenges such as implementation of the ACA. The association develops model insurance laws and regulations affecting managed care—such as the Utilization Review Model Act—which are adopted by the states. In addition, the NAIC is responsible for creating the statutory accounting and risk-based capital standards used by MCOs and other insurers in financial reporting to the agencies. The NAIC also provides the insurance regulatory agencies with opportunities to coordinate financial and market conduct reviews of MCOs that operate on a national basis.

CONCLUSION

States continue to exercise significant control over the operations of managed care organizations and the provision of managed care to individuals. These requirements concern almost every aspect of managed care, from the types of organizations that may be licensed as MCOs, to the products offered to enrollees, to the premium rates that may be charged for insured coverage.

An increasing number of federal laws regulate the operations of managed care organizations. These laws directly govern MCOs, define how managed care may be provided, and regulate the employers and unions that contract with MCOs to administer their benefits plans. The federal requirements affect almost all aspects of managed care and MCO operations, including standards for how insurance coverage must be provided to individuals and employers, provisions affecting health benefits and group health plans, tax preferences for individual and group health coverage, and protections for health information.

Glossary of Terms and Acronyms*

AAAHC—See Accreditation Association for Ambulatory Health Care.

AAC—See Actual Acquisition Cost.

AAHC—See American Accreditation HealthCare Commission.

Abandonment Rate—The percentage of calls where the caller hangs up before reaching a service representative due to lengthy average speed to answer times.

ABN—See Advanced Beneficiary Notice of Noncoverage.

Abuse or Healthcare Abuse—A term that is not as well defined as fraud, abuse typically occurs if an activity abuses the healthcare system; for example, using billing codes that are related to, but pay higher than, the service actually provided, or charging outrageous fees.

ACA—See Patient Protection and Affordable Care Act.

Access Fee—A fee charged by a PPO or HMO for access to its provider network, including its payment terms, by an employer or another payer. See also Rental PPO.

---

* These are working definitions of common terms and acronyms in the health insurance and managed healthcare industry and related healthcare sectors. In such a dynamic industry, it is not possible to list every term or acronym in use because new ones come into use faster than any publication can keep up with them. Other terms may become obsolete or fall out of use, especially in the case of governmental agencies and programs. The entries included here are operational—not legal—definitions, and the reader must look to appropriate laws and regulations when legal matters are at issue. Some definitions in this glossary may also be disputed by others in the industry, and the author is open to receiving suggestions or different points of view from any such nitpickers.

Access Standards—Also called Network Adequacy Standards, these are Standards specifying the minimum number of providers in a specific geographic area that an HMO or other type of health plan must have to be able to market and sell in that area. Alternatively, drive times may be used to set the access standards. Access standards differ for PCPs and specialists, general and specialty hospitals, and urban and rural areas. For physicians, only those with open practices may be counted.

Accountable Care Organization (ACO)—A term coined by CMS and MedPAC, and used in the ACA, to describe an organized group of physicians, possibly including a hospital, that are supposed to coordinate the care for beneficiaries with high medical costs who are in traditional FFS Medicare. Those beneficiaries are not locked in or required to use the ACO. CMS assigns or attributes them to the ACO through statistical means. An overall target cost is calculated, and the ACO shares in savings if costs are less than the target, but pays back a portion of what it was paid if costs exceed the target. Despite being specifically addressed in the ACA, it is not known yet at the time of publication whether ACOs will work as intended.

Accreditation—Certification by a qualified neutral agency that an organization meets defined criteria for participation in a program. For payers, this means accreditation by NCQA, URAC, or (less commonly) AAAHC. For healthcare facilities, it most commonly means accreditation by The Joint Commission (TJC) or, for ambulatory facilities, TJC or AAAHC. Other agencies exist for different types of facilities such as rehabilitation, osteopathy, and so forth. See also Deeming.

Accreditation Association for Ambulatory Health Care (AAAHC)—An accreditation agency that focuses on ambulatory facilities such as ASCs, endoscopy centers, dialysis centers and so forth. It is also one of three accreditation agencies certified by CMS to accredit MA plans, along with NCQA and URAC.

Accrete—The process of adding new Medicare enrollees to a plan. See also Delete.

Accrual—The amount of money that is set aside to cover expenses. The accrual is the plan's best estimate of what those expenses are and (for medical expenses) is based on a combination of data from the authorization system, the claims system, lag studies, and the plan's prior history.

Accrual Accounting—Use of accruals for purposes of counting assets and debits. It differs from cash accounting, which is what you do when you balance your checkbook (assuming you do balance your checkbook).

ACD—See Automated Call Distributor.

ACGs—See Ambulatory Care Groups.

ACO—See Accountable Care Organization.

ACR—See Adjusted Community Rate.

Actual Acquisition Cost (AAC)—The actual cost a pharmacy or provider paid to acquire a drug or a device, as opposed to a published average.

Actuarial Assumptions—The assumptions that an actuary uses in calculating the expected costs and revenues of a healthcare plan. Examples include utilization rates, age and sex mix of enrollees, and cost for medical services.

Actuarial Equivalent—(1) In the ACA, an aggregate level of cost sharing. For example, a Silver Plan has the actuarial equivalent of 30% cost sharing, meaning the total of all deductibles, copayments, and coinsurance for an average member adds up to 30%. (2) Under Medicare Advantage, a health benefit plan that offers coverage similar to that provided by a standard benefit plan. Actuarially equivalent plans will not necessarily have the same premiums, cost-sharing requirements, or even benefits, but the expected average amount of cost-sharing by enrollees in the different plans will be the same.

Acuity—How sick a person is; typically used most often in the context of multiple chronic illnesses, but it can also be used in the context of a single costly illness.

ADGs—See Ambulatory Diagnostic Groups.

Adjudication—The management, processing, and final disposition of claims by a payer or health insurance company.

Adjusted Average per Capita Cost (AAPCC)—The amount of money spent on health care in a given area or by a given population.

Adjusted Community Rate (ACR)—A form of premium rating that does not take health status into account and that is instead based on factors such as age and geographic location. The ACA requires individual and small group health insurance to use adjusted community rates, with age-related adjustments limited to a 3 to 1 difference.

Administrative Contract Services (ACS)—See Administrative Services Only.

Administrative Services Only (ASO)—A contract between an insurance company or health plan administrator and a self-funded plan in which the insurance company or administrator performs administrative services only and does not assume any risk. Services usually include claims processing and member services, but may include other services such as actuarial analysis and utilization review. See also ERISA.

Admitted Asset—A financial asset of a health plan that can be converted to cash on short notice. See also Nonadmitted Asset, Net Worth, and Risk-Based Capital.

Advanced Beneficiary Notice of Noncoverage (ABN)—A form designated by CMS for use by providers and suppliers for all situations where Medicare payment is expected to be denied.

Adverse Selection—The problem of attracting members who are sicker than the general population (specifically, members who are sicker than was anticipated when the budget for medical costs was developed).

Affordable Care Act (ACA)—See Patient Protection and Affordable Care Act.

Age Band or Age-Banding—Putting individuals into different age groups for purposes of premium rate adjustments, with younger individuals paying lower premiums than older ones; applicable primarily to the individual and small group insurance markets. Under the ACA, the maximum difference between the lowest and highest age-banded premiums was 3 to 1 as of 2014.

Agency for Healthcare Research and Quality (AHRQ)—A federal agency charged with addressing a wide array of quality-related issues and evidence-based standards of care. An excellent resource for the most current thinking on these topics.

Agent—A person who is authorized by an HMO or an insurer to act on its behalf to negotiate, sell, and service coverage contracts. May be self-employed, employed by an agency, or employed by a broker.

AHIP—See America's Health Insurance Plans.

AHP—See Association Health Plan.

AHRQ—See Agency for Healthcare Research and Quality.

All Payer—A system in which the government—state or federal—sets payment rates for defined health services, which all payers, public and private, must follow. Potentially applies to hospitals and/or physicians. Used in many European nations but not (so far) in the United States, with the exception of Maryland where it applies to hospitals only. Also referred to as all payer rates or all payer fee schedule.

Allowed Charge—The maximum charge that a payer (such as Medicare, Medicaid, or a commercial health plan) will cover for a specific service, even if the amount billed is greater than the allowed charge.

ALOS—See LOS.

Alternative Medicine—See Complementary and Alternative Medicine.

Ambulatory Care Group (ACG)—A method of categorizing outpatient episodes that are based on resource use over time, modified by principal diagnosis, age, and sex. See also Ambulatory Diagnostic Group, Enhanced Ambulatory Patient Group, and Ambulatory Patient Classification.

Ambulatory Diagnostic Group (ADG)—A method of categorizing outpatient episodes. See also Enhanced Ambulatory Care Groups and Ambulatory Patient Group.

Ambulatory Patient Classification (APC)—A methodology used by CMS to pay facilities for ambulatory services. Like DRGs, APCs bundle various charges into a single payment. Unlike DRGs, they are based primarily on procedures, not diagnoses. They also differ from DRGs in that they can be added together, while DRGs are used in a hierarchy for purposes of calculating payment. APCs are an outgrowth of APGs.

Ambulatory Patient Group (APG)—See Enhanced Ambulatory Patient Group (EAPG).

Ambulatory Surgical Category (ASC)—A term used by Medicare in its Hospital Outpatient Prospective Payment System (HOPPS) program. It specifically refers to a payment term using CMS's methodology.

Ambulatory Surgical Center (ASC)—A facility for ambulatory procedures. The term may be applied to several types of outpatient facilities, not all of which are actually surgical, such as dialysis facilities and endoscopy facilities.

American Accreditation HealthCare Commission (AAHC)—A name once used by URAC, but now obsolete. See also URAC.

American National Standards Institute (ANSI)—An organization that develops and maintains standards for electronic data interchange. HIPAA mandates the use of ANSI X 12N standards for electronic transactions in the U.S. healthcare system.

America's Health Insurance Plans (AHIP)—The primary trade organization of health insurers and managed care organizations. Its areas of focus include legislative and lobbying efforts, education, certification of training in managed healthcare operations, and representation of the health insurance industry to the public. Initially there were three groups—Group Health Association of America (GHAA), American Managed Care and Review Association (AMCRA), and Health Insurance Association of America (HIAA)—that represented different types of health plan constituencies. GHAA and AMCRA merged to form the American Association of Health Plans (AAHP), which in turn merged with HIAA to form AHIP.

Ancillary Services—Healthcare services that are ordered by a physician, but provided by some other type of provider—for example, diagnostic testing or physical therapy. Does not apply to inpatient care, ambulatory procedures, or pharmacy.

Annual Limit—An archaic term referring to the maximum amount of coverage that a health plan would provide in a year; for example, coverage ends when costs exceed $1 million in a year). Under the ACA, annual limits were phased out for all benefits plans as of 2014.

ANSI—See American National Standards Institute.

Any Willing Provider (AWP)—A state law that requires a payer to accept any provider willing to meet the terms and conditions in the payer's contract, whether or not the payer wants or needs that provider in its network. Considered to be an expensive form of anti-managed care legislation.

APC—See Ambulatory Patient Classification.

APG—See Enhanced Ambulatory Patient Group.

Appeal—A formal appeal by a member of a denial of coverage. It requires a response within a fixed time frame. Under the ACA, a member can appeal at least twice—once for an internal review and once for an external review. It is not the same as a grievance.

ASA—See Average Speed to Answer.

ASC—See Ambulatory Surgical Center (facility term) or Ambulatory Surgical Category (payment term).

ASO—See Administrative Services Only.

ASP—See Average Sales Price.

Assignment of Benefits—A form signed by a patient directing the insurer to pay a nonparticipating provider directly, rather than reimbursing the member. The member is still liable for whatever a nonparticipating provider bills versus what the plan pays. Health plans, especially Blue Cross and Blue Shield plans, long refused to directly pay nonparticipating providers because direct payment is a valuable reason to participate due to difficulties collecting from patients, including who receive a check from the insurer. To counter this, providers successfully lobbied state legislatures in several states to require it.

Association Health Plan—An association made up of smaller businesses that group together for purposes of providing health benefits to employees. This may be done by purchasing group health insurance in which all of the businesses in the association participate equally, or it may be done by creating a pool of employees sufficiently large so as to self-insure, thereby avoiding state benefits mandates and premium taxes. See also Multiple Employer Welfare Association or Multiple Employer Trust.

Attachment Point—A reinsurance contract term that refers to the size that a claim must be before any reinsurance coverage applies. For example, an 80/20 reinsurance contract with an attachment point of $100,000 means that if any individual incurred claims adding up to more than $100,000 in the contract period (usually a year), reinsurance would pay 80% of any amount in excess of $100,000.

Authorization—In the context of managed care, the need to obtain authorization before certain types of healthcare services are covered. Most commonly used in "gatekeeper"-type HMOs in which a PCP must authorize a referral to a specialist or else the HMO will not pay for the specialist visit. Sometimes referred to as preauthorization; sometimes used synonymously with precertification. Although no clear distinction is actually made, by convention authorization is applied more often to specialty referral services, while precertification is applied more often to facility-based services.

Auto-adjudication—The complete processing of a claim without any manual intervention. May also be applied to claims processing following claims data entry—called claims capture. Claims capture is not a trivial cost, so comparisons of auto-adjudication rates between payers must use a consistent definition.

Automated Call Distributor (ACD)—A computerized system that automatically routes calls or contacts coming into a call center based on programmed distribution instructions.

Average Handle Time—The length of time it takes a customer service representative to resolve or complete a call or contact from a member.

Average Sales Price (ASP)—A method to determine the amount that Medicare or a payer will pay for drugs, particularly biological or injectable drugs, or in some cases a device. It is based on the average price for which the manufacturer sells the drug, not what is charged by whoever is administering it. Payment for administering the drug is usually the ASP plus 6%.

Average Speed to Answer (ASA)—The average time it takes to answer a call, typically measured in seconds; it is commonly used in measuring the performance of a customer service representative.

Average Wholesale Price (AWP)—Commonly used in pharmacy contracting, a price that is generally determined through reference to a common source or sources of information.

Avoidable Readmission—The unplanned readmission of a patient to a hospital within 30 (or 60) days of discharge for the same medical problem or one related to the first admission, and that could have been prevented through intervention. For example, a patient with a chronic condition who does not receive office-based follow-up care from his or her doctor or does not comply with his or her medications and is then rehospitalized would be considered an avoidable readmission.

AWP—See Average Wholesale Price or Any Willing Provider.

BAA—See Business Associate Agreement.

Balance Billing—The practice of a provider billing a patient for all charges not covered by the benefits plan. Managed care plans and service plans generally prohibit contracted providers from balance billing except for allowed copayments, coinsurance, and deductibles.

Balanced Budget Act of 1997 (BBA '97)—A sweeping piece of legislation, part of which created the Medicare+Choice program (since replaced by Medicare Advantage) as well as demonstration MSAs.

BCBS—Blue Cross Blue Shield.

BD/K—See Bed Days per Thousand.

Bed Days per Thousand (BD/K)—Also called bed days per thousand per year; a standard method of measuring inpatient utilization on an annualized basis. It is the number of hospital days that are used in a year for each 1,000 covered lives. It may be applied to differing time periods such as a single day, month to date, and year to date.

Behavioral Shift—A change in the behavior of an individual with health insurance or managed care coverage based on the design of the benefits. For example, higher cost sharing may reduce unnecessary visits to the emergency department for nonurgent care. A related meaning includes a change or loss of coverage resulting in postponing or not even seeking necessary care due to high costs and inability to pay.

Benefit Buy Down—Increasing employee cost sharing so as to reduce an employer's benefits costs. This term is most often used by actuaries, underwriters, and benefits consultants.

Benefit Design—The exercise of designing a benefits package to effectively compete in the market by balancing the level of benefits and the costs.

Benefit Waiver—A part of most case management programs under which the case manager can authorize coverage for something that is not normally a covered benefit so as to keep a member out of the hospital. For example, a plan may pay for a hospital bed in the home even though it does not cover durable medical equipment if it allows a member to receive home care rather than inpatient care.

Biologics—A type of specialty pharmacy drug that is biologic in nature; it is usually created by recombinant DNA and administered via injection. Biologics exist for the treatment of cancer, rheumatoid arthritis, anti-inflammatory diseases, and a host of other conditions. They are usually extremely expensive, and are often the focus of specialized utilization management by specialty pharmacy companies. Most types of insulin also fall into this category, but by convention they are not treated like other biologics from a benefits standpoint.

Biosimilar—A generic biologic drug, or a biologic drug that is similar enough to another one that it may be used in its place.

Blank—A state financial filing form. There are numerous specific types of blanks, sometimes called schedules, such as annual reports and surplus reports.

Book Rate—A premium rate developed using the experience of all individuals or groups in a specific block or pool; also called a manual rate or a base rate. The book rate is used as the basis for calculating various market rates such as family rates, single rates, and so forth. See also Community Rating.

BPO—See Business Process Outsourcing.

Bridge—See Doughnut Hole.

Bronze Level of Benefits or Bronze Plan—As defined in the ACA, a qualified health benefits plan with the actuarial equivalent or average of 40% cost sharing, when accounting for deductibles, copayments, and coinsurance as applied to in-network services.

Bundled Payment—An all-inclusive payment for all facility and professional services associated with an episode of care.

Business Associate—Under the privacy provisions of HIPAA, a person or organization that, on behalf of a covered entity (health plan, healthcare clearinghouse, or healthcare provider) or organized healthcare arrangement, performs or assists in the performance of activities involving the use or disclosure of protected health information (PHI). A business associate is not an employee of the covered entity. See also Protected Health Information.

Business Associate Agreement (BAA)—A contract between a covered entity under HIPAA and one of its business associates, requiring the business associate to comply with the privacy and security requirements for covered entities.

Business Process Outsourcing (BPO)—A form of outsourcing to a third party that focuses on one or more administrative processes of a payer such as claims or enrollment. See also Outsourcing.

Buy Down—See Benefits Buy Down.

"Cadillac" Plan—A high-cost health plan, also called a high-value plan, which exceeds cost levels defined under the ACA and, therefore, is subject to an additional tax.

Cafeteria Plan—An informal term for a flexible benefits plan.

CAHPS—See Consumer Assessment of Healthcare Providers and Systems.

Call Center—See Contact Center.

CAM—See Complementary and Alternative Medicine.

Capitated Risk Pool—See Risk Pool (Capitation).

Capitation—A set amount of money received or paid out; it is based on membership rather than on services delivered and usually is expressed in dollars per member per month (PMPM). The amount may vary based on such factors as age and sex of the enrolled member.

Captive or Captive Insurer—A restricted insurance company that provides coverage only for subsidiaries of its parent company or companies, not to the marketplace at large—for example, a national employer with a subsidiary providing long-term care insurance benefits to its employees. Captives are not subject to the same degree of regulation as regular insurers, and are often based offshore and subject to minimal regulation. Captives often do not have adequate reserves, putting them at more risk of failure; however, this is typically offset by having reinsurance from a commercial reinsurer. See also Fronting Insurer.

CAQH—A nonprofit alliance of health plans, networks, and trade associations, that seeks to foster industry collaboration on initiatives that would simplify healthcare administration, including credentialing of providers. Once called the Council for Affordable Quality Healthcare, it changed its name to CAHQ.

Care Continuum Alliance—The organization for disease management, formerly called the Disease Management Association of America.

Care Management—A broad term that is sometimes used synonymously with utilization management. Also, an umbrella-like term that refers to the combination of utilization management, disease management, case management, condition management, and so forth.

Carve-out—(1) In relation to payment terms, something that is carved out of the basic payment methodology; for example, the cost of implantable devices might be carved out of hospital or ambulatory case rates and charged for separately. (2) In relation to plan benefits, a set of benefits that are carved out and contracted for separately; for example, mental health/substance abuse services may be separated from basic medical/surgical services.

Case Management—A method of managing the provision and coverage of health care services to members with high-cost medical conditions. The goal is to coordinate the care so as to improve continuity and quality of care as well as lower costs. It is generally a dedicated function in the utilization management department. According to the Certification of Insurance Rehabilitation Specialists Commission, "Case management is a collaborative process which assesses, plans, implements, coordinates, monitors, and evaluates the options and services required to meet an individual's health needs, using communication and available resources to promote quality, cost-effective outcomes" and "occurs across a continuum of care, addressing ongoing individual needs" rather than being restricted to a single practice setting. When focused solely on high-cost inpatient cases, it may be referred to as large case management or catastrophic case management.

Case Mix—The mix of illness and severity of cases for a provider; the mix of cases in an inpatient setting, accounting for differences in potential or real cost and outcomes. Case mix adjustment refers to use of case mix to evaluate performance of a provider or project potential costs.

Cat Claim—A catastrophic claim. See also Shock Claim.

CCIIO—See Center for Consumer Information and Insurance Oversight.

CCIP—See Chronic Care Improvement Program.

CCO—Corporate compliance officer. See also Corporate Compliance.

CCP—See Coordinated Care Plan.

CDH/CDHP—See Consumer-Directed Health Plan.

Census—In the context of health care, the number of filled inpatient beds, in whole numbers or as a percentage of a hospital's capacity. Payers may use this term to refer to the number of members who are inpatients at one hospital, or to the number of hospitalized members overall.

Center for Consumer Information and Insurance Oversight (CCIIO)—An agency within CMS, responsible for ensuring compliance with the ACA's market rules and medical loss ratio rules. It assists states in reviewing insurance rates; provides guidance and oversight for state-based insurance exchanges; and compiles and maintains data on insurance.

Center for Medicare and Medicaid Innovation (CMMI)—See CMS Innovation Center.

Centers for Medicare & Medicaid Services (CMS)—The federal agency within the Department of Health and Human Services responsible for Medicare and (with the states) Medicaid and implementation of the ACA.

CER—See Comparative Effective Research.

Certificate of Authority—A license issued by a state to an HMO that meets regulatory requirements; this form of state licensure is required for HMOs and differs from the insurance licenses that health insurers are issued.

Certificate of Coverage—See Evidence of Coverage.

Certificate of Need (CON)—The requirement that a healthcare organization obtain permission from an oversight agency before making changes; it generally applies only to facilities or facility-based services, and varies on a state-to-state basis.

CHAMPUS—Civilian Health and Medical Program of the Uniformed Services. See also TRICARE.

Chargemaster—The list of every charge that a hospital has can make on a pure fee-for-service basis. What a hospital is actually paid by a payer, Medicare, or Medicaid rarely matches the charges listed on the chargemaster. Even when payment is not directly based on the chargemaster, it generally forms the basis upon which hospital payments are negotiated or paid one way or another.

Chase and Pay—A term used during coordination of benefits that means determining which carrier is primary and which is secondary before paying anything. Also called Pursue and Pay. The antonym of Chase and Pay is Pay and Chase. See also Coordination of Benefits and Pay and Chase.

CHIP—See State Children's Health Insurance Program.

Chronic Care Improvement Program (CCIP)—A requirement of the MMA, part of a MA plan that identifies enrollees with multiple or sufficiently severe chronic conditions who meet the criteria for participation and employs a mechanism for monitoring enrollees' participation; a form of a disease management program under MA.

Churning—The practice of a provider seeing a patient more often than is medically necessary, primarily to increase revenue through delivery of an increased number of services. Churning may also apply to any performance-based payment system where there is a heavy emphasis on productivity (in other words, rewarding a provider for seeing a high volume of patients whether through FFS or through an appraisal system that pays a bonus for productivity).

Civilian Health and Medical Program of the Uniformed Services (CHAMPUS)—The old name for the federal program providing healthcare coverage to families of military personnel, military retirees, certain spouses and dependents of such personnel, and certain others. The program is now called TRICARE. See also Military Health System and TRICARE.

Claim—A bill for services from a healthcare provider to the organization or person responsible for payment. Claims can be paper or electronic.

Claims Capture—The process of entering claims data into a claims processing system. Electronic claims without errors and containing all required data are captured quickly and at very little cost. Standardized paper claims such as the CMS-1450 and the CMS-1500 are usually scanned in via optical character recognition programs, with the data then manually reviewed and corrected as needed. Member-submitted claims may also be scanned in or may require manual key entry, all of which are very expensive.

Claims Clearinghouse—A company that accepts claims or other transactions from providers, formats them according to HIPAA-compliant standards, and electronically transmits them to the payer.

Claims Made Reinsurance or Insurance—A common type of reinsurance, and one of two primary types of professional liability insurance; it applies to professional malpractice insurance for physicians, but is applicable to directors' and officers' liability policies as well. "Claims made" means that the insurer has liability only when the event occurred and the insurer was informed of the potential for liability while the insurance was in force. If informed after the policy has lapsed, the insurer has no liability. See also Claims Paid Reinsurance and Occurrence Insurance or Reinsurance.

Claims Paid Reinsurance—A reinsurance policy that applies to claims paid in a specific time period (e.g., one year). The coverage is for any claims paid during the contract period. After the period of coverage has ended, there is no further coverage for costs even if they were incurred during the period when the reinsurance was in force but claims were not actually paid by the benefits plan. Coverage may extend to claims incurred for a defined period before and/or after the policy period if such coverage is purchased ahead of time. Not to be confused with claims made reinsurance/insurance, in which notification of the potential for liability, not necessarily the payment of a claim, is sufficient to activate coverage.

Claims Repricing—An activity in which a rental PPO receives claims submitted by the participating providers, reprices them using the PPO fee schedule, and then transmits the repriced claim to the payer or insurance company for final processing.

Clawback—When the government takes back some of the money it paid out to an organization or an individual.

Clean Claim—A claim that has no errors and contains all required data. This term can apply to either paper or electronic claims, but is increasingly being used only for electronic claims.

Closed Panel—A managed care plan that contracts with physicians on an exclusive basis. Examples include staff and group model HMOs, or health systems that offer a commercial health plan that is staffed primarily by their employed physicians. Note that even closed-panel plans contract with private physicians for services that the group or staff physicians are not able to provide.

CMP—See Competitive Medical Plan.

CMS—See Centers for Medicare & Medicaid Services. Also stands for contract management system when used in the context of network management systems support.

CMS-1450—A paper claim form used by hospitals and facilities, which has standardized by CMS. It replaced the UB-92 form. It does not apply to electronic claims. CMS discourages paper claims, but if an institution submits one to any type of payer, this is what it uses. Also called the UB-04.

CMS-1500—A paper claims form used by professionals to bill for their services. It was developed for Medicare, but is also used in the commercial sector. It does not apply to electronic claims. CMS no longer accepts paper claims, although most commercial health plans do.

CMS Innovation Center—A branch of CMS created under the ACA and charged with identifying, testing, and ultimately spreading new ways of delivering and paying for care in Medicare and Medicaid. It was previously called the Center for Medicare and Medicaid Innovation (CMMI).

CMS-Hierarchical Condition Categories System (CMS-HCC)—A system based on the diagnosis codes used in inpatient and outpatient settings as well as physician settings of care. The codes are assigned to groups of diagnoses called condition categories. The condition categories are ranked in a hierarchy, such that a higher category trumps a lower category for a patient whose diagnoses map to both categories. Each category is assigned a value (risk adjustment factor) based on the statistical relationship between that category and the following year's claim costs, and is used to adjust payments to MA plans.

COA—See Certificate of Authority.

COB—See Coordination of Benefits.

COBRA—See Consolidated Omnibus Budget Reconciliation Act.

Code Sets—Sets of codes used by providers to bill for services. As a practical matter, the official codes that must be used for any electronic transaction covered under HIPAA. These code sets are ICD-9-CM (until October 1, 2015) and ICD-10 (after October 1, 2015), CPT-4, NDC, HCPCS, and the Code on Dental Procedures and Nomenclature.

Coinsurance—A cost-sharing provision in a member's coverage that is based on a percentage of covered charges paid by the plan. Coinsurance may vary in some plans depending on whether a service was received from an in-network versus out-of-network provider (e.g., 80% for in-network care, 60% for out-of-network care), but are always based on what the plan covers, not necessarily what the provider charges. Any additional costs are paid by the member out of pocket.

Commercial Health Plan—Health insurance or HMO coverage for subscribers who are not covered by virtue of a governmental program such as Medicare, Medicaid, or SCHIP. May be an insured or a self-funded plan.

Commission—The money paid to a sales representative, broker, or other type of sales agent for selling the health plan. May be a flat amount of money or a percentage of the premium.

Community Rating—A form of premium rating required by the ACA for all individual and small group coverage. With this system, the HMO or insurer obtains the same amount of money per member for all members in the appropriate coverage group; for example, all individuals and/or all small groups. Some states require community rating for groups that are slightly larger than the definition used by the ACA. Community rating is usually calculated as adjusted community rating. See also Adjusted Community Rating and Experience Rating.

Comparative Effective Research (CER)—The use of scientific studies to determine how effective one type of treatment or procedure is compared to another.

Complementary and Alternative Medicine (CAM)—Treatment modalities other than traditional allopathic medicine. Examples include acupuncture, chiropractic medicine, homeopathy, and various forms of "natural healing."

Compliance—See Corporate Compliance.

Compounding Pharmacy—A pharmacy that combines different drugs or solutions for administration—for example, mixing small amounts of a chemotherapeutic drug with a solution for injection into an organ. May be considered a form of specialty pharmacy.

Computer Telephony Integration (CTI)—In a payer's call center or contact center, the use of information input by a member at the beginning of a call to access relevant data in the transaction system, route the call to the most appropriate customer service representative (CSR), and provide decision support to the CSR.

Computerized Physician Order Entry (CPOE)—A system in which a physician enters medical orders into an electronic medical record or transactional system such as a drug dispensing program. It is supposed to lower the error rate caused by illegible handwriting. CPOE systems may also be partially or completely automated for certain things, such as routine or standing orders for a patient admitted to the ICU.

CON—See Certificate of Need.

Concurrent Review—Utilization management that takes place during the provision of services. This term is mostly used with inpatient hospital stays, but also may apply to certain extended types of treatment such as long-term rehabilitation.

Condition Management—A term that may be used interchangeably with disease management, or to refer to the management of those patients with multiple chronic conditions, meaning a sort of multidisease management. See also Disease Management.

Consolidated Omnibus Budget Reconciliation Act (COBRA)—Legislation that, among other things, allows for a limited continuation of healthcare coverage for people who lose their eligibility for coverage through an employer group's medical plan. See also Conversion.

Consumer Assessment of Healthcare Providers and Systems (CAHPS)— A rating system begun by the federal government for use in Medicare and Medicaid managed care plans, but which is now also used by commercial health plans. It is maintained by the AHRQ and participation is required as part of the NCQA accreditation process. Its initial focus was on managed healthcare plans, but is being expanded to ambulatory providers, hospitals, and the Medicare prescription drug program. The hospital version is called the Hospital Consumer Assessment of Healthcare Providers and Systems (HCAHPS) survey.

Consumer-Directed Health Plan (CDH/CDHP)—A type of health plan that combines a qualified HDHP with a pretax fund such as a health reimbursement account (HRA) or a health savings account (HSA). The HRA or HSA is used to pay for qualified services on a first-dollar basis, but is not large enough to cover the entire deductible, the so-called doughnut hole. CDHPs also provide information such as cost data and decision-support tools to consumers to promote greater involvement on the part of the consumer in making health care choices.

Consumer-Operated and -Oriented Plan (CO-OP) Program—Under the ACA, a new type of consumer-operated, nonprofit payer organization offering coverage through a state health insurance exchange.

Consumer Portal—See Portal.

Contact Center—The place within a payer that supports inbound inquiries across a broad array of media (most frequently, inbound telephone calls), blended with outbound contact and outreach transactions.

Contract Management System (CMS)—A computer program or database management system that keeps track of the various provider contracts and their terms. A CMS may also sometimes be used to track employer group master contracts and benefits terms, but that system is usually separate from the provider system.

Contract Year—The 12-month period that a contract for services is in force. It is not necessarily tied to a calendar year.

Contributory Plan—A group health plan in which the employees must contribute a certain amount toward the premium cost, with the employer paying the rest.

Convenient (or Convenience) Care Clinic (CCC)—See Retail Clinic.

Conversion—The conversion of a member covered under a group master contract to coverage under an individual contract. This option is offered to subscribers who lose their group coverage (e.g., through job loss, death of a working spouse) and who are ineligible for coverage under another group contract. Since 2014, it is used almost entirely for COBRA conversions because there is little reason to consider other forms of conversion.

Co-op—See Healthcare Cooperative.

Coordinated Care Plan (CCP)—Network-based Medicare Advantage plans that include HMOs, PPOs (both regional and local), IDSs that operate like HMOs, and HMOs with point-of-service products. CCPs can require enrollees to use a network of providers for coverage of Medicare services.

Coordination of Benefits (COB)—An agreement that uses language developed by the NAIC to prevent double payment for services when a subscriber has coverage from two or more sources. For example, one parent may have Blue Cross Blue Shield insurance through work, and the other parent may have elected to join an HMO through her or his place of employment; if both parents elected to cover dependents, then their child or children would be covered under two plans. The agreement specifies which organization has primary responsibility for payment and which organization has secondary responsibility for payment. The respective primary and secondary payment obligations of the two carriers are determined by the order of benefits determination (OOBD) rules contained in the NAIC Model COB Regulation, as interpreted and adopted by the various states. See also Other Party Liability.

Copayment—That portion of a claim or medical expense that a member must pay out of pocket. It is usually a fixed amount, such as $20 in many HMOs.

Corporate Compliance—The function in a health plan or provider charged with ensuring compliance with federal rules and regulations. There are many compliance areas for Medicare; specific compliance requirements exist for privacy and security under HIPAA and financial requirements under the Sarbanes-Oxley Act. Regulations for Medicare and HIPAA also require the existence of a corporate compliance officer.

Corporate Practice of Medicine (CPM) Law—A state law that prohibits a corporation (other than a professional corporation, or PC) from practicing medicine or employing a physician to provide professional medical services. Some states with CPM laws allow certain corporations such as hospitals or HMOs to employ physicians, however.

Cost Sharing—Any form of coverage in which the member pays some portion of the cost of providing services. Usual forms of cost sharing include deductibles, coinsurance, and copayments.

Cost Shifting—A situation in which a provider cannot cover the cost of providing services under the payment received, so the provider raises the prices to other payers to cover that portion of the cost.

Council for Affordable Quality Healthcare—See CAHQ.

Coverage Gap—See Doughnut Hole.

Covered Entity—A person or organization that must meet the HIPAA standards for transactions, code sets, privacy, and security; defined as a provider (professional or facility), a health plan, or a claims clearinghouse.

CPM Law—See Corporate Practice of Medicine Law.

CPOE—See Computerized Physician Order Entry.

CPT-4—See Current Procedural Terminology, Fourth Edition.

Credentialing—Obtaining and reviewing the documentation of professional providers. Such documentation includes licensure, certifications, insurance, evidence of malpractice insurance, malpractice history, and so forth. It generally includes both reviewing information provided by the provider and verifying that the information is correct and complete.

Credentialing Verification Organization (CVO)—An independent organization that performs primary verification of a professional provider's credentials. The managed care organization may then rely on that verification rather than requiring the provider to provide credentials independently. This lowers the cost and "hassle" for credentialing. NCQA has issued certification standards for CVOs.

Credibility—An insurance term of art that refers to how much weight is given to a group's prior experience for purposes of calculating premium rates. The larger the group and the longer the history, the more credibility it is given.

Creditable Coverage—Healthcare benefits coverage from any source that meets the ACA's minimum standards to be creditable. In the context of a special enrollment period, it also refers to proof that an individual had creditable coverage up until 60 days or less prior to obtaining new coverage or a coverage extension. See also Special Enrollment Period.

Critical Paths—Defined pathways of clinical care that provide for the greatest efficiency of care at the greatest quality. Critical paths are also an ever-changing activity as science and medicine evolve. This term is being replaced through common usage with the term "clinical guidelines."

CRM—See Customer Relationship Management.

C-SNP—A chronic care special needs plan for beneficiaries with one or more severe or disabling chronic conditions.

CSR—See Customer Service Representative.

CTI—See Computer Telephony Integration.

Current Procedural Terminology, Fourth Edition (CPT-4)—A set of five-digit codes that apply to medical services delivered. It is frequently used for billing by professionals and is maintained by the American Medical Association. See also Healthcare Common Procedural Coding System.

Custodial Care—Care provided to an individual that consists primarily of assistance with the basic activities of living. It may be medical or nonmedical, but the care is not meant to be curative or to serve as a form of medical treatment; it is often lifelong. Custodial care is not a covered benefit in any form of group health insurance, HMO, or Medicare. Only long-term care insurance policies (which are property/casualty policies, not health plans) or, for the indigent, Medicaid, provides any coverage for custodial care.

Customer Relationship Management (CRM)—Originally, all of the processes and information systems used by an organization in regard to its interactions with its customers, such as telephone calling systems and customer databases. Today this term is used more broadly to include the use of the same processes and technology in regard to any external constituency, such as a payer's nonroutine interactions with its providers.

Customer Service Representative (CSR)—An individual in the member services function who has direct communications with members. There are usually different levels of CSRs consistent with these individuals' different levels of experience, training, and authority.

Customer Services—See Member Services.

CVO—See Credentialing Verification Organization.

CWW—Clinic Without Walls. See also Group Practice Without Walls.

Data Transparency—The practice in which a payer or governmental agency makes data about healthcare costs and quality available to consumers, usually via the Internet.

The Databank—The federal data repository that includes both the National Practitioner Data Bank and the Healthcare Integrity and Protection Data Bank.

Date of Service—The date on which medical services were rendered. It is usually different from the date a claim is submitted.

DAW—See Dispense as Written.

Days per Thousand—See Bed Days per Thousand.

DCG—See Diagnostic Care Group.

Death Spiral—An insurance term that refers to a vicious spiral of high premium rates and adverse selection, generally in a free-choice environment (typically, an insurance company or health plan in an account with multiple other plans, or a plan offering coverage to potential members who have alternative choices). One plan ends up having continually higher premium rates such that the only members who stay with the plan are those whose medical costs are so high that they far exceed any possible premium revenue. The losses from underwriting mount faster than the premiums can ever cover, and the account eventually terminates coverage, leaving the carrier in a permanent loss position and possibly resulting in the insurer's bankruptcy.

Deductible—That portion of a subscriber's (or member's) covered healthcare expenses that must be paid out of pocket before any insurance coverage applies, commonly $500 to $1,000. It may apply only to the out-of-network portion of a point-of-service plan. It may also apply only to one portion of the plan coverage (e.g., there may be a deductible for pharmacy services or hospital care, but not for anything else).

Deeming—The practice in which an organization that is accredited by the appropriate accreditation agency as meeting defined requirements is deemed to be in compliance with the requirements of a governmental agency. For payers, accreditation by NCQA, URAC, or (less commonly) AAAHC is deemed by CMS as meeting at least some requirements for participation in Medicare Advantage. Many states also deem plans as being in compliance with certain requirements of licensure. Accreditation by The Joint Commission for facilities and accreditation by AAAHC for ambulatory facilities are usually deemed as being in compliance with certain state and Medicare requirements.

Defined Benefit—An insurance practice in which an employer provides a benefit that is the same regardless of the cost to provide that benefit. Under the ACA, only defined benefits plans can be considered as creditable health plans.

Defined Contribution—An insurance practice in which an employer designates a fixed amount of money for use in purchasing insurance or for funding a retirement account. Generally speaking, defined contribution plans do not meet the ACA's requirement for creditable coverage.

Delete—The term used by CMS for the process of removing Medicare enrollees from a plan. See also Accrete.

Demand Management—Services or support that a payer provides to members in an effort to lower the demand for acute care services. It includes self-help tools, nurse advice lines, and preventive services.

Dental Content Committee of the American Dental Association—A designated standards maintenance organization under HIPAA that focuses on coding standards for dental procedures.

Dental Health Maintenance Organization (DHMO)—An HMO organized strictly to provide dental benefits.

Department of Health and Human Services (DHHS)—The U.S. Cabinet-level federal agency that oversees many healthcare-related programs, including the CMS, which is responsible for Medicare and Medicaid (in conjunction with individual states), as well as HIPAA and other related federal legislation.

Department of Labor (DOL)—The U.S. Cabinet-level federal agency that regulates coverage offered to employees when employers retain the insurance risk through self-funding pursuant to ERISA, either on a stand-alone basis or through a multiple employer welfare arrangement. Certain ERISA requirements are also applicable to insured plans and, therefore, are regulated by the DOL as well.

Dependent—A member who is covered by virtue of a family relationship with the member who has the health plan coverage. For example, one person may have health insurance or an HMO through work, and that individual's spouse and children, the dependents, may also therefore be eligible for coverage under the same contract.

Designated Standards Maintenance Organization (DSMO)—An organization designated in HIPAA that is charged with making recommendations to

DHHS regarding updates to existing standards as well as the addition of new standards to the transactions and code sets.

DFRR—See Disclosure of Financial Relationships Report.

DHHS—See the Department of Health and Human Services.

DHMO—See Dental Health Maintenance Organization.

Diagnosis-Related Groups (DRGs)—The initial version of the statistical system of classifying any inpatient stay into groups for purposes of payment. DRGs may be primary or secondary, and an outlier classification also exists. This is the form of payment that the CMS used to pay hospitals for Medicare recipients. It was also used by a few states for all payers and by many private health plans for contracting purposes. CMS replaced DRGs with MS-DRGs in 2008–2009, and most commercial plans that used DRGs have followed suit. See also MS-DRG.

Diagnostic Care Group (DCG)—A methodology commissioned by the CMS to look at how to adjust prospective payments to health plans based on retrospective severity. It was replaced by the CMS-Hierarchical Condition Categories.

Direct Access—See Open Access.

Direct Contract Model—A managed care health plan that primarily contracts directly with private practice physicians in the community, rather than through an intermediary such as an independent practice association or a medical group. A common type of model in open-panel HMOs.

Direct Contracting—(1) Contracting directly with private practice physicians for specialty services not available through a contracted group or an IPA. (2) A system in which a provider or integrated healthcare delivery system contracts directly with an employer rather than using an insurance company or managed care organization. This option occasionally works when the employer is large enough and employees are mostly located in one geographic region. This approach often does not last for long because it almost always ends up being more costly than working through an existing health plan, though there are exceptions.

Direct-Pay Subscriber—An individual subscriber to a health plan who is not covered under a group policy, but rather pays the health plan directly. This term is usually not used to describe Medicare or Medicaid subscribers because part or all of their premiums are paid via a governmental agency.

Discharge Planning—That part of utilization management that is concerned with arranging for care or medical needs to facilitate discharge from the hospital.

Disclosure of Financial Relationships Report (DFRR)—A mandatory hospital disclosure form applicable to Medicare. It was created by CMS to report any financial relationships between hospitals and physicians, and to measure compliance with physician self-referral statutes and regulations.

Disease Management—The process of intensively managing members with one or more particular diseases. This approach differs from large case management in that it goes well beyond a given case in a hospital or an acute exacerbation of a condition, and it typically focuses on a defined set of specific conditions such as diabetes, cardiac disease, and so forth. Disease management encompasses all settings of care, and it places a heavy emphasis on prevention and maintenance. See also Condition Management.

Disenrollment—The process of termination of coverage. Voluntary termination would include a member quitting because he or she simply wants out. Involuntary termination would include a person leaving the plan because he or she takes a new job or loses eligibility for coverage. A rare and serious form of involuntary disenrollment is when the plan terminates a member's coverage against the member's will. This step is usually allowed (under state and federal laws) only for gross offenses such as fraud, abuse, or nonpayment of premiums or copayments.

Dispense as Written (DAW)—The written instruction from a physician to a pharmacist to dispense a brand-name pharmaceutical rather than a generic substitution.

Dispensing Fee—The fee paid to a pharmacy for that part of the cost of a prescription that is not the ingredient cost. Usually a flat dollar amount, not tied to the cost of the drug.

Disproportionate Share Hospital (DSH) Payment—An amount added to payments by Medicare and Medicaid to help defray the costs of uncompensated care or for having a disproportionately high percentage of low income or indigent patients. It differs for each hospital and state and is based on a complex formula. DSH payments were significantly reduced as of 2014 under the ACA because of coverage expansions through subsidized commercial health insurance and the Medicaid expansion; hospitals in states that have not expanded Medicaid took a hit because they no longer receive DSH payments but still provide uncompensated care.

Distribution Channel or Distribution—The various ways that a payer sells its products—for example, brokers, consultants, employed sales force, and electronic sales portals.

DME—See Durable Medical Equipment.

DOL—See Department of Labor.

Doughnut Hole—Also called a Coverage Gap, it is the difference between when first-dollar coverage stops and insurance begins; also may be referred to as a bridge. This term may be applied in a CDHP plan to the gap between the health reimbursement account/health savings account and the point at which the high-deductible insurance plan starts to cover costs. A doughnut hole also exists in the basic Medicare Part D drug benefit passed under the MMA, but under the ACA it is being partially phased out by 2020.

Downstream Risk—When a capitated provider subcapitates another provider to assume a portion of the capitated provider's risk. For example, a large medical group is paid capitation for all professional services, and in turn subcapitates (capitates) a specialty medical group for all services related to that specialty.

DRGs—See Diagnosis-Related Groups.

Drive Time—The average amount of time it takes for a member to get to a provider. It is often used as a measure of network accessibility.

Drug Utilization Review (DUR)—Utilization management applied to the pharmaceutical benefit. It relies mostly on prospective review but does use some concurrent review as well.

DSH—See Disproportionate Share Hospital Payments.

DSMO—See Designated Standards Maintenance Organization.

DSM-V (or DSM-5)—*Diagnostic and Statistical Manual of Mental Disorders, Fifth Edition.* The manual used to provide a diagnostic coding system for mental and substance abuse disorders. See also ICD-9-CM.

D-SNP— Dual-eligible special needs plan for beneficiaries who are eligible for both Medicare and Medicaid ("dual eligibles" or "duals").

Dual Choice—An archaic term, sometimes also referred to as Section 1310 or mandating. That portion of the original HMO Act that required any employer that met certain criteria—25 or more employees who reside in an HMO's service area, pays minimum wage, and offers health coverage—to offer a federally qualified HMO as well. This provision of the HMO Act became obsolete in 1995.

Dual Eligibles or Duals—Individuals who are entitled to both Medicare and Medicaid coverage. Sometimes referred to as "Medi-Medi's."

Dual Option—This once referred to offering both an HMO and a traditional insurance plan by one carrier. It now refers to offering two different health plans, regardless of type, or to a POS plan that has only in-network and out-of-network benefits (i.e., there is no associated PPO as a middle option).

Duplicate Claims—A situation in which the same claim is submitted more than once, usually because payment has not been received quickly. It can lead to duplicate payments and incorrect data in the claims file, and at the very least it can clog up the claims system.

DUR—See Drug Utilization Review.

Durable Medical Equipment (DME)—Medical equipment that is not disposable (i.e., is used repeatedly) and is related to care for a medical condition. Examples include wheelchairs, insulin pumps, and orthotics.

EAP—See Employee Assistance Program.

EAPGs—See Enhanced Ambulatory Patient Groups.

Early and Periodic Screening, Diagnostic, and Testing (EPSDT)—A defined set of screening benefits provided to children covered under Medicaid.

Earned Premium—That portion of the premium attributable to coverage for a time period that has already passed. A premium that is paid in advance is considered an unearned premium until the time period that the premium is meant to cover has passed.

e-Business—See e-Commerce.

e-Commerce—The use of electronic communications to conduct business; also called e-business.

ED—See Emergency Department.

EDI—See Electronic Data Interchange.

Edit—A term used in claims processing. See also Suspend.

Effective Date—The day that health plan coverage goes into effect or is modified.

EFT—See Electronic Funds Transfer.

EHR—See Electronic Health Record.

Electronic Data Interchange (EDI)—The exchange of data through electronic means rather than by using paper or the telephone. Prior to the rise of the

Internet, EDI was applied primarily to direct electronic communications via proprietary means. EDI now encompasses electronic data exchange via both proprietary channels as well as the Internet.

Electronic Funds Transfer (EFT)—Getting paid by electronic transfer of funds directly to one's bank instead of receiving a paper check.

Electronic Health Record (EHR)—An expansive type of electronic record encompassing more than the care provided by a single provider or entity to a single patient.

Electronic Medical Record (EMR)—An electronic version of the type of health record that a physician or a hospital keeps on a single patient, though it could apply to any patient-specific clinical record.

Eligibility—The condition in which an individual meets the criteria for coverage under a plan. It is also used to determine when an individual is no longer eligible for coverage (e.g., a dependent child reaches a certain age and can no longer receive coverage under his or her parent's health plan). The same term may be used with groups.

Emergency—See Emergency Medical Condition.

Emergency Department (ED)—The location or department in a hospital or other institutional facility that is focused on caring for acutely ill or injured patients. In earlier times, this was often a room or set of rooms; hence the older designation emergency room (ER). These days, at least in busy urban and suburban hospitals, volume is high, physicians are specially trained in emergency care, and emergency care has grown to be an entire department.

Emergency Medical Treatment and Active Labor Act (EMTALA) 1986. 42 USC 1395 dd (1986), Pub. L. No. 99-272, 9121— "Antidumping" legislation that dictates all patients presenting to any hospital emergency department must have a medical screening exam performed by qualified personnel, usually the emergency physician. The medical screening exam cannot be delayed for insurance reasons, either to obtain insurance information or to obtain preauthorization for examination. This legislation also provides a definition of emergency medical condition that is used both for EMTLA purposes and, using a prudent layperson standard, as part of the ACA.

Employee Assistance Program (EAP)—A program that a company puts into effect for its employees to provide them with help in dealing with personal problems such as alcohol or drug abuse, mental health issues, and stress issues.

Employee Retirement Income Security Act (ERISA)— Federal legislation that allows self-funded plans to avoid paying premium taxes, complying with state-mandated benefits, or otherwise complying with most state laws and regulations that apply to health insurance. Another provision requires that plans and insurance companies provide an explanation of benefits (EOB) statement to a member or covered insured in the event of a denial of a claim, explaining why the claim was denied and informing the individual of his or her rights of appeal; this aspect was significantly strengthened under the ACA. Numerous other provisions in ERISA are very important for a managed care organization to know.

Employer Coverage Mandate—A provision of the ACA that requires employers with 50 or more full-time employees to offer affordable coverage or face a financial penalty.

EMR—See Electronic Medical Record.

EMTALA—See Emergency Medical Treatment and Active Labor Act.

Encounter—An outpatient or ambulatory visit by a member to a provider. This term applies primarily to physician office visits, but may encompass other types of contacts as well. In FFS plans, an encounter also generates a claim. In capitated plans, the encounter is still the visit, and a claim may even be generated, but it does not result in a claims payment.

End-Stage Renal Disease (ESRD)—A clinical condition involving failure of the kidneys. Medicare treats beneficiaries with ESRD differently than other individuals for purposes of enrollment in Medicare and in MA plans.

Enhanced Ambulatory Patient Group (EAPG)—A payment methodology developed by 3M Health Information Systems for CMS, but also used by some commercial health plans and by many state Medicaid agencies. EAPGs are a more comprehensive successor to APGs. EAPGs are to outpatient procedures what MS-DRGs are to inpatient days. EAPGs provide for a fixed payment to an institution for outpatient procedures or visits based on diagnoses, the procedure or procedures performed, and condition or procedure intensity. Like MS-DRGs, they are also subject to modifiers. EAPGs significantly reduce unbundling of ancillary services. See also Ambulatory Diagnostic Group and Ambulatory Patient Classification.

Enrollee—An individual enrolled in a managed healthcare plan. Usually the subscriber or person who has the coverage in the first place rather than his or her dependents, although the term is not always used that precisely.

Enrollment Period—A period in which individuals can join or change health plans, as defined in the ACA and applicable to the mandated open enrollment requirements that began in 2014. See also Open Enrollment Period.

Entitlement Program—A governmental program such as Medicare or Medicaid, though there are others as well, for which people who meet eligibility criteria have a right to benefits, and in which changes to eligibility criteria and benefits require legislation. The government is required to spend the funds necessary to provide benefits for individuals in these programs; in contrast, spending for discretionary programs is set by Congress through the appropriations process. Enrollment in entitlement programs cannot be capped, and neither states nor the federal government may establish waiting lists for joining the programs.

EOB—See Explanation of Benefits.

EOC—See Evidence of Coverage.

EPO—See Exclusive Provider Organization.

e-Prescribing—When a physician uses electronic means to prescribe drugs.

EPSDT—See Early and Periodic Screening, Diagnostic, and Testing.

Equity Model—A form of for-profit, vertically integrated healthcare delivery system in which the physicians are owners or have an ownership-like interest (e.g., through a leasing arrangement).

ER—Emergency room. See Emergency Department.

ERA—Electronic remittance advice; used in conjunction with EFT payments.

ERISA—See Employee Retirement Income Security Act.

ERISA Preemption—ERISA preempts state laws pertaining to employee benefits except for insurance, banking, or securities; however, the U.S. Supreme Court further defined the ERISA preemption as limiting any actions or remedies against an insurer to what is defined under ERISA. For example, lawsuits about benefits coverage can award only the cost of the coverage, not additional penalties. For self-funded benefits plans, ERISA preempts state laws in general.

ESRD—See End-Stage Renal Disease.

Essential Health Benefits—A benefits design under the ACA that includes ambulatory patient services; pediatric services, including oral and vision care; emergency services; hospitalization; maternity and newborn care; mental health and substance use disorder services; prescription drugs; rehabilitative and habilitative services and devices; laboratory services; preventive and wellness services; and chronic disease management. The specific definitions of each category be determined by each individual state using DHHS guidelines. As many as four different levels of cost sharing may be applied depending on the level of coverage.

Ethics in Patient Referrals Act—A law prohibiting physicians from referring patients to diagnostic, therapeutic, or supply services in which the physician has a financial interest. Also known as the Stark Laws after Fortney "Pete" Stark, a now-retired congressional representative from California. The so-called Stark regulations are actually two sets of regulations: Stark I and Stark II. These regulations are not for amateurs to handle, and competent legal counsel is required for any provider system doing business with federal or state governments.

Evergreen Contract—A contract that continues in force unless one or both parties give notice of cancellation.

Evidence-Based Medicine (EBM) or Medical Guidelines—Clinical practices or guidelines that are based on scientific studies, not habits, hope, or hype. The "gold standard" for EBM guidelines is a randomized clinical trial comparing one treatment to another treatment (or no treatment at all). Evidence-based medical guidelines are not the same as consensus-driven professional standards, which are fallback standards if no EBM guidelines are available.

Evidence of Coverage (EOC)—Also known as a certificate of benefits. A document that describes in detail which healthcare benefits are covered by the health plan, what is excluded, and how benefits are affected by utilization management requirements, medical necessity definitions, and so forth.

Evidence of Insurability—A form that documents whether an individual is eligible for health plan coverage when the individual is not enrolling during an open enrollment period—for example, when an individual applies for an extension of coverage under COBRA.

e-Visit—Electronic visit; an interaction between a provider (usually a physician) and a patient using a secure electronic communications channel rather than face-to-face or via telephone.

Exchange—See Health Insurance Exchange.

Exclusion—As used in managed care and health insurance, a service or condition for which there will be no (or very limited) coverage.

Exclusion period—See Waiting Period.

Exclusive Provider Organization (EPO)—A healthcare plan that is similar to an HMO in that it has a limited provider panel, uses an authorization system, and requires members to remain within the network to receive benefits. Unlike HMOs, EPOs usually do not require members to access care through a PCP. EPOs are not common and are used mostly by self-funded plans and governmental agencies for their employees.

Experience Rating—The method of setting premium rates based on the actual healthcare costs of a group or groups.

Experimental and Investigational Treatment—A term used by payers and insurance companies to refer to medical care that is not yet proven, or that may be the subject of clinical investigation. Most plans will not cover such treatments unless the patient is enrolled in a qualified investigational trial, and the ACA requires coverage only for such qualified trials.

Explanation of Benefits (EOB)—A statement mailed to a member or covered insured explaining how and why a claim was or was not paid; the Medicare version is called an explanation of Medicare benefits (EOMB). See also ERISA.

External Review—The second part of a formal appeal of a denial of benefits coverage, in which a panel of physicians who do not work for the payer organization review the appeal and make a decision that is binding on the payer. It is often required by states and addressed in ERISA, and is required for all plans under the ACA.

Extracontractual Benefits—Healthcare benefits beyond what the member's actual policy covers. These benefits are provided by a plan to reduce utilization. For example, a plan may not provide coverage for a hospital bed at home, but it might be more cost-effective for the plan to provide such a bed rather than keep admitting a member to the hospital.

Facility Fee or Facility Add-on Fee—A fee added on to a physician office visit by a hospital or facility owner. Adding a facility fee to a charge is generally prohibited if the physician owns or leases the office because payments for office visits include that cost (and are specifically built in to the RBRVS payment system). The facility fee is an additional charge that hospitals now bill for care provided by hospital-employed physicians, without lowering the physician's office visit fee. These fees may or may not be covered by health insurance, and payers seek to include clauses in their contracts with hospitals to prohibit add-on fees.

Faculty Practice Plan (FPP)—A form of group practice organized around a teaching program. It may be a single group encompassing all the physicians providing services to patients at the teaching hospital and clinics, or it may be multiple groups drawn along specialty lines (e.g., psychiatry, cardiology, or surgery).

FAR—See Federal Acquisition Regulations.

Fast Track ED—A pathway in the ED allowing minor ailments to be managed quickly, at lower cost, often by nonphysician practitioners.

Favored Nation Clause—See Most Favored Nation Clause.

Federal Acquisition Regulations (FAR)—The regulations applied to the federal government's acquisition of services, including healthcare services, excluding Medicare. See also Federal Employee Health Benefit Acquisition Regulations.

Federal Employee Health Benefit Acquisition Regulations (FEHBARs)—The regulations applied to the Office of Personnel Management's purchase of healthcare benefits programs for federal employees.

Federal Employee Health Benefits Program (FEHBP)—The program that provides health benefits to federal employees. See also Office of Personnel Management.

Federal Qualification—A term once applied to HMOs and competitive medical plans that met federal standards regarding benefits, financial solvency, rating methods, marketing, member services, healthcare delivery systems, and other standards. Not used since 1995.

Federally Qualified Health Center—A health center approved by the government to provide health care to low-income individuals in medically underserved areas.

Fee-for-Service (FFS)—A payment arrangement in which a patient sees a provider, the provider bills the health plan or patient, and the provider gets paid based on that bill. In the case of a contracted provider, the maximum payment may be limited to the fee schedule.

Fee Schedule—A listing of the maximum fees that a health plan will pay for certain services, based on CPT billing codes. Also referred to as fee maximums, maximum allowable charges, or a fee allowance schedule.

FEHBARs—See Federal Employee Health Benefit Acquisition Regulations.

FFS—See Fee-for-Service.

Fiduciary—A term that applies to employer self-funded benefits plans, the fiduciary is a person or controlling party that manages the assets of the benefits plan and has discretionary powers, and must act solely for the benefit of the plan's beneficiaries, not on behalf of the employer or itself.

File-and-Use Rating Laws—State-based laws that permit insurers to adopt new premium rates without the prior approval of the insurance department. Usually insurers submit their new rates with supporting statistical data to the state's insurance department.

Financial Services Modernization Act of 1999—Also called the Gramm-Leach-Bliley Act, legislation that repealed the Glass-Steagall Act of 1933. The Glass-Steagall Act prohibited most U.S. commercial banks from performing investment banking activities such as bringing new debt and equity issues to market, or other such underwriting, and from functioning as insurance companies. In addition to the repeal of Glass-Steagall, the 1999 act allows affiliations between securities firms, banks, and insurance companies.

First-Call Resolution—The percentage of contacts resolved on the first call. Typically used in call centers by member services.

First-Dollar Coverage—Benefits coverage that has no cost sharing of any type. Under the ACA, benefits for wellness and prevention must be first-dollar coverage, even if cost-sharing applies to other benefits.

First-Pass Rate—The percentage of claims auto-adjudicated to completion the first time they go through the claims processing system.

Fiscal Intermediary—A company that processes administrative transactions on behalf of Medicare or Medicaid. The arrangement with such a company may be limited to adjudication and payment of claims, or it may encompass other activities as well.

Flexible Benefits Plan—A benefits plan at a company that allows an employee to select from different options up to a set amount of money, and always includes an FSA. Also called a cafeteria plan or a Section 125 plan.

Flexible Spending Account (FSA)—A financial account funded with pretax dollars via payroll deduction by an employer. Funds may be used to reimburse the employee for qualified expenses not covered under insurance. FSAs exist for health care and, separately, for childcare services. Unused FSA funds do not roll into following years; they are "use it or lose it" funds except that in some cases, unused FSA funds can roll over into a health savings account.

Formulary—A listing of drugs that a health plan provides coverage for, but almost always at differing levels, called tiers. For example, drugs considered to be in

Tier 1 in the formulary may be covered with a $10 copayment, Tier 2 drugs may have a $40 copayment, and Tier 3 drugs may have a $100 copayment. A formulary may also list drugs that require precertification for coverage, or that are subject to other coverage limitations. Formularies are either open, meaning there is at least some level of coverage for drugs not listed in the formulary, or they are closed, meaning there is no coverage for nonformulary drugs.

Foundation—As applied to managed health care, a not-for-profit form of integrated healthcare delivery system. A foundation model system is usually formed in response to tax laws that affect not-for-profit hospitals, or in response to states with laws prohibiting the corporate practice of medicine. The foundation purchases both the tangible and intangible assets of a physician's practice; the physicians then form a medical group that contracts with the foundation on an exclusive basis for services to patients seen through the foundation.

FPP—See Faculty Practice Plan.

Fraud and Abuse—A term that has been succeeded by the more expansive term Fraud Waste and Abuse. See Fraud Waste and Abuse. See also Abuse or Healthcare Abuse; Fraud or Healthcare Fraud; and Fraud, Waste, and Abuse.

Fraud or Healthcare Fraud—When someone misrepresents or falsifies a fact related to healthcare services to receive payment from a health plan or the government. Abuse may be considered fraud when someone knowingly misrepresents significant details in delivery of healthcare services or supplies in order to be paid significantly more money. Soliciting, paying bonuses for, or receiving any compensation for referrals or use of goods or services—for example, getting a kickback for referring a patient to a specialist or receiving a bonus in return for using a manufacturer's device—are also forms of fraud.

Fraud, Waste, and Abuse (FWA)—Not the name of a law firm or a rock band, this term is used collectively to cover fraud, abusive practices, and wasteful practices by either providers or health plans; a handy catch-all for casting general blame at an industry sector. See also Abuse or Healthcare Abuse; Fraud and Abuse; and Fraud or Healthcare Fraud.

Fronting or Fronting Insurer—A commercial insurer that has a market rating and meets state insurance requirements, and that "fronts" for a nonrated insurer or captive insurer while typically taking only 10–20% of the risk.

FSA—See Flexible Spending Account.

Full Professional Risk Capitation—A physician group or organization that receives capitation for all professional expenses, not just for the services they provide themselves; it does not include capitation for institutional services. The group is then responsible for subcapitating (also called downstream risk) or otherwise paying other physicians for services to their members.

FWA—See Fraud, Waste, and Abuse.

Gag Clause—A clause in a provider contract that prevents a physician from telling a patient about available clinical treatment options (i.e., a "gag"). Gag clauses are like the Sasquatch—legendary, big, and scary, but nobody has ever actually found one. Nevertheless, gag clauses are banned under the ACA as well as by many states. Most or all contracts between payers and physicians do contain clauses that prohibit the physician from revealing business secrets such as payment schedules, but this is a different matter. In some cases in the past, contracts required a physician to contact the payer before initiating a treatment option, which may have been interpreted or treated as such a clause, but the majority of contracts actually require the physician to actively discuss options with the patient.

Gatekeeper—An informal, though widely used term that refers to a primary care case management model health plan. In this model, all care from providers other than the primary care physician, except for true emergencies, must be authorized by the primary care physician before care is rendered. This is a predominant feature of most (but not all) HMOs.

Generic Drug—A drug that is equivalent to a brand-name drug, but is usually less expensive. Most managed care organizations that provide drug benefits cover generic drugs, but may require a member to pay a higher copayment for a brand-name drug.

Genetic Information Nondiscrimination Act (GINA)—Legislation passed in 2008 that prohibits discrimination in health coverage and employment based on genetic information. GINA, plus certain provisions of HIPAA, generally prohibit health insurers or health plan administrators from requesting or requiring genetic information of an individual or the individual's family members. This act also prohibits using genetic information for decisions regarding coverage, rates, or preexisting conditions.

GINA—See Genetic Information Nondiscrimination Act.

Glass-Steagall Act—See Financial Services Modernization Act of 1999.

GLB—Gramm-Leach-Bliley Act. See Financial Services Modernization Act.

Global Capitation—A situation in which an organization receives capitation for all medical services, including institutional and professional services.

Global Payment—A single fixed payment for an episode of care. Most commonly used for well-defined types of care such as maternity or surgery. When combined with facility payment, it may still be called a global payment but is more likely to be referred to as a bundled payment. See also Bundled Payment.

Gold Level of Benefits or Gold Plan—As defined in the ACA, a qualified health benefits plan with the actuarial equivalent or average of 20% cost sharing, when accounting for deductibles, copayments, and coinsurance as applied to in-network services.

Grace Period—The amount of time that a payer or insurance company must allow a group or individual that has not paid a premium to make good on the payment before the plan can cancel the policy. If the delinquent company or individual pays up during the grace period, the policy is said to be reinstated and coverage is considered unbroken.

Gramm-Leach-Bliley (GLB) Act—See Financial Services Modernization Act.

Grandfathered Plan—A health benefits plan meeting certain criteria that is exempt from some, but not all, of the new requirements under the ACA. A grandfathered plan loses that exemption if it changes in any substantial way.

Grievance—A formal complaint by a member about a payer, requiring a response within fixed timelines. It does not apply to appeals of benefits coverage denials (also referred to simply as appeals), which also follow a formal process.

Group—The members of a health plan who are covered by virtue of receiving coverage at a single company.

Group Health Insurance—A commercial health insurance or HMO policy that is sold to an employer to provide coverage to its employees. This term does not apply to conversion policies or direct-pay policies, nor to Medicare or Medicaid plans.

Group Model HMO—An HMO that contracts with a medical group for the provision of healthcare services. The relationship between the HMO and the medical group is generally very close, although there are wide variations in the relative independence of the group from the HMO. A form of closed-panel health plan.

Group Practice—According to the American Medical Association, three or more physicians who deliver patient care, make joint use of equipment and personnel, and divide income by a prearranged formula.

Group Practice Without Walls (GPWW)—A group practice in which the members of the group come together legally, but continue to practice in private offices scattered throughout the service area. Sometimes called a clinic without walls (CWW).

Guaranteed Availability, Issue, or Renewal—A law that requires insurers to offer and renew coverage, without regard to health status, use of services, or preexisting conditions. The ACA requires these conditions apply to all individuals and employer groups, although the requirement may be limited to open enrollment periods or following a life event.

HBP—See Hospital-Based Physician.

HCAHPS—Hospital Consumer Assessment of Healthcare Providers and Systems Survey. See also Consumer Assessment of Healthcare Providers and Systems (CAHPS).

HCFA—See Health Care Financing Administration.

HCFA-1500—See CMS-1500.

HCPCS—See Healthcare (previously HCFA) Common Procedural Coding System.

HDHP—High-deductible health plan. See also High-Deductible Health Insurance.

Health Care—The services that a healthcare professional or institution provides to customers (services from a physician, at a hospital, from a physical therapist, and so on) as well as medical goods such as prescription drugs and durable medical equipment; it is this meaning of the term that is intended when discussing care management. A broader definition encompasses services from nontraditional providers and, more importantly, the health care that individuals self-administer, which is actually the majority of health care most people receive. When individuals use the term "health care" in its broadest sense, they frequently use the term "medical care" to refer to what is considered the narrow meaning.

Health Care Anti-Fraud Association—A public–private partnership founded in 1985 to combat fraud in health care.

Health Care Financing Administration (HCFA)—The older name of the Centers for Medicare & Medicaid Services.

Health Information Exchange (HIE)—An entity to facilitate the electronic exchange of health information between physicians, hospitals, laboratories, payers, and so on. By informal convention, the acronym "HIE" is used for Health Information Exchange, while "HIX" is used for Health Insurance Exchange.

Health Insurance—Technically, health benefits plans for which an insurer is at risk for costs. More broadly, any type of health plan. Technically HMOs are not considered health insurance, as they are licensed differently than are insurers and are subject to different regulations, but the general public often includes HMOs as a form of health insurance. This term is even used to describe self-funded benefits plans in which the employer is at risk for expenses, not an insurance company or an HMO (a legal distinction that is rarely made by most individuals covered by a self-funded plan).

Health Insurance Exchange (HIX or "Exchange")—Under the ACA, state-level health insurance exchanges where individuals and small group employers may purchase qualified health plans. The exchange used by small businesses is referred to as the Small Business Health Options Program (SHOP). States may set up and run their own exchanges, they may partner with the federal government to do so, or they may choose not run their own exchange. If a state does not create an exchange, the federal government steps in to administer the HIX. Provisions in the ACA also allow for multistate health insurance exchanges. By informal convention, the acronym "HIX" is used for Health Insurance Exchange, while "HIE" is used for Health Information Exchange.

Health Insurance Portability and Accountability Act (HIPAA)—Enacted in 1997, part of HIPAA provides benefits coverage issue and continuation rights that have since been made obsolete by provisions of the ACA. More importantly, HIPAA's administrative simplification provisions mandate the use of certain standardized electronic transactions by covered entities, privacy and security requirements, and use of standardized identifiers by covered entities. See also Covered Entities.

Health Insuring Organization (HIO)—An organization that contracts with a state Medicaid agency as both a fiscal intermediary and to manage the beneficiaries covered by the HIO. The term may less commonly, and more loosely, be used to refer to health insurers generally.

Health Level 7 (HL7)—A designated standards maintenance organization under HIPAA that focuses on electronic connectivity standards for clinical information.

Health Maintenance Organization (HMO)—The definition of an HMO has changed substantially, at least in common use. Originally, an HMO was defined as a prepaid organization that provided health care to voluntarily enrolled members in return for a preset amount of money on a per member per month (PMPM) basis. That, however, was based on group model HMOs of the time, so years ago it was replaced by language similar to that found in the NAIC Model HMO Act: "Health Maintenance Organization means a person that undertakes to provide or arrange for the delivery of basic health care services to covered persons on a prepaid basis, except for a covered person's responsibility for copayment, coinsurance or deductibles." With the increase in self-insured business, or with financial arrangements that do not rely on prepayment, even that definition is no longer accurate. A working definition of an HMO in the current environment could also include the following: It is licensed by the state under a certificate of authority; it is one of the few types of payers that may enter into risk-sharing payment arrangements with providers (although the ACA's Shared Savings Program for the traditional FFS Medicare program includes risk, so this aspect of the definition is now a little shaky); it must meet network access needs that are more stringent than most other types of payer; it must have strong "hold harmless" language in its provider contracts; it usually (but not always) requires members to go through their PCP to access specialty services; it allows direct access to all types of PCPs and OB/GYNs; and it has policies and procedures for utilization and quality management that exceed that found in most other types of payer.

Health Outcomes Survey (HOS) or Medicare Hospital Outcomes Survey (MHOS)—A survey that health plans with a Medicare Advantage risk contract must conduct to look at clinical outcomes of covered Medicare beneficiaries. CMS arranges and pays for administration of the CAHPS, while Medicare Advantage health plans are responsible for administering the HOS.

Health Plan—Technically, the health plan is the benefits plan, including its sponsor, not necessarily the administrator of the plan. Said another way, from a technical standpoint, for fully insured policies, the health plan is the insurer or HMO; for self-funded benefits plans, it is the employer and that plan's fiduciary that are considered the health plan, though this distinction is not always made by providers and patients. See also Fiduciary.

Health Plan Identifier (HPID)—A uniform health plan identification number required under HIPAA. Originally scheduled for a 2014 implementation date, at the time of publication it has been postponed indefinitely.

Health Reimbursement Account/Arrangement (HRA)—A financial account associated with a consumer-directed health plan that is used to pay for first-dollar qualified healthcare expenses up to a preset limit using pretax funds provided solely by an employer; it is regulated under tax laws. Unused HRA funds typically may roll into the next year, but they do not follow an individual when he or she changes employment. An HRA is always associated with a high-deductible health plan.

Health Risk Appraisal (HRA)—An instrument designed to elicit or compile information about the health risk of any given individual. Initially these tools were fairly uniform, but some are now specialized and targeted toward particular populations with distinctive risk profiles (e.g., Medicare, Medicaid, underserved, commercial population).

Health Savings Account (HSA)—Created under the MMA, a financial account containing pretax dollars intended to cover current or future qualified medical expenses, retirement, or long-term care premium expenses. Unused funds typically roll into HSAs for following years. This type of consumer-directed health plan is funded and used by individuals; it always associated with a qualified high-deductible health plan; and it is regulated under tax laws.

Healthcare Common Procedural Coding System (HCPCS, previously HCFA)—A set of codes used by Medicare and other payers that describes services and procedures. The HCPCS is divided into two parts: Level I is comprised of CPT codes maintained by the AMA; Level II is everything else (more or less) and is maintained by CMS. While HCPCS is nationally defined, there is provision for local use of certain codes. Many HCPCS Level II codes will be replaced by special codes in ICD-10, but not HCPCS Level I codes.

Healthcare Cooperative—One of the earliest forms of health plans and a forerunner of managed care; a nonprofit organization operated by its members for providing care to its members. Healthcare cooperatives generally look like prepaid group health plans. Once more common, examples of well-known existing co-ops include Group Health Cooperative of Puget Sound and Group Health Cooperative of Southern Wisconsin. See also CO-OP for its use as defined in the ACA.

Healthcare Effectiveness Data and Information Set (HEDIS)—An ever-evolving set of data reporting standards developed by NCQA with considerable input from the employer, provider, and managed care communities. HEDIS is designed to provide some standardization in performance reporting of financial, utilization, membership, and clinical data, and more. Medicare and many states accept or require HEDIS data as meeting certain regulatory requirements. Employers and consumers then can compare the performance of various plans, if a plan reports HEDIS data. Originally called the Health Plan Employer Data Information Set, these standards initially focused on HMOs, but they have since become used by many PPOs and other types of plans. They have also become much more varied, and different versions now exist for commercial, Medicare Advantage, and managed Medicaid plans.

Healthcare Integrity and Protection Data Bank (HIPDB)—An electronic data bank established under HIPAA that records information about providers related to fraud and abuse, criminal convictions, civil judgments, injunctions, licensure restrictions, and exclusion from participation in any governmental programs. Now combined with the National Practitioner Data Bank and called simply "The Databank."

HEDIS—See Healthcare Effectiveness Data and Information Set.

HHS—See Department of Health and Human Services.

HIE—See Health Information Exchange.

High-Deductible Health Insurance/High-Deductible Health Plan (HDHP)—A health insurance policy with very high minimum and maximum annual deductibles; for example, for 2015 the minimum single and family deductibles are $1300 and $2600, respectively, while single and family maximum deductibles are $6450 and $12,900, respectively. The specific deductible amounts are determined each year by the Treasury Department.

High-Risk Pool—Programs that were found in some, but not all, states designed to provide health insurance to residents who are considered medically uninsurable and are unable to buy coverage in the individual market. The ACA provided extra funding for states to expand eligibility for uninsurable individuals. Beginning in 2014, guaranteed issue requirements under the ACA made such pools unnecessary for the most part. High-risk pools still exist here and there, however, especially in states that did not expand Medicaid under the ACA and therefore have a group of low-income individuals who have no coverage but who have significant medical problems. Coverage through High-Risk Pools is usually limited compared to regular health coverage.

High-Value Plan—A high-cost health plan that exceeds cost levels defined under the ACA and, therefore, is subject to an additional tax. Also referred to informally as a "Cadillac" health plan.

HIO—See Health Insuring Organization.

HIPAA—See Health Insurance Portability and Accountability Act.

HIPDB—See Healthcare Integrity and Protection Data Bank.

HIX—See Health insurance exchange.

HL7—See Health Level 7.

HMO—See Health Maintenance Organization.

HMO Act of 1973 (42 U.S.C. § 300e)—A law passed by Congress in 1973 to promote the expansion of HMOs by putting aside state anti-HMO laws and requiring large employers to offer at least one closed-panel and one open-panel HMO. This act also required HMOs to offer then-rare comprehensive benefits and abide by community rating requirements. Some elements of the HMO Act are no longer in effect, although the law itself is.

Hold Harmless Clause—A contractual clause between a provider and a payer that prohibits the provider from billing a member for charges associated with covered services, other than copayments, coinsurance and/or deductible, even if the payer does not pay anything (i.e., the provider holds the member harmless in the event of nonpayment by the payer).

HOPPS—See Hospital Outpatient Prospective Payment System.

HOS—See Health Outcomes Survey.

Hospice—A program or facility dedicated to palliative care at the end of life. It may consist of a combination of a home-care program, an outpatient facility, and/or an inpatient facility.

Hospital-Based Physician (HBP)—A specialty physician who practices primarily within a hospital or ambulatory surgical center in one of five clinical areas: anesthesia, radiology, pathology, emergency department, or as a hospitalist. Traditionally, this term is not applied to hospital-employed physicians except if they fit into one of these categories. See also RAPs.

Hospital-Employed Physician—The direct employment of a physician by a hospital or health system. The term could be applied to an HBP, but the more common usage is for other specialties such as primary care, cardiology, and so forth. Employment may be direct, or may be done through an intermediate organization such as a captive medical group.

Hospital Outpatient Prospective Payment System (HOPPS)—The overall term used by CMS for its different methods of prospective payment to facilities for outpatient care such as surgery, dialysis, and drug administration.

Hospitalist—A physician who concentrates solely on hospitalized patients.

HPID—See Health Plan Identifier.

HRA—See Health Risk Appraisal or Health Reimbursement Account, depending on the context.

HSA—See Health Savings Account.

IBNR—See Incurred But Not Reported.

ICD-9-CM—International Classification of Diseases, Ninth Revision, Clinical Modification. ICD-9-CM classifies diseases by diagnosis using six-digit numbers. It will be replaced by ICD-10 by October 1, 2015.

ICD-10—International Classification of Diseases, Tenth Revision. ICD-10 will replace ICD-9-CM and several other codes sets on October 1, 2015. It has up to seven alphanumeric characters, allowing coding of up to 16,000 different diseases, procedures, patient complaints, and other clinical data.

IDN—See Integrated Delivery System.

IDS—See Integrated Delivery System.

Impaired Insurer—An insurer that is in financial difficulty to the point where its ability to meet its financial obligations or regulatory requirements is in question.

Imputed Premium—Applies to self-funded plans where no actual premium is paid (other than reinsurance premium) because the self-funded plan bears the risk for costs rather than the insurer. However, even a self-funded plan must budget for expected costs and must determine the amount that should be deducted from an employee's paycheck for his or her portion of the cost of the plan; therefore, an imputed premium is calculated for these purposes. Also called premium equivalent.

In-Office Ancillary Services Exception (IOASE)—A loophole that allows physicians to bill Medicare for ancillary services they provide as long as those services are provided in the physician's office. Provisions in the ACA require physicians who own and order certian costly "in-office" services, such as CT or PET scanners, to disclose their ownership to Medicare, and to provide their patients with a disclosure form that also lists alternative providers.

In-Sourcing—Bringing back into the payer a process or activity that was once outsourced.

Incurred But Not Reported (IBNR)—The amount of money that the plan should accrue for medical expenses for which no claims have yet been received, but will need to paid once they do come in. Inadequate claims reserves due to faulty or unaccounted for IBNRs have torpedoed more managed care plans than any other cause. Typical causes for inadequate IBNRs include inexperienced managers, faulty information systems, claims backlogs, and delusional optimism.

Indemnity Insurance—Insurance that "indemnifies" the policyholder from losses to at least some degree. In health insurance, this applies to providing financial coverage for healthcare costs. Once common, pure health insurance indemnity plans are quite rare now due to their high costs, though any out-of-network coverage may be considered a form of indemnity insurance.

Independent Practice Association (IPA)—An organization that has a contract with a managed care plan to deliver services in return for a single capitation rate. The IPA, in turn, contracts with individual providers to provide the services either on a capitation basis or on a FFS basis. The typical IPA encompasses all specialties, but an IPA can be solely for primary care, or it may be single specialty. An IPA may also be the "physician organization" part of a physician–hospital organization.

Independent Review Organization—An independent group with which a state or a payer contracts to provide a secondary external review of coverage denials based on medical reasons. The use of an IRO for external review is required in most states, and is required for all payers and health plans under the ACA.

Individual Mandate or Penalty—An ACA requirement that all individuals, except for those with a low income, obtain health insurance. The individual mandate is the other side of the guaranteed issue requirement, so that all individuals, not just the sick ones, will contribute funds to the overall risk pool.

Individual Policy—See Direct Pay.

Information Technology (IT)—A blanket term referring to all of the computer hardware and software systems that support the operations of a health plan.

Virtually all operational functions of a health plan are supported by IT in one way or another. An older term that is still used by some is Management Information System (MIS).

Integrated Delivery System (IDS)—Also referred to as an integrated healthcare delivery system or an integrated delivery network (IDN). An organized system of healthcare providers spanning a broad range of healthcare services. In its full flower, an IDS should be able to access the market on a broad basis, optimize cost and clinical outcomes, accept and manage a full range of financial arrangements to provide a set of defined benefits to a defined population, align financial incentives of the participants (including physicians), and operate under a cohesive management structure. See also Accountable Care Organization, Equity Model, Foundation Model, Independent Practice Association, Management Service Organization, Physician–Hospital Organization, and Staff Model.

Intelligent Call Routing or Skill-Based Routing—A computer system in a call center or contact center that sends the contact to the customer service representative (CSR) group best prepared to handle the contact. Criteria for routing may include the issue type, severity of the issue, past history of interaction with a specific CSR or set of CSRs, employer group, or other business rules into which have been programmed into the switch (i.e., the computerized telephone system). See also Switch.

Intensivist—A type of hospitalist who focuses solely on care provided in the intensive (or critical) care unit.

Intermediary—See Fiscal Intermediary.

Investigational Treatment—See Experimental and Investigational Treatment.

IOASE—See In-Office Ancillary Services Exception.

IPA—See Independent Practice Association.

IRO—See Independent Review Organization.

IS—Information systems. See Information Technology.

I-SNP—Institutional special needs plan for beneficiaries who are institutionalized in a skilled- or intermediate-care nursing facility, or an assisted living facility.

IT—See Information Technology.

JCAHO—See The Joint Commission.

J-Codes—A subset of the HCPCS codes used by Medicare, Medicaid, and commercial payers to identify injectable drugs and oral immunosuppressive drugs. May be created on the fly by CMS when a new drug first appears.

The Joint Commission (TJC)—A not-for-profit organization that performs the majority of accreditation reviews on hospitals, ambulatory facilities, and other types of clinical facilities. Most managed care plans require any hospital under contract to be accredited by The Joint Commission or a similar type of accreditation organization acceptable to Medicare. The old name was the Joint Commission for the Accreditation of Healthcare Organizations (JCAHO).

Lag Study—A report related to IBNRs that tells managers how old the claims are when they are processed and how much is paid out each month (both for that month and for any earlier months) and compares these to the amount of money that was accrued for expenses each month as IBNRs. This powerful tool is used to monitor whether the plan's reserves are adequate to meet all expenses. It is often automated. Plans that fail to perform lag studies properly may find themselves descending into the abyss.

Lag Table—The tool used by financial personnel to manage the lag study manually.

Lapse—To drop coverage. This may refer to an individual who stops paying premiums, thereby allowing his or her policy to lapse, subject to a grace period. When used as a ratio, it is the opposite of a persistency ratio (i.e., the percentage of commercially enrolled groups that drop the health plan).

Laser or Lasering—Actuarial and underwriting reinsurance slang referring to reducing or eliminating a very specific benefit—in other words, a benefit reduction that is focused like a laser. The more formal term used by reinsurers is a "special limitations" clause. Lasering is used only in self-funded employee benefits plans because it is prohibited in state-regulated health insurance, but reinsurance is not technically health insurance. Examples of a laser might include placing very high deductibles or significant limits on claims incurred by a single individual (e.g., an employee with a disabled dependent), specific conditions (e.g., hemophilia), or types of treatments (e.g., transplants). A laser does not, however, mean that the self-funded employee benefits plan can also reduce benefits in the same way, which would likely be considered discriminatory under ERISA. Only the reinsurer can apply the laser, while the employer remains liable for benefit costs.

Length of Stay (LOS)—The total number of days spent in the hospital for an inpatient admission.

Levels of Coverage—Cost-sharing levels defined in the ACA as falling into four categories: Platinum (90% coverage), Gold (80%), Silver (70%), and Bronze (60%). Cost sharing includes all out-of-pocket expenses such as copayments, coinsurance, and deductibles. It applies only to services provided by in-network providers.

Life Event—An event in a person's life that makes him or her eligible for coverage outside of the usual eligibility periods—for example, childbirth or adoption of a child, or losing coverage as a consequence of losing employment. See also Special Enrollment Period.

Lifetime Maximum—A term no longer applicable in health insurance for the maximum benefit available under a benefits plan; once that maximum is reached, there would be no additional coverage. A common example would have been a $2 million lifetime maximum, so that if an individual with extremely high healthcare costs reached a point where that much coverage had been spent, that individual had no more coverage. Lifetime maximums are now prohibited under the ACA. See also Annual Limit.

Limited Benefits Plan—Very low-cost health "insurance" that offers significant limits on benefits by capping the amount that the insurer pays out. For example, it may cap coverage at only $10,000 or $20,000 per year, and may cover outpatient care only up to a set amount of dollars per visit regardless of charges. These plans do not provide adequate coverage for any serious illness or injury and are not considered as qualified plans under the ACA. Also called a "Mini-Med" plan.

Line of Business (LOB)—A health plan such as a health maintenance organization, exclusive provider organization, or preferred provider organization that is set up as a line of business within another, larger organization, such as an insurance company. This legally differentiates it from a free-standing company or a company set up as a subsidiary. It may also refer to a unique product type (e.g., Medicaid) within a health plan.

LIS—See Low-Income Subsidy.

LOB—See Line of Business.

Lock-in Period—The period of time during which a member cannot switch to another plan. For example, MA annual open enrollment begins in the fall each year and coverage begins on January 1, but beneficiaries can change plans until April 1 when the lock-in period begins.

Long-Term Care—Services needed by people to live in the community, such as home health and personal care, as well as institutional care such as nursing homes. Long-term care is not covered by any commercial or self-funded health plan or by Medicare. It is paid for either through special long-term care insurance policies, out of pocket, or by Medicaid for low-income individuals.

LOS/ELOS/ALOS—Length of stay/estimated length of stay/average length of stay. See also Length of Stay.

Loss Ratio—See Medical Loss Ratio.

Low-Income Subsidy (LIS)—A subsidy provided for dual-eligible (Medicare–Medicaid) individuals for the Part D drug benefit.

MA Local Plan—A Medicare Advantage managed care plan that does not provide services throughout an entire region as designated by CMS.

MA Regional Plan—A Medicare Advantage PPO plan that provides services throughout an entire region as designated by CMS.

MAC—See Maximum Allowable Charge or Cost.

MACPAC—See Medicaid and CHIP Payment and Access Commission.

Major Medical—An old but still used term that refers to health insurance covering physician and many other nonhospitalization services. It can be traced back to the 1940s through the early 1960s when employer-sponsored group health coverage usually covered "hospitalization," meaning hospital costs only. Commercial insurers of the time were essentially mimicking Blue Cross and Blue Shield plans with their historical roots in coverage of services provided by hospitals and physicians, respectively. The term was never applicable to self-funded plans or HMOs, and became a relic in 2014 when the ACA's qualified health benefit plans went into effect.

Managed Behavioral Healthcare Organization (MBHO)—A third party that manages the behavioral health services benefits for a payer. It may also contract directly with an employer. An MBHO may be at financial risk, or it may manage the services under an administrative contract only. A form of clinical outsourcing.

Managed Care Organization (MCO)—A generic term applied to all types of managed care plans. It arose because many thought that it held less negative connotation than did the term HMO. This term was then broadened to encompass plans other than HMOs, such as POS plans, PPOs, EPOs, CDHPs, or any other type of plan that uses elements of managed health care.

Managed Health Care—A somewhat nebulous term referring to a system of healthcare financing, benefits management, and delivery (closed-panel HMOs and IDSs only) that tries to manage the cost of health care benefits, quality, and access. Common denominators include a panel of contracted (or in some cases, employed) providers that is less than the entire universe of available providers, some type of limitations on benefits to members who use noncontracted providers (unless authorized to do so), and some type of authorization or precertification system.

Management Information System (MIS)—An older term for information technology (IT). See Information Technology.

Management Service Organization (MSO)—A form of integrated health delivery system. Sometimes similar to a service bureau, the MSO may actually purchase certain hard assets of a physician's practice, and then provide services to that physician at fair market rates. MSOs are often formed as a means to contract more effectively with managed care organizations, although their simple creation does not guarantee success.

Mandated Benefits—Benefits that a health plan is required to provide by law. This term applies to some benefits required in the ACA such as first dollar coverage for prevention or in-network coverage levels for emergency care. More commonly, however, it applies to condition- or treatment-specific coverage required by a state, with high variability from state to state. Common examples include in vitro fertilization and other special-condition treatments. Self-funded plans are exempt from most mandated benefits under ERISA, but even the federal government gets into the act with a mandatory two-day length of stay for childbirth and mental health parity provisions under HIPAA and the ACA that apply to both insured and self-funded plans.

Manual Rate—See Book Rate.

MAO—See Medicare Advantage Organization.

Margin—The amount of money left over, or lost, after costs are subtracted from revenues. There are two different types: operating margin and underwriting margin.

Market Segment—A portion of the total market that may be defined two different ways—by the source of funding and by size. The two entitlement programs, Medicare and Medicaid, each make up a market segment, with the commercial market making up a third segment. Within the commercial market segment, segments are further divided by size into the individual market segment; the small group market segment, meaning employers with at least 1 but no more than 100 full-time equivalent employees (states may reduce this to 50 or more employees); and the large group market.

Markup Fee—A type of add-on provider fee in which the cost of something is marked up by a percentage amount. For example, a physician administering intravenous chemotherapy in the office may charge for the office visit, for the administration of the chemotherapy, and for the drugs and IV solutions at cost plus 50%. Medicare and many commercial health plans limit the markup fee to approximately 6%.

Master Group Contract—The actual contract between a health plan and a group that purchases coverage. The master group contract provides specific terms of coverage, rights, and responsibilities of both parties.

Master Member Index (MMI)—A database used to identify in a reliable manner each member, or in medical management to identify each patient receiving care from a particular physician.

Maximum Allowable Cost (MAC)—The maximum that a vendor may charge for something. MAC is a term that is often used in pharmacy contracting; a related term, used in conjunction with professional fees, is maximum allowable charge or fee maximum.

Maximum Out-of-Pocket Cost—The most amount of money a member will ever need to pay out of pocket for covered services during a contract year. The maximum out-of-pocket expenditure includes deductibles, copayments and coinsurance. Once this limit is reached, cost-sharing stops.

MBHO—See Managed Behavioral Healthcare Organization.

McCarran-Ferguson Act of 1945—Federal legislation that established (by default) that states had the authority and responsibility to regulate the business of insurance without federal government interference, and that allows states to establish mandatory licensing requirements. This act also contains a limited antitrust exemption allowing insurers to share certain underwriting information for purposes of rate development, but that aspect is not particularly relevant to health insurers or payers.

MCE—See Medical Care Evaluation.

MCO—See Managed Care Organization.

MEC—See Minimum Essential Coverage.

Medicaid—The federal entitlement program under Social Security Act Title XIX that is funded jointly by the states and the federal government, and which provides health and long-term care coverage to certain categories of low-income Americans; it was enacted in 1965 at the same time as Medicare. States may design their own programs within broad federal guidelines. Medicaid eligibility was expanded under the ACA, but states are not required to comply. See also Medicaid Expansion.

Medicaid and CHIP Payment and Access Commission (MACPAC)—A commission created by the ACA to focus on Medicaid payment policy. MACPAC is similar to MedPAC, which focuses on Medicare payment policy.

Medicaid Expansion—The portion of the ACA that increased eligibility for Medicaid coverage by requiring states to expand Medicaid eligibility standards to a consistent level, with the federal government assuming 100% of the cost until 2016, after which the federal government will assume 90% of the cost. The U.S. Supreme Court, along with ruling that the ACA was constitutional, removed Medicaid expansion as a requirement for states. Consequently, some states have not undertaken this expansion of coverage.

Medicaid Management Information System (MMIS)—The mechanized claims processing and information retrieval system that states are required to have, unless this requirement is waived by the Secretary of Health and Human Services.

Medicaid Waivers—Also known as a Section 1115 waiver; a section of federal law allowing a state to opt out of the standard Medicaid fee-for-service program and adopt a managed care approach to financing and providing healthcare services to Medicaid-eligible recipients. It usually requires that some of the savings be applied to broaden coverage of who is eligible for Medicaid.

Medical Care Evaluation (MCE)—A component of a quality assurance program that looks at the process of medical care. The term is now archaic, but was used specifically when HMOs were federally qualified.

Medical Home—See Patient-Centered Medical Home.

Medical Loss Ratio (MLR)—The ratio between the amount paid out for medical benefits and the amount of money that was taken through premium payments. It applies only to fully insured or at-risk business. See also Medical Loss Ratio Limitations.

Medical Loss Ratio (MLR) Limitations—The ACA sets limits on the MLR of 80% for individual and small group coverage, and 85% for large groups. If the MLR is below those levels, the plan must rebate the difference; if it is above these levels, the plan must absorb any losses that may result and may not recover it later by raising rates. The MLR depends on the amount of money brought in as well as the cost of delivering care; thus, if the rates are too low, the ratio may be high, even though the actual cost of delivering care is not really out of line.

Medical Policy or Medical Payment Policy—From an operational point of view, the internal rules about what will be paid for as medical benefits. Routine medical policy is linked to routine claims processing, and is typically automated. For example, the plan may pay only 50% of the fee of a second surgeon, or it may not pay for two surgical procedures done during one episode of anesthesia.

Medical Savings Account (MSA)—A specialized savings account into which a consumer can put pretax dollars for use in paying medical expenses in lieu of purchasing a comprehensive health insurance or managed care product. MSAs were created as a demonstration under BBA '97 and updated in the MMA. They require a catastrophic health insurance policy as a "safety net" to protect against very high costs. They still exist, in both commercial form and for Medicare, but have been supplanted by HSAs and HRAs in consumer-directed health plans that are similar in approach but have additional features that make them more attractive to the market.

Medically Necessary or Medical Necessity—The policies used for benefits determinations when medical services or products may or may not be covered depending on certain criteria. Typical criteria used include being necessary to protect or preserve the health of an individual; being based on evidence-based clinical standards of care; not being primarily for the convenience of the patient or physician; not more costly than an alternative service or sequence of services at least as likely to produce equivalent results; not experimental or investigational care, except in defined circumstances; not considered custodial care or care that is essentially assistance with acts of daily living; and not considered medically appropriate by generally accepted standards of medical practice. "Medically necessary" is defined in the evidence of coverage document for all benefits plans; although those definitions are generally similar, they are typically not exactly the same.

Medicare—The federal entitlement program under Social Security Act Title XVIII under which health benefits coverage is provided by the federal government for citizens older than the age of 65 as well as some others, such as individuals with end-stage renal disease. Regular Medicare is a fee-for-service type of insurance; *Part A* covers hospital care and is the only mandatory part of the Medicare benefit, while *Part B* covers professional services. *Part C* authorizes private plans such as Medicare Advantage. *Part D*, passed under the MMA, provides a drug benefit. Traditional fee-for-service Medicare is administered by intermediaries on behalf of CMS, while Parts C and D come through various forms of private plans.

Medicare Advantage (MA)—Created as part of the MMA, a program that replaced the prior term Medicare+Choice and expanded other forms of Medicare managed care. MA plans may be HMOs, PPOs, or PFFS plans; they may also be local or regional. Special needs plans were also created to focus on specific types of beneficiaries. MA medical savings accounts are also overseen under MA.

Medicare Advantage MSA Plan (MA MSA)—A non-network-based Medicare Medical Savings Account plan. See also Medical Savings Account.

Medicare Advantage Organization (MAO)—CMS's overall term used to refer to the various types of MA plans.

Medicare+Choice—The old name for Medicare private insurance options, created under BBA '97; most often applied to Medicare HMOs. The name was replaced by Medicare Advantage under the MMA.

Medicare Improvements for Patients and Providers Act of 2008 (MIPPA)—A law that reduced overpayments to the MA plan, required MA private FFS plans to establish networks, changed Part D marketing practices, and added preventive benefits (pre-ACA), among other things.

Medicare Modernization Act of 2003 (MMA)—The federal act originally titled the Medicare Prescription Drug Improvement and Modernization Act of 2003. The MMA is the basis for both the Medicare Part D drug benefit and for the variety of Medicare Advantage (MA) plans described elsewhere, including MA Local, MA Regional, and MA PFFS.

Medicare Payment Advisory Commission (MedPAC)—An independent congressional agency established by the Balanced Budget Act of 1997 to advise Congress on issues affecting the Medicare program. The Commission's statutory mandate is to advise Congress on payments to providers in Medicare's traditional fee-for-service program and private health plans participating in Medicare, and to analyze access to care, quality of care, and other issues affecting Medicare.

Medicare Recovery Audit Contractors (RAC)—Auditors under contract with CMS to review the appropriateness of data supporting payment.

Medicare Severity Diagnosis-Related Groups (MS-DRGs)—A system implemented by Medicare to replace traditional DRGs. MS-DRGs not only are based on the diagnosis and procedures performed, but also take into account other chronic conditions and comorbidities, including those that are major. The intent in developing this system was to reduce the number of cases classified as outliers.

Medicare Shared Savings Program (MSSP)—A payment methodology in traditional fee-for-service Medicare in which an accountable care organization (ACO) is paid as usual, but an overall cost target is calculated for a cohort of individuals with high medical costs who are "assigned" to the ACO, and the ACO shares in a portion of any savings compared to that target. The ACO also shares risk in that it must repay a portion of any costs in excess of the target. Unlike in an HMO, there is no lock-in, meaning beneficiaries are not required to use the ACO for care.

Medication Therapy Management (MTM)—A program to ensure optimal therapeutic outcomes and reduced adverse events for targeted beneficiaries through improved medication use. MTM is required under the MMA for Part D sponsors.

MediGap Insurance—A form of state-licensed supplemental insurance that covers much of what Medicare does not. MediGap policies are subject to minimum standards under federal law and are restricted to 12 different benefits plans, labeled A through L, sold and administered by private companies. MediGap has been further restricted under the MMA.

MedPAC—See Medicare Payment Advisory Commission.

Member—An individual covered under a managed care plan. May be either the subscriber or a dependent. See also Subscriber.

Member-Months—The total number of members covered each month, added together. For example, if a plan had 10,000 members in January and 12,000 members in February, the total member-months for those two months would be 22,000.

Member Services—The department that directly interacts with members, not including the actual provision of health care. Examples of member services include resolving problems, managing disputes by members about coverage issues, and managing the grievance and appeals processes. Member services may also function in a proactive manner, reaching out to members with educational programs, self-service capabilities, and the like. Known in other industries as customer services.

Mental Health Parity Act of 1996—The initial federal legislation that required annual or lifetime dollar limits on mental health benefits to be no lower than dollar limits for medical and surgical benefits offered by a group health plan. This act did not apply to benefits for substance abuse or chemical dependency, however. See also Mental Health Parity and Addiction Equity Act of 2008.

Mental Health Parity and Addiction Equity Act of 2008—Federal legislation that requires group health plans and health insurance issuers to ensure that financial requirements (such as copayments and deductibles) and treatment limitations (such as visit limits) for mental health or substance use benefits are no more restrictive than those used for medical/surgical benefits. Provisions of this act were strengthened under the ACA, which also eliminated the annual and lifetime limit for all benefits, including mental health and addition services.

Messenger Model—A type of integrated delivery system (IDS), usually a physician–hospital organization, that simply acts as a messenger between a payer and the providers participating in the IDS in regard to contracting terms. It does not have the power to collectively bargain, thus avoiding antitrust violations.

MET—Multiple employer trust. See Multiple Employer Welfare Association.

MEWA—See Multiple Employer Welfare Association.

MFN—See Most Favored Nation Clause.

MHOS—See Hospital Outcome Survey.

MHS—See Military Health System.

Midlevel Practitioner (MLP)—Physician's assistants, clinical nurse practitioners, nurse–midwives, and the like; nonphysicians who deliver medical care, generally under the supervision of a physician but for less cost. The term has been declining in use over the past several years.

Military Health System (MHS)—A large and complex healthcare system designed to provide, and to maintain readiness to provide, medical services and support to the armed forces during military operations and to provide medical services and support to members of the armed forces, their dependents, and others entitled to Department of Defense medical care. See also TRICARE.

Mini-Med—See Limited Benefits Plan.

Minimum Creditable Coverage—The minimum level of health benefits coverage from any source necessary for an individual to be considered insured under the requirements of the ACA.

Minimum Essential Coverage (MEC)—A term that is roughly equivalent to minimum creditable coverage.

Minimum Premium Plan—A once-common type of insurance plan for large employer groups that closely resembles self-funding, in which the employer is responsible for claims costs up to a certain level, which is usually very high. After that, the insurer is at risk, similar to reinsurance. With the advent of ERISA, minimum premium plans have largely been replaced with self-funded plans and reinsurance.

MIPPA—See Medicare Improvements for Patients and Providers Act of 2008.

MIS—See Management Information System.

Mixed Model—A managed care plan that mixes two or more types of delivery systems. This term has traditionally been used to describe an HMO that has both closed-panel and open-panel delivery systems.

MLP—See Midlevel Practitioner.

MLR—See Medical Loss Ratio.

MMA—See Medicare Modernization Act.

MMI—See Master Member Index.

MMIS—See Medicaid Management Information System.

Modified Adjusted Gross Income (MAGI)—How an individual's income is determined under the ACA for purposes of coverage subsidies and/or eligibility for Medicaid coverage.

Moral Hazard—In the context of insurance, changes in the behavior of an insured individual (or organization) caused by the existence of insurance itself, such that the behavior change may increase costs to the insurer. The word moral refers to a state of mind (e.g., "moral support"), and hazard may refer to a dice game that is the forerunner of craps. A description of the many ways moral hazard can occur is beyond the scope of any simple glossary, but examples include buying coverage only when you need it so that the benefits you receive always outweigh the cost you pay in (e.g., the cost of a gallbladder removal is around 25 times higher than the cost of 3 months of premiums), operating under the principle of induced demand (e.g., you do not burn down your house because it's insured, but you do go to the doctor because you're insured), or receiving benefits simply because you do not have to pay for them, or in the case of providers, ordering a service simply because it is profitable (e.g., a physician overordering costly scans using a scanner that he or she owns and profits from).

Most Favored Nation (MFN) Clause—A clause in a contract between a payer and a health system that requires the health system to give the payer the best rate; in other words, a clause that prohibits the health system from giving any nongovernmental payer a more favorable rate than it gives the payer. Once commonly used by large hegemonic payers such as Blue Cross and Blue Shield plans that had most of the business in a state, MFN clauses are now illegal in many states, although they are not actually considered anticompetitive.

MSA—See Medical Savings Account.

MS-DRG—See Medicare Severity Diagnosis-Related Groups.

MSO—See Management Service Organization.

MSSP—See Medicare Shared Savings Program.

MTM—See Medication Therapy Management.

Multiple Employer Trust (MET) or Multiple Employer Welfare Association (MEWA)—A group of employers that band together for purposes of creating a self-funded health benefits plan to avoid state mandates, premium taxes, and insurance regulation. By virtue of ERISA, such entities are regulated little, if at all by the states. However, they are subject to the ACA in the same manner as any self-funded benefits plans. Many MEWAs have enabled small employers to obtain less costly health coverage compared to purchasing health insurance, but some have not had the financial resources to withstand the risk of medical costs and have failed, leaving their employees and their dependents without coverage. They also risk having employer groups with low costs leave the MEWA to avoid subsidizing the cost of coverage for employer groups with high costs, putting the MEWA into a death spiral. MEWAs and METs are also more susceptible to fraud than traditional insurance or a single employer self-funded benefits plan. See also Association Health Plan and Death Spiral.

Mutual Insurance Company, Mutual Insurer, or Mutual—Companies with no capital stock, which are owned by policyholders. The earnings of the company—over and above the payments of the losses, operating expenses, and reserves—are the property of the policyholders.

NADDI—See National Association of Drug Diversion Investigators.

NAIC—See National Association of Insurance Commissioners.

National Association of Drug Diversion Investigators (NADDI)—A nonprofit organization that facilitates cooperation between law enforcement, healthcare professionals, state regulatory agencies, and pharmaceutical manufacturers in the prevention and investigation of prescription drug diversion.

National Association of Insurance Commissioners (NAIC)—An organization that represents all of the state insurance departments and that formulates model insurance laws and regulations. Provisions of the ACA require the Secretary of Health and Human Services to seek the recommendations of the NAIC for many elements of the U.S. healthcare insurance system.

National Committee on Quality Assurance (NCQA)—A nonprofit organization that performs accreditation reviews on HMOs and other types of managed care plans. NCQA also now accredits credentialing verification organizations, preferred provider organizations, certain types of disease management programs, and so forth. NCQA developed and maintains the HEDIS standards.

National Council for Prescription Drug Programs (NCPDP)—An organization that developed and maintains accepted electronic data interchange standards for pharmacy claims transmission and accelerated adjudication adoption of pharmacy e-commerce. These standards permit the submission of pharmacy claims and the adjudication of those claims in a real-time interactive mode. The NCPDP standards are recognized by ANSI and addressed under HIPAA.

National Drug Code (NDC)—The national classification system for identifying prescription drugs.

National Health Plan Identifier—See Health Plan Identifier.

National Practitioner Data Bank (NPDB)—A data bank established under the federal Health Care Improvement and Quality Act of 1986, which electronically stores information about physician malpractice suits successfully litigated or settled and disciplinary actions upon physicians. The NPDB is accessible by hospitals and health plans under controlled circumstances as part of the credentialing process. Hospitals and health plans must likewise report disciplinary actions to the data bank. It is now combined with the Healthcare Integrity and Protection Data Bank and called simply "The Databank."

National Provider Identifier (NPI)—An identification number mandated under HIPAA, which replaced most other types of provider identifiers regardless of the type of customer (e.g., commercial health plan, Medicare, Medicaid, TRICARE). The NPI does not replace the DEA number or the tax ID number of a provider, however.

National Quality Forum (NQF)—A not-for-profit, public–private organization created to develop and implement a national strategy for healthcare quality measurement and reporting. This voluntary consensus standards-setting organization addresses quality measurements in patient care, electronic health records, patient safety, and so forth.

Navigator—Under the ACA, a qualified entity that helps consumers and employers understand their options and select coverage through state health insurance exchanges.

NCPDP—See National Council for Prescription Drug Programs.

NCQA—See National Committee on Quality Assurance.

NDC—See National Drug Code.

NDP—See Notice of Denial of Payment.

Net Worth—See Statutory Net Worth.

Network Adequacy, or Network Adequacy Standards—See Access Standards.

Network Model HMO—Also called a true network model HMO; a health plan that contracts with multiple physician groups, usually large ones, to deliver health care to members. It is distinguished from group model plans that contract with a single medical group, independent practice associations that contract through an intermediary, and direct contract model plans that contract with individual physicians in the community. Note, however, that open-panel plans of any type are often referred to as network model plans, making this term less precise than the other HMO model types.

Never Events—See Serious Reportable Events.

NHCAA—See Health Care Anti-Fraud Association.

NIO—See Non-investor Owned.

Nonadmitted Asset—An asset owned by an insurer or HMO that does not count toward its statutory net worth under SAP rules. The understanding of this term may vary slightly from state to state, but it usually is applied to assets that cannot be readily converted into cash in the event of a health plan failure. It may also apply to only a portion of such an asset; for example, no more than 5% of a plan's statutory net worth can consist of such assets as computers, real estate, and so forth.

Non-investor Owned (NIO)—An insurer that is not a for-profit company, but is not technically a nonprofit charitable organization. It is most often a type of mutual insurer or mutual reserve company.

Nonpar—Slang that is short for a nonparticipating (non-contracted) provider.

Notice of Denial of Payment (NDP)—A form that CMS requires MA plans to use when notifying a beneficiary that a payment for a service is being denied, why it is being denied, and what the beneficiary's appeal rights are.

NPDB—See National Practitioner Databank.

NPI—See National Provider Identifier.

Null Claim—A claim submitted by a capitated provider that is used only to collect encounter data, not for purposes of payment.

Occurrence Insurance or Reinsurance—One of two primary types of professional liability insurance. This term applies to professional malpractice insurance for physicians as well as to directors' and officers' liability policies and to reinsurance. Occurrence means that the insurer has liability if the policy was in force when the event occurred, regardless of whether the professional has notified the insurer. It differs substantially from the other common form of professional liability known as claims made, and from a third type of reinsurance called claims paid. See also Claims Made Reinsurance or Insurance and Claims Paid Reinsurance.

OCR—See Office for Civil Rights or Optical Character Recognition, depending on the context.

Office for Civil Rights (OCR)—A department within the U.S. Department of Health and Human Services charged with enforcing HIPAA privacy and security standards, among other things.

Office of the Inspector General (OIG)—The federal agency responsible for conducting investigations and audits of federal contractors or any system that receives funds or payment from the federal government. There are actually several OIG departments in different federal programs; examples pertinent to managed health care would include DHHS, DOL, TRICARE, CMS, and the FEHBP.

Office of Personnel Management (OPM)—The federal agency that administers the FEHBP. A health insurance or managed care plan must contract with the OPM in order to be offered to federal employees.

OIG—See Office of the Inspector General.

Open Access—An HMO that does not use a primary care physician "gate-keeper" model to manage access to specialty physicians. In other words, a member may self-refer to a specialty physician rather than seeking an authorization from their PCP. HMOs that use an open-access model typically have a significant copayment differential depending on the physician from whom care is received. Also called direct access.

Open Enrollment Period—The period when an employee may change health plans, a Medicare Beneficiary can enroll in or change Medicare Advantage (MA) plans, or an individual or small group can apply for coverage under guaranteed issue. Open enrollments usually occur once per year. Open enrollment takes place for all individual and small group guaranteed issue, all MA, and about half of all large employer group coverage in the fall of each year for an effective date of January 1. The ACA leaves it to the states to define when that will happen each year, however, including the possibility of more than one open enrollment period.

Open-Panel HMO—A managed care plan that contracts (either directly or indirectly) with private physicians to deliver care in their own offices. Examples would include a direct contract HMO and an IPA-model HMO.

Operating Margin—The amount of money left over, or lost, after subtracting the cost of medical benefits and the cost of operations from revenues. It generally does not include the cost of taxes, but does include the revenue from investments; it also may or may not include margin contribution from subsidiaries.

OPL—See Other Party Liability.

OPM—See Office of Personnel Management.

Opt Out—(1) A managed care benefits design in which a member can opt out of using the plan's network and still receive some coverage for medical services. For example, a point-of-service plan may be considered an HMO with an opt-out benefit. (2) A brief period after the MA open enrollment period during which a Medicare beneficiary can opt out of an MA plan and go back to the traditional Medicare FFS plan.

Optical Character Recognition (OCR)—A system of hardware and software that is able to recognize written characters scanned in from a paper source and convert those characters into standard data. This technology is used in any processing systems in which paper forms (e.g., claims and enrollment forms) may be submitted. Data scanned in via OCR are usually checked by clerks for accuracy and to correct errors; however, this approach is still more efficient than keying the data in manually.

Organization Provider—The term used by NCQA and some other organizations to describe healthcare facilities—for example, hospitals, ambulatory care centers, dialysis centers, and so forth.

Out-of-Pocket—Any amount of money spent by a member on benefits. This term is usually synonymous with cost sharing, but some sources include payroll deductions in the category as well. See also True-Out-of-Pocket Cost.

Other Party Liability (OPL)—A condition in which another party is responsible for paying for costs. The most common examples are worker's compensation and automobile liability policies. See also Coordination of Benefits.

Other Weird Arrangement (OWA)—Some type of benefits plan, product design, payment scheme, or network contract that some bright person or consultant has created but for which there is no precedent, no track record, and no easy means of implementation.

Outlier—Something that is outside of a range; something that is significantly more or less than expected. This term is most often applied to hospital payment arrangements in which inpatient cases that exceed a certain cost, usually based on chargemaster fees, receive additional payments based on a discount to chargemaster fees. It may also refer to a provider who is using medical resources at a much higher rate than his or her peers.

Outsourcing—An arrangement in which a process or activity that a payer provides is handled by a contracted third party. It is somewhat broader than the term Business Process Outsourcing, which includes such activities as contracting with an off-shore company to manually enter data from images of paper claims. Outsourcing may also include medical management functions such as managing behavioral health utilization, or network management such as contracting and managing a provider network.

OWA—See Other Weird Arrangement.

P4P—See Pay for Performance.

PACE—See Programs for All-Inclusive Care for the Elderly.

Package Pricing—An older term for bundled payment. See also Bundled Payment.

Part D—The drug benefit created under the MMA and provided by a private, free-standing prescription drug plan (PDP) or included in an MA plan as an MA-PDP.

Partial Hospitalization—A hospital stay that lasts between 4 and 23 hours.

Participating Provider—A contracted provider.

Patient-Centered Medical Home (PCMH)—The term used by CMS and others to refer to a form of coordinated care through the use of designated clinical teams. The medical home concept put forth by a joint statement by the AAFP, ACP, AAP, and AOA emphasizes four primary care elements—accessibility, continuity, coordination, and comprehensiveness—which research shows positively affect health outcomes, satisfaction, and costs. Most well-run group-model HMOs have offered PCMHs for decades. Without substantial organizational changes, the PCMH concept's long-term utility, durability, and replicability is unknown. Sometimes called a primary care medical home or simply medical home.

Patient Protection and Affordable Care Act (ACA or PPACA; Public Law 111-148)—An act signed into law by President Barack Obama in 2010 that provides for a sweeping overhaul of the rules under which health insurance may operate and requirements for all types of health benefits plan. Some requirements apply only to fully insured plans, while others apply to both fully insured and to self-funded plans. The ACA also contains many provisions beyond those that directly affect health coverage, including changes in funding for primary care, payments to hospitals, and changes to Medicare Advantage and to Medicaid.

Patient Safety and Quality Improvement Act of 2005 (PSQIA)—A law providing federal privilege and confidentiality protections for patient safety information (called a patient safety work product) that includes information collected and created during the reporting and analysis of patient safety events. This act was created in response to the difficulty in collecting information about patient safety problems due to the threat of such information being used as the basis for a lawsuit.

Patient Safety Organization (PSO)—A new type of organization described by federal rules in which clinicians and healthcare providers can work to collect, aggregate, and analyze data within a legally secure environment of privilege and confidentiality protections to identify and reduce patient care risks and hazards. AHRQ administers provisions governing PSO operations, and DHHS's Office for Civil Rights enforces confidentiality provisions. The same acronym was used in the past for the now archaic term "provider-sponsored organization."

Patient's Bill of Rights (PBR)—A law or policy that describes the rights a patient has regarding his or her health care and how he or she should be treated, and that may be applied to either a provider or a payer. A voluntary PBR is often posted by hospitals. Some states also have PBR legislation regarding health insurers. In the 1990s, the U.S. Congress made several attempts to pass a PBR, but never succeeded. With the passage of the ACA, various provisions falling under the broad category of consumer protections are now called a Patient's Bill of Rights.

Pay and Chase, or Pay and Pursue—A term commonly used in coordination of benefits that refers to the health plan paying for the claim and then trying to recover all or some of the costs from the other insurance company. The antonym is pursue and pay, or "chase" and pay. See also Chase and Pay and Coordination of Benefits.

Pay for Performance (P4P)—The provision of financial incentives to providers (hospitals and/or physicians) to improve compliance with standards of care and to improve outcomes and patient safety.

Payer or Payor—Generic term applicable to any commercial health insurer or benefits administrator that pays medical claims.

Payment—The term that should be used instead of "reimbursement" when referring to provider payment.

PCCM—See Primary Care Case Manager.

PCMH—See Patient-Centered Medical Home.

PCP—See Primary Care Physician.

PDP—See Prescription Drug Plan.

Peer Review Organization (PRO)—The old name for organizations charged with reviewing quality and cost for Medicare; it has since been replaced by Quality Improvement Organization (QIO).

PEL—See Provider Excess Loss.

Pend or Pended—A term used in claims processing referring to a claim being held while additional information is sought before final adjudication. Some payers use *pend* to refer to claims put on hold by a claims examiner, and *suspend* for claims put on hold by the system. As a practical matter, pend and suspend are nearly the same. See also Suspend.

PEPM—Abbreviation for Per Employee per Month.

Per Diem Payment—Payment of an institution, usually a hospital, based on a set rate per day rather than on charges. Per diem payment can be varied by service (e.g., medical/surgical, obstetrics, mental health, and intensive care) or by day (e.g., first day per diem is higher than remaining days) or can be uniform regardless of the intensity of services.

Per Member per Month (PMPM)—The total revenue, cost, or unit of utilization during a time period, averaged across all enrolled members on a monthly basis. To use a simple example, if an HMO has 100 members and during the course of the year one member has $70,000 in hospital expenses, one has $50,000 in hospital expenses, and one has $45,000 in hospital expenses, the HMO's hospital costs would be $137.50 PMPM [(($70,000 + $50,000 + $45,000) ÷ 12) ÷ 100].

Per Member per Year (PMPY)—The total revenue, cost, or unit of utilization during a time period, averaged across all enrolled members on an annual basis (i.e., do not divide by 12 in the PMPM example).

Per Thousand Members per Year (PTMPY)—A common way of reporting utilization. The most common example is hospital utilization, expressed as days per thousand members per year or simply bed days per thousand (BD/K).

Persistency—The tendency of a commercial group to stay with a payer organization from year to year. A persistency of 90 would mean that 90% of covered groups do not change insurers.

Personal Health Record (PHR)—A record, often created by a health plan, of an individual's health-related data. The sources of those data include claims from providers, prescription drugs the plan paid for, demographic data, and so forth. Clinical data such as results of diagnostic lab tests or imaging may be provided if the plan has access to it, and the member can add other data such as drug allergies or the results of a health risk appraisal. The purpose is to provide at least a usable subset of important health-related information in an electronically portable or transmittable format to improve continuity of care and emergency care.

PFFS—See Private FFS Plan.

PHI—See Protected Health Information.

PHO—See Physician–Hospital Organization.

PHR—See Personal Health Record.

PHSA—See Public Health Service Act.

Physician–Hospital Organization (PHO)—An organization that represents hospitals and the attending medical staff, developed for the purpose of contracting with managed care plans. A PHO may be open to any members of the staff who apply, or it may be closed to staff members who fail to qualify or who are part of an already overrepresented specialty.

Physician Incentive Program (PIP)—A generic term referring to a payment methodology under which a physician's income from a payer (or an integrated delivery system) is affected by the physician's performance or the overall performance of the plan (e.g., utilization, medical cost, quality measurements, member satisfaction). This term has a very specific usage by the CMS, which limits the degree of incentive or risk allowed under a Medicare HMO. CMS essentially bans "gainsharing" via a PIP altogether in an IDS receiving payment under Medicare. Some states also now have laws and regulations regarding limits on PIPs and requirements for disclosure of incentives to members enrolled in payers. See also Significant Financial Risk.

Physician Practice Management Company (PPMC)—An organization that manages physicians' practices, and in most cases either owns the practices outright or has rights to purchase them in the future. PPMCs concentrate only on physicians and not on hospitals, although some have also branched into joint ventures with hospitals and insurers. Most PPMCs in the late 1980s through the 1990s failed, but some still exist, particularly for single specialties. Others morphed into management service organizations.

Physician Quality Reporting System (PQRS)—A program under Medicare in which physicians report data on selected measures of quality and receive an incentive payment.

PIP—See Physician Incentive Program.

Platinum Level of Benefits or Platinum Plan—As defined in the ACA, a qualified health benefits plan with the actuarial equivalent or average of 10% cost sharing, when accounting for deductibles, copayments, and coinsurance as applied to in-network services.

PMPM—See Per Member per Month.

PMPY—See Per Member per Year.

POD—See Pool of Doctors. Alternatively, see *Invasion of the Body Snatchers*, starring Kevin McCarthy and Dana Wynter (1956), that has nothing to do with health care, but does have pod people.

Point of Service (POS)—A benefits plan design that combines features of an HMO with a PPO and/or indemnity plan, known as triple option and dual option, respectively. Members must use the HMO system to obtain the highest level of benefits; out-of-network services are also covered but require more cost sharing.

Pool of Doctors (POD)—A system in which a plan groups physicians into units smaller than the entire panel, but larger than individual practices. Typical PODs have between 10 and 30 physicians. This arrangement is often used for performance measurement and compensation. The POD is typically not a legal entity, but rather a grouping.

Pooling—See Risk Pool.

Portability—The ability of people to obtain coverage as they move from job to job or in and out of employment.

Portal—A single Internet website providing access to multiple other sites and/ or functionalities. For example, payers in a region may jointly offer a single sign-on portal for providers to use for checking a patient's coverage eligibility. The ACA also required DHHS to create a consumer portal for health insurance (found at www.healthcare.gov), and state health insurance exchanges also have consumer portals. Also called an Internet portal.

POS—See Point of Service.

PPACA—See Patient Protection and Affordable Care Act.

PPMC—See Physician Practice Management Company.

PPO—See Preferred Provider Organization.

PPS—See Prospective Payment System.

PQRI—Physician Quality Reporting Initiative; the pilot program replaced by the Physician Quality Reporting System.

PQRS—See Physician Quality Reporting System.

Preauthorization—See Authorization. See also Precertification.

Precertification—The process of obtaining certification or authorization from the health plan for routine hospital admissions or for ambulatory procedures. It often involves an appropriateness review against criteria and assignment of length of stay. Failure to obtain precertification often results in a financial penalty to either the provider or the subscriber. Also known as preadmission certification, preadmission review, and pre-cert.

Preexisting Condition—A medical condition for which a member has received treatment during a specified period of time prior to becoming covered under a health plan. Prior to 2014, preexisting conditions disqualified people from purchasing individual health insurance, but that practice is now prohibited by the ACA.

Preferred Provider Organization (PPO)—A plan that contracts with independent providers at a discount for services. The panel is limited in size and usually has some type of utilization review system associated with it. A PPO may be risk bearing, like an insurance company, or may be non-risk bearing, like a physician-sponsored PPO that markets itself to insurance companies or self-insured companies via an access fee. See also Rental PPO.

Premium—The money paid to a health plan for coverage by the insurer; i.e., the insurer is at risk for medical costs. This term may be applied on an individual basis or a group basis. See also Imputed Premium.

Premium Compression or Premium Rate Compression—The result of a law or regulation placing limits on how much difference is allowable between the highest and lowest premiums. The ACA allows no more than a threefold difference in rates charged to individuals. Premium rate compression is a means of subsidizing the cost of covering less healthy individuals.

Premium-Cost Compression—The reduction in the difference between what a health plan is able to charge in premiums and what it costs to pay for medical benefits. This situation may be a result of regulatory or competitive market forces. It not only reduces the plan's ability to generate a positive underwriting margin, but also reduces the ability to withstand errors or cost overruns.

Premium Equivalent—See Imputed Premium.

Premium Insufficiency—An insurer's failure or inability to charge enough in premiums to cover medical benefits and administrative costs. Out-of-control administrative costs can cause this gap, but it typically occurs when benefits costs rise higher than the level expected when the premium rates were originally calculated. This situation is particularly dangerous because an insurer must live with a premium insufficiency for the entire year that policy is in place, so losses mount each month the policy or policies remain in force.

Premium Tax—A tax levied by a state on health insurance premiums for policies sold in that state. Employers that self-fund their health benefits plan, as well as Medicare Advantage plans, are not subject to state premium taxes. The same term may be used for a tax fee imposed on all types of health benefits plans under the ACA.

Premium Tax Credits—The subsidies provided to low-income individuals to help offset the premium cost of health insurance purchased through a health insurance exchange.

Prepaid or Prepayment—Payment for services before they are incurred. Capitation is a form of prepayment, in that the provider is paid before the month in which services will be provided. HMOs and early Blue Cross plans were once called prepaid health plans because premiums were paid in advance of the HMO or the hospital providing the service. The term "prepayment" can also be applied to the prepayment of any type of insurance premium, although health plans sometimes prefer to call it unearned premium revenue. It never applies to self-funding except when self-funded plans pay capitation to providers.

Prescription Drug Plan (PDP)—A private, free-standing plan that provides drug coverage to Medicare beneficiaries under MA. It does not provide coverage for other services.

Preventive Care—Health care that is aimed at preventing complications of existing diseases or preventing the occurrence of a disease.

Primary Care Case Manager (PCCM)—A term used in Medicaid managed care programs. It refers to the state designating primary care physicians to be case managers who function as "gatekeepers," but paying those PCPs using traditional Medicaid fee-for-service plus an ongoing nominal management fee such as $5 or $10 PMPM.

Primary Care Physician (PCP)—Generally, an internist, pediatrician, family physician, or (rarely) a general practitioner, and occasionally an obstetrician/gynecologist.

Private Fee-for-Service Plan (PFFS)—A type of Medicare Advantage plan in which a private insurance company accepts risk for enrolled beneficiaries, but pays providers on a FFS basis that does not have any risk component to the provider. PFFS plans originally did not use networks, but are now required to have them. Because of new network requirements and reductions in payment from CMS, PFFS plans have sharply declined in numbers.

Private Health Insurance Exchange—An insurance exchange run by an insurer or a benefits management consulting firm that may be used by employers to offer different options to their employees, or by insurers to offer options to employer groups. It is not the same as a health insurance exchange under the ACA.

Private Inurement—What happens when a nonprofit business operates in such a way as to provide more than incidental financial gain to a private individual; for example, if a not-for-profit hospital pays too much money for a physician's practice, or fails to charge fair market rates for services provided to a physician. This practice is prohibited by the Internal Revenue Service.

PRO—See Peer Review Organization.

Producer—In health insurance and managed care, a broker or agent who sells a plan's policies to businesses and individuals.

Professional Services Agreement (PSA)—A contract between a physician or medical group and an integrated delivery system or payer for the provision of medical services.

Profiling—Measurement of a provider's performance on selected measures, with that performance then being compared to the performance of similar providers. Profiling is usually applied to physicians. It may be used for purposes of network selection or tiering, feedback reports, and/or P4P programs, but is very complicated to perform properly.

Programs for All-Inclusive Care for the Elderly (PACE)—A federally funded program to facilitate community resources to help seniors who are state certified as needing nursing home care, but who can live safely in their communities with assistance.

Prospective Payment System (PPS)—Medicare's terminology for determining fixed pricing for payment of hospitals and facilities for care. The most well-known examples of PPS are DRGs, MS-DRGs, and APCs. Prospective payment may be used by commercial plans, as it applies to payment of facilities using the same methodologies.

Prospective Review—A review intended to determine whether a medical service will be covered before the care is rendered. See also Precertification.

Protected Health Information (PHI)—That information that reveals medical information or data about an individual. PHI is addressed specifically by HIPAA in the Privacy and Security sections.

Provider—The generic term used to refer to anyone providing medical services. In fact, it may even be used to refer to any*thing* that provides medical services, such as a hospital. Most often, however, this term is used to refer to physicians.

Provider Excess Loss (PEL)—A stop-loss or reinsurance insurance policy purchased by risk-bearing provider organizations, full-risk-bearing medical groups, or integrated delivery systems in an effort to limit their exposure to catastrophic claims costs.

Provider-Sponsored Organization (PSO)—An archaic term referring to an entity allowed under the BBA '97. A PSO was a risk-bearing managed care organization owned and operated by providers that contracted directly with CMS (HCFA at the time) to cover Medicare enrollees. PSOs were the result of a belief by providers and legislators that there were fat profits to be had through "cutting out the middleman"—that is, by removing the HMO from the equation. With a few small exceptions, PSOs failed utterly and lost considerable amounts of money. The federal waiver authority for PSOs expired quietly in 2002. CMS recycled the PSO acronym and it now stands for "patient safety organization."

Prudent (or Reasonable) Layperson Standard—According to the ACA, "a medical condition manifested by acute symptoms of sufficient severity (including severe pain) such that a prudent layperson, who possesses an average knowledge of health and medicine," could reasonably expect "to result in: a) placing the patient's health in serious jeopardy; b) serious impairment to bodily functions; or c) serious dysfunction of any bodily organ or part." The ACA requires health plans to provide unrestricted in-network benefits regardless of whether the provider is in- or out-of-network under this definition of an emergency.

PSA—See Professional Services Agreement.

PSO—See Patient Safety Organization (first definition) or Provider-Sponsored Organization (second and older definition).

PTMPY—See Per Thousand Members per Year.

Public Health Service Act of 1944 (PHSA)—A federal law that established the role of the federal government in preventing transmittable diseases. It has been amended constantly since then, and many other laws derive their authority from the PHSA—for example, considerable portions of HIPAA, the ACA, and numerous medically related laws.

Pursue and Pay—See Pay and Pursue.

QA or QM—Quality assurance or quality management.

QBP—See Quality Bonus Program.

QHP—See Qualified Health Plan.

QIO—See Quality Improvement Organization.

QIP—See Quality Improvement Program.

QISMC—See Quality Improvement System for Managed Care.

Qualified Health Plan (QHP)—As defined in the ACA, a health plan that is certified by a state health insurance exchange, provides the ACA-defined essential health benefits and cost-sharing limitations, is licensed by the state, and offers at least one Gold-level and one Silver-level benefits plan through the exchange. See also Essential Health Benefits and Health Insurance Exchange.

Quality Bonus Program (QBP)—The star-rating bonus program for MA plans. It covers multiple measures in five broad areas: (1) wellness and prevention, including screenings, tests, and vaccines; (2) managing chronic conditions; (3) member experience and satisfaction; (4) member complaints and plan performance changes; and (5) customer service.

Quality Improvement Expenses—Under the ACA, health plan costs associated with improving quality may be considered as a medical cost instead of an administrative cost, for purposes of calculating the MLR.

Quality Improvement Organization (QIO)—An organization under contract to CMS to conduct quality reviews of providers, respond to beneficiary complaints about care, measure and report performance of providers, ensure that payment is made only for medically necessary services, and carry out other functions. Its work applies to all types of plans and services, not just managed care.

Quality Improvement Program (QIP)—The quality improvement program put in place by CMS for Medicare Advantage plans of all types. The QIP uses data from HEDIS, HOS, and CAHPS, as well as financial and member disenrollment data. Accreditation by NCQA is also considered under the QIP.

Quality Improvement System for Managed Care (QISMC)—A now-discontinued CMS program focusing on quality of care and member satisfaction for Medicare risk plans. It was replaced by the Quality Improvement Program.

Qui Tam Sui—A provision in tort law that allows a citizen to file suit on behalf of the (federal) government, and to collect one-third of the proceeds of that lawsuit. Such suits are usually also subject to treble damages, making success a lucrative endeavor.

RAC—See Medicare Recovery Audit Contractors.

RAP—Radiology, Anesthesia, Pathology. Three common types of hospital-based physicians that often have near-monopoly control over their specialties within a hospital, and that patients/members have little ability to choose from.

Rate Band—Premium rates charged to all individuals within a specific age group, such as all individuals between the ages of 41 and 50. Rate banding was designed to provide low rates to the young and healthy, thereby enticing these individuals to buy coverage, and then progressively rise consistent with higher costs incurred by older people. The ACA does not prohibit rate banding, but restricts the rate spread to a maximum of 3:1.

Rate Spread—The difference between the highest and lowest premium rates within a risk pool—for example, all individual subscribers or small employer groups. The ACA prohibits a rate spread greater than 3:1, and even then the difference may be based only on age.

Rating—The process by which the health plan develops its premium rates.

RBC—See Risk-Based Capital.

RBRVS—See Resource-Based Relative Value Scale.

Rebate—In general usage, the return of some money to a purchaser. Under the ACA, a system in which a health insurer must return to consumers or employers the difference in its actual medical costs and the medical loss ratio (MLR). For large employer groups, the minimum MLR is 85%, and for individuals and small employer groups it is 80%. Another common use applies to pharmaceutical manufacturers rebating some part of the purchase price to PBMs, plans, employers, or government based on volume.

Rebundlers—Software programs that roll up and reprice fragmented bills as well as apply industry-standard claims adjudication conventions.

Reference Pricing—A pricing scheme in which benefits coverage is based on the lowest available market price, not necessarily what was charged. Such pricing is usually applied to biologics and other pharmaceuticals, as well as devices, but is sometimes used for facility services.

Regional Health Information Organization (RHIO)—A nongovernmental entity that facilitates the flow of electronic health information between different organizations such as physicians, hospitals, and payers. At the time of publication and for more than 20 years, most RHIOs' operations consisted primarily of committee meetings. See also Health Information Exchanges.

Reimbursement—A term commonly but incorrectly used to refer to payment of healthcare providers. Reimbursement is more applicable to something like an employer covering an employee's out-of-pocket travel costs. The relationship of what it actually costs to provide care and how much a provider is paid is approximate at best, and payers (e.g., Medicare, Medicaid, HMOs, and PPOs) do not all pay the same amount for the same provider billing code. The more accurate term in health care, therefore, is payment, not reimbursement.

Reinstatement—The situation in which an insurance or managed care policy is restored after payment for delinquent premiums during a defined grace period. See also Grace Period.

Reinsurance—Insurance purchased by a health plan, self-funded employer group, or at-risk provider system to protect it against extremely high-cost cases. See also Stop Loss.

Relative Value Units (RVUs)—Numeric values used as multipliers to calculate the payment to a provider. RVUs may be used for time units such as for anesthesia, but their most common use is as part of the Resource-Based Relative Value Scale.

Relative Value Scale Update Committee (RUC)—A committee of the American Medical Association that reviews the weights placed on the relative value units in the Medicare RBRVS every 5 years. CMS usually uses its recommendations to adjust payment rates.

Rental PPO—A PPO network owned and managed by a third party that rents access to the network (and often services such as claims repricing) to a payer or health insurance company. It is not the same as a risk-bearing PPO that combines a network with the insurance function.

Rescission—The retroactive rejection of an issued insurance policy "for cause." The ACA places severe restrictions on rescissions, limiting it mostly to instances of fraud.

Reserves—The amount of money that a health plan puts aside to cover healthcare benefits costs. It may apply to anticipated costs such as IBNRs, or it may apply to money that the plan does not expect to have to use to pay for current medical claims, but keeps as a cushion against future adverse healthcare costs. Reserves can include only admitted assets under Statutory Accounting Principles (SAP), not Generally Accepted Accounting Principles (GAAP). See also Admitted Assets, Nonadmitted Assets, and Risk-Based Capital.

Resource-Based Relative Value Scale (RBRVS)—A relative value scale developed for the CMS for use by Medicare. The RBRVS assigns relative value units (RVUs) to each CPT code based on the level of skill and complexity required for that procedure, including office visits. Smaller RVUs are also assigned based on costs associated with the setting in which the care was provided, and for the cost of malpractice insurance. The RVUs are then added together and multiplied by a dollar-amount conversion factor to calculate the actual payment. Commercial versions exist as well to cover procedures not typically used by Medicare.

Retail Clinic—A type of urgent care clinic, usually located in a drug store or grocery store, that is often staffed by nonphysician primary care providers who provide care for routine illnesses (e.g., sore throat), but are limited in what they can do. Such care is often less expensive than a physician office visit, and it reduces primary care providers' income. Also called a convenient care clinic (CCC).

Retention—(1) That portion of a health insurance premium that goes toward administrative costs and reserves, not medical claims costs (most common use). (2) Persistency (less common use).

Retrospective Review—A review of healthcare costs or utilization after the care has been rendered. Several forms of retrospective review are possible. One form looks at individual claims for medical necessity, billing errors, or fraud. The other form looks at patterns of costs and utilization rather than individual cases.

RHIO—See Regional Health Information Organization.

Rider—An add-on to the core insurance or HMO policy—for example, coverage for vision services.

Risk Adjustment—A methodology to account for the health status of patients when predicting or explaining costs of health care for defined populations or for evaluating retrospectively the performance of providers who care for them. Risk adjustment is also used by CMS in the payment of MA plans. Also known as severity adjustment and acuity adjustment. Case mix is a related term.

Risk-Based Capital (RBC)—A formula embodied in the Risk-Based Capital for Health Organizations Model Act, created under the auspices of the NAIC. RBC takes into account the fluctuating value of plan assets; the financial condition of plan affiliates; the risk that providers may not be able to provide contracted services; the risk that amounts due may not be recovered from reinsurance carriers; and general business risks (i.e., expenses may exceed income). The RBC formula gives credit for provider payment arrangements that reduce underwriting risk, including capitation as well as provider withholds, bonuses, contracted fee schedules, and aggregate cost arrangements. While not required in all states, RBC is the primary agreed-upon standard for an insurance department to determine whether a health plan meets the minimum financial solvency requirements.

Risk Contract—A contract between a health plan and the CMS under Medicare Advantage under which the health plan is at risk for the cost of medical services to voluntary Medicare beneficiaries, and receives a monthly payment in return. Also known as a Medicare risk contract.

Risk Corridor—The upper and lower limits of financial risk for a health plan or provider that is at risk for medical costs. Both limits must exist for the arrangement to be considered a risk corridor. A risk corridor of 20%, for example, would mean that the plan or provider can have financial losses or gains of no more than 10% of the baseline payment.

Risk Management—(1) As applied to the management of a health plan's operations, steps taken to reduce the risk of litigation or regulatory sanctions—for example, working with a member who has experienced a negative event in which the health plan may have had a role. (2) Steps taken to manage the overall risk of healthcare costs (i.e., managing the insurance risk). (3) Obtaining various forms of liability insurance (unrelated to medical claims costs) for financial protection in case of a lawsuit. (4) Reducing medical errors (provider only).

Risk Pool (Capitation)—In the context of capitation, a pool of funds that may be drawn against to cover medical costs, with any unused funds being paid to a provider or providers under capitation. See also Rule of Small Numbers.

Risk Pool (Premiums)—In the context of premiums, a group of individuals (e.g., all individual subscribers, employees in a group, or Medicare enrollees) who all put in the same amount of money, thereby spreading out the risk even though some are healthier and some are sicker. Also called pooling. Risk pools for premiums are addressed specifically in the ACA.

RUC—See Relative Value Scale Update Committee.

Rule of Small Numbers—The notion that predictions that are based on large numbers are usually reasonably accurate, but as the numbers get smaller, chance plays a far more important role until eventually chance completely outweighs predictability.

RVU—See Relative Value Unit.

Safe Harbor—The circumstances under which a hospital or other healthcare entity can provide something to a physician or other health entity and not violate the anti-kickback portion of the Stark laws and regulations. See also Ethics in Patient Referrals Act.

SBC—See Summary of Benefits Coverage.

Schedule of Benefits—The listing in the evidence of coverage document of what is and what is not covered by a health plan, and under which circumstances.

SCHIP—See State Children's Health Insurance Program.

SCP—See Specialty Care Physician.

Second Opinion—An opinion obtained from another physician regarding the necessity for a treatment that has been recommended by another physician. It may be required by some health plans for certain high-cost procedures. Once commonly used, requirements for second opinions are now rare.

Section 125 Plan—A plan that allows employees to receive specified benefits, including health benefits, on a pretax basis. Section 125 plans enable employees to pay for health insurance premiums on a pretax basis, whether the insurance is provided by the employer or purchased directly in the individual market. See also Flexible Benefits Plan.

Section 1115 Waiver—See Medicaid Waiver.

Self-Care—The series of steps that "lay" individuals take to assess and treat an illness or injury, typically without the benefit of higher levels of training in the theory or science of medicine and with little or no consultation with a medical professional.

Self-Insured or Self-Funded Plan—A health plan where the risk for medical cost is assumed by the employer rather than an insurance company or managed care plan. Self-funding makes up the majority of employer-sponsored coverage. Under ERISA, self-funded plans are exempt from most state laws and regulations such as premium taxes and mandatory benefits. State and municipal employee benefits plans are also often self-funded, though under state laws, not ERISA. Self-funded plans are also exempt from some, but not all, of the requirements created under the ACA. Self-funded plans typically contract with insurance companies or third-party administrators to administer the benefits. See also Administrative Services Only.

Self-Referral—The practice in which a physician refers a patient for a costly service or procedure that uses a facility or equipment in which the physician has a financial interest, thereby profiting by increasing its utilization above levels seen when a physician has no financial interest. In the earliest days of HMOs, self-referral meant a member's consultation of a specialist without getting a PCP authorization, but that use of the term is now archaic.

Sentinel Effect—The phenomenon that when it is known that behavior is being observed, that behavior changes, often in the direction the observer is looking for. For example, utilization management systems and profiling systems often lead to reductions in utilization before much intervention even takes place, simply because the providers know that someone is watching.

Serious Reportable Events (SREs)—Also called Never Events, medical errors that occur in a facility (hospital or ambulatory surgical center) that should never happen. An example of a "never event" is amputation of the wrong limb. Maintained by the National Quality Forum, definitions of serious reportable events are grouped into seven categories: surgical, product or device, patient protection, care management, environmental, radiologic, and criminal. Medicare as well as most payers will not pay for care required as a result of a "never event."

Service Area—The geographic area in which managed care plans provides access to medical care through contracted providers. The service area is usually specifically designated by the regulators (state or federal), and the HMO is prohibited from marketing outside the service area. It may be defined by county or by ZIP code. An HMO might potentially have more than one service area, and the service areas might be either contiguous (i.e., they border each other) or noncontiguous (i.e., there is a geographic gap between them). Also referred to as Network Adequacy. Service area is also a term used by Blue Cross and Blue Shield plans to apply to the geographic locations in which they may market and sell using the BCBS marks and signs.

Service Bureau—(1) A weak form of integrated delivery system in which a hospital or other organization provides services to a physician's practice in return for a fair market price; it may also try to negotiate with managed care plans, but is generally not considered to be an effective negotiating mechanism. (2) An older term used for a service plan.

Service-Level Agreement (SLA)—The part of a contract specifying performance standards such as average speed to answer telephone calls or percentage of claims processed within 14 days. An SLA is often part of an administrative services-only contract between a large self-funded employer group and a payer. It is also commonly found in a contract between a payer and a company providing outsourced services.

Service-Level Percentage—A measurement in a call center of the specific percentage of calls to be answered within a given timeliness goal.

Service Plan—A prepaid health plan made up of contracting providers, but that is not necessarily a managed care plan. The archetypal service plans are traditional (i.e., nonmanaged care) Blue Cross and Blue Shield plans, although a few non-Blue service plans do exist. The contract applies to direct billing of the plan by providers (rather than billing of the member), a provision for direct payment of the provider (rather than reimbursement of the member), a requirement that the provider accept the plan's determination of usual, customary, or reasonable charges and not balance bill the member in excess of that amount, and a range of other terms. A service plan is virtually indistinguishable from a health insurer.

SFR—See Significant Financial Risk.

Shadow Pricing—The practice of setting premium rates at a level just below the competition's rates, whether or not those rates can be justified. This practice is generally considered unethical and, in the case of community rating, possibly illegal.

Shared Savings—See Medicare Shared Savings Program.

SHMO—See Social Health Maintenance Organization.

Shock Claim—A very costly episode of care for an individual member; also referred to as a catastrophic claim or "cat claim" for short. Shock claims are taken into account by actuaries to varying degrees when they determine the trends for medical costs because shock claims, while costly, are infrequent and have a certain amount of randomness to them.

Shoe Box Effect—A practice in which beneficiaries save up their receipts of self-paid claims to file for reimbursement at a later time (e.g., by saving those receipts in a shoe box). Those receipts are sometimes lost, or the beneficiary never sends them in, in which case the insurance company does not have to reimburse the member.

SHOP—See Small Business Health Options Program.

Significant Financial Risk (SFR)—A term used by the CMS that refers to the total amount of a physician's income at risk in a Medicare HMO. Such financial risk is considered "significant" when it exceeds a certain percentage of the total potential income that physician could receive under the payment program. SFR most commonly is defined as any physician incentive payment program that allows for a variation of more than 25% between the minimum amount and the maximum amount of potential payment.

Silent PPO—A form of rental PPO that a payer did not clearly identify by having the PPO's name or logo on the member's ID card. A provider without a contract with the payer would bill for full charges, but the rental PPO's payment terms would be applied to pay the claim, resulting in unanticipated reductions in the provider's booked revenue. This practice, which is now rarely used, is considered either unethical or illegal, and payers that use rental networks typically now include that PPO's logo somewhere on the ID card. See also Rental PPO.

Silver Level of Benefits or Silver Plan—As defined in the ACA, a qualified health benefits plan with the actuarial equivalent or average of 30% cost sharing, when accounting for deductibles, copayments, and coinsurance as applied to in-network services.

Single-Payer System—A healthcare system in which the government, or an intermediary functioning on behalf of the government, pays for all healthcare services. It is financed through taxes and/or healthcare premiums collected by the government or intermediary. It is usually combined with some type of socialized health insurance. Unless the government owns the facilities and/or employs providers directly, the providers and the government negotiate payment rates that are then used by all. Canada uses a single-payer system. See also the related but differing terms All Payer, Social Insurance, and Socialized Medicine.

Single-Specialty Hospital—A hospital that provides services focusing on a single specialty such as cardiac procedures or orthopedics. Physicians often have an equity interest in them.

Skill-Based Routing—See Intelligent Call Routing.

SLA—See Service-Level Agreement.

Slice Business—A large employer group that offers more than one insurer and/or HMO to its employees.

Small Business Health Options Program (SHOP)—That part of a state health insurance exchange that provides access to health insurance for small businesses as defined in the ACA.

SNP—See Special Needs Plan.

SOC—See Summary of Benefits Coverage.

Social Health Maintenance Organization (SHMO)—A type of demonstration Medicare HMO that went beyond the medical care needs of its membership, to include their social and custodial needs as well. Authorized as demonstration projects under Medicare, SHMOs were always rare and Congress ended the Medicare demonstration project in 2008; though at the time of publication, four legacy SHMOs remain. See also Programs for All-Inclusive Care for the Elderly (PACE).

Social Insurance—A form of national financing in which the government provides benefits to all for such things as health care, disability, old age or retirement, long-term care, unemployment, and so forth. It is funded through mandatory taxes on all citizens and residents. An example in the United States is Social Security.

Social Security Administration (SSA)—The federal agency that manages eligibility and enrollment for both Social Security and Medicare benefits.

Socialized Medicine—A type of social insurance in which the government not only pays for health care as a single payer system, but also owns and operates, or has control over the budgets of, significant portions of the healthcare provider system—for example, owning and operating the hospitals, controlling regional funding of all healthcare services, and paying the physicians as a single payer. See also Single Payer and Social Insurance.

Solvency—Having sufficient assets to be eligible to transact insurance business and meet liabilities. For insurers and HMOs, solvency is based on statutory net worth. See also Statutory Net Worth.

Special Enrollment Period—A defined period of time following a life event during which an individual is eligible to apply for coverage or to change coverage outside of an established open enrollment period.

Special Limitations Clause—See Laser or Lasering.

Special Needs Plan (SNP)—A type of MA plan that may exclusively enroll, or enroll a disproportionate percentage of, Medicare beneficiaries with special needs. Individuals with special needs include beneficiaries entitled to both

Medicare and Medicaid ("dual eligibles"), institutionalized beneficiaries, and individuals with severe or disabling chronic conditions.

Special Qualifying Period—See Special Enrollment Period.

Specialty Care Physician (SCP)—A physician who is not a primary care physician (i.e., a specialist). Occasionally referred to by the acronym "SCP," but that acronym is not used nearly as often as is "PCP."

Specialty Network Manager—A single specialist or a specialist organization that accepts capitation to manage a single specialty. Specialty services typically are supplied by many different specialty physicians, but the network manager has the responsibility for managing access and cost, and is at economic risk. This is a relatively uncommon model.

Specialty Pharmacy—Very specialized and very costly drugs that include biopharmaceuticals, meaning injectable drugs created through recombinant DNA; drugs for rare conditions; drugs that require special handling or monitoring; drugs that are available only through limited supply channels; and/or any drug that exceeds some cost threshold such as $500 or $1000 per month to use. See also Compounding Pharmacy.

Specialty Pharmacy Benefits Manager (SPBM)—A pharmacy benefits manager that focuses on managing specialty pharmacy benefits. It may be part of a pharmacy benefits manager or a separate company.

Specialty Pharmacy Distributor (SPD)—A company that distributes specialty pharmacy products from the manufacturer to the provider and/or directly to the patient, so as to address the unique distribution, storage, and utilization issues around these types of injectable drugs. It may be part of a pharmacy benefits manager or a separate company.

SREs—Serious reportable events. See also Never Events.

SSA—See Social Security Administration.

Staff Model HMO—A closed-panel HMO that employs providers directly, and those providers see members in the HMO's own facilities.

Stark Laws or Stark Regulations—See Ethics in Patient Referrals Act.

Stars Program—An unofficial name for the Quality Bonus Program (QBP) for MA plans. See also Quality Bonus Program.

State Children's Health Insurance Program (SCHIP or CHIP)—A program created by the federal government to provide a "safety net" and preventive-care level of health coverage for children, funded through a combination of federal and state funds, and administered by the states in conformance with federal requirements.

State Insurance Exchanges—A means for individuals and small employer groups to access coverage from qualified health plans as provided for in the ACA. States are to create and operate exchanges, but in those states that either could not or would not create and operate their own exchange, the federal government then does it on behalf of the state.

State Licensure—The insurance license, or the certificate of authority (COA) issued by a state to a health plan that allows an insurer or HMO to write business in the state. It may be based on having a license in a different state. See also State of Domicile.

State of Domicile—The state in which an insurance company or HMO is licensed as its primary location. For example, a payer may have its state of domicile in Virginia, but also be licensed and doing business in Maryland and the District of Columbia. In many states, the insurance commissioner will defer primary regulation to the insurance department in the state of domicile as long as all of the minimum state standards are met.

Statutory Net Worth, Statutory Surplus, or Statutory Reserves—The total net worth of an insurer or HMO as defined under Statutory Accounting Principles (SAP) rules. For purposes of health insurance and managed care, net worth is what a health plan has in cash or in assets that can immediately be converted into cash in the event of plan failure. States have net worth minimum requirements for licensed health plans that vary with the size of the potential liability. States define the minimum statutory net worth that an insurer or HMO must have before it is considered to be financially impaired. See also Nonadmitted Asset and Risk-Based Capital.

Stop Loss—A form of reinsurance that provides protection for medical expenses above a certain limit, generally on a year-by-year basis, and may be specific and/or aggregate. Specific coverage applies to individual cases, while aggregate coverage applies to the total costs rather than a specific case. HMOs may also provide a form of stop loss protection to capitated providers, but it is not an actual insurance policy. See also Capitation and Reinsurance.

Subordinated Note—Essentially an irrevocable promise from a qualified lender such as a bank that a health plan can borrow money up to the limit of the note if necessary to pay claims, with the holder of the note being repaid only after all claims costs are settled; in other words, repayment of the lender is subordinate to payment of claims. This subordination allows the plan to claim the note for purposes of net worth since it is immediately convertible to cash. A note or loan for which the plan must pay the note holder regardless of the plan's inability to pay claims is not subordinated and cannot be counted as part of its net worth.

Subrogation—The contractual right of a health plan to recover payments made to a member for healthcare costs after that member has received such payment for damages in a legal action. Subrogation is illegal in some states but is required in others.

Subscriber—The individual or member who has the health plan coverage by virtue of being eligible on his or her own behalf, rather than as a dependent. See also Member.

Summary of Benefits Coverage (SBC or SOC)—A brief and easily understandable standardized four- to six-page document summarizing benefits, requirements, and rights. Under the ACA, payers are required to provide the SBC before enrollment, each time a policy is renewed, and whenever there is a substantial change in the policy.

Surplus—The amount of money that an insurer or HMO has that is not earmarked for claims payment. A surplus may be used to boost reserves, to keep rate increases down, or to invest in operational improvements. In nonprofit plans, it equates to the profit margin in a for-profit plan, but it may not be distributed like profits or dividends to shareholders or executives.

Suspend—What happens when a claim is being processed but cannot be completed due to missing or inconsistent information; it is suspended until manual intervention allows it to be completed. Claims suspensions may also be called edits or pends. As a practical matter, the terms "pend" and "suspend" are often used synonymously, but some payers differentiate between claims that examiners place on hold (pends) and those that are placed on hold automatically by one or more systems edits (suspends).

Sutton's Law—"Go where the money is!"—the reply attributed to the Depression-era bank robber Willy Sutton, when asked why he robbed banks (it is not clear that he actually said it, but he did agree with it). It is a good law to use when determining what needs attention in a health plan, or any aspect of any business for that matter.

Switch—The computer that handles the telephone calling system; a charming holdover from the days when calls were routed by using a mechanical switchboard.

Taft-Hartley Plan—A type of association health plan under ERISA that is provided by a union to its members, typically using funds contributed by more than one employer or company. It is also eligible to be a type of MA plan. Also called a Taft-Hartley Trust.

TANF—See Temporary Assistance to Needy Families.

TAT—See Turnaround Time.

Tax Equity and Fiscal Responsibility Act of 1982 (TEFRA)—A federal law that prohibits employers and health plans from requiring full-time employees between the ages of 65 and 69 to use Medicare rather than the group health plan. TEFRA also first enabled federally qualified HMOs to offer plans to Medicare beneficiaries if they met certain other requirements as well.

TCM—See Transitional Case Management.

TEFRA—See Tax Equity and Fiscal Responsibility Act of 1982.

Temporary Assistance to Needy Families (TANF)—A government program that provides assistance and work opportunities to needy families by granting states the federal funds and wide flexibility to develop and implement their own welfare programs. Medicaid coverage is typically one component of the TANF program.

Third-Party Administrator (TPA)—A firm that performs administrative functions such as claims processing, membership, and the like for a self-funded plan or a start-up managed care plan. By convention, it is used for free-standing administrators, not for insurers that also provide administrative services to self-funded accounts. See also Administrative Services Only.

Tiering—Categorizing coverage into different tiers, or benefits levels. In pharmacy tiering, for example, Tier 1 drugs require lower copayments than to Tier 2 drugs, Tier 3 drugs, and so forth. When it is applied to providers, members accessing Tier 1 providers have less (or even no) cost sharing than if they use a Tier 2 provider.

Time Loss Management—The application of managed care techniques to worker's compensation treatments for injuries or illnesses so as to reduce the amount of time lost on the job by the affected employee.

TJC—See The Joint Commission.

Total Capitation—See Global Capitation.

TPA—See Third-Party Administrator.

Transitional Case Management (TCM)—A program to facilitate the discharge of a patient with complex medical problems or who is otherwise at risk for post-discharge complications and/or an avoidable readmission. TCM programs function much like traditional case management, but focus on the immediate post-discharge period. Also called transitional care management. See also Avoidable Readmission.

Transparency—The practice of making data available to the public. Also called pricing transparency when such data consist of the prices for services from different providers of care.

Treaty—A reinsurance agreement between the reinsured company and the reinsurer, usually for one year or longer, which stipulates the technical particulars applicable to the reinsurance of some class or classes of business. Used in place of the term "policy" because not all reinsurance is actually issued by insurance companies.

Triage—In health plans, the process of sorting out requests for services by members into those who need to be seen right away, those who can wait a little while, and those whose problems can be handled with advice over the phone. The origins of this term are grim: The process of sorting out wounded soldiers into those who need treatment immediately, those who can wait, and those who are so severely injured they cannot be saved and are given pain relief only.

TRICARE—The U.S. Department of Defense's worldwide managed healthcare program. TRICARE was initiated in 1995, integrating healthcare services provided in the direct care system of military hospitals and clinics with services purchased from civilian providers for anyone eligible for coverage (e.g., retirees and dependents). There are a variety of TRICARE benefits programs. The nonmilitary treatment facility portion of TRICARE is administered by private managed care companies in three regions in the United States. See also Military Health System.

Triple Option—Most common meaning is a POS plan that combines an HMO, a PPO, and indemnity coverage to provide three coverage options to members whenever they seek services. Using the HMO system has little cost-sharing, using the PPO system has a cost-sharing amount typical for PPOs in general, and using providers that do not contract with the plan in any way incurs the most cost-sharing.

TrOOP—See True-Out-of-Pocket Cost.

True-Out-of-Pocket Cost (TrOOP)—The full amount of out-of-pocket costs paid by an individual before any annual limits on out-of-pocket costs apply. This term is used for MA plans in applicable regulations, and it may be used for commercial plans.

Turnaround Time (TAT)—The amount of time it takes a health plan to process and pay a claim from the time it arrives.

UB-04—See Universal Billing Form 04.

UB-92—No longer in use. See also CMS-1450 and Universal Billing Form 04.

UCR—See Usual, Customary, or Reasonable.

UM—See Utilization Management.

Unbundling—The practice of a provider billing for multiple components of service that were previously included in a single fee. For example, if dressings and instruments were included in a fee for a minor procedure, the fee for the procedure remains the same, but there are now additional charges for the dressings and instruments.

Uncompensated Care—Healthcare services that are not paid for by the patient or by insurance. These uncompensated costs are partly shifted into higher prices charged to private insurers, absorbed in part by healthcare providers, and are factored in to Medicare and Medicaid payments called Disproportionate Share Hospital (DHS) payments. Under the ACA, DHS payments have been reduced for most hospitals. See also Disproportionate Share.

Underwriting—(1) Bearing the risk for something (i.e., a policy is underwritten by an insurance company). (2) The analysis of a group that is done to determine rates and benefits, or to determine whether the group should be offered coverage at all. (3) The practice of conducting health screening of each individual applicant for insurance and then refusing to provide coverage for people with preexisting conditions, which is now prohibited under the ACA.

Underwriting Margin—The amount of money left over, or lost, after medical costs are subtracted from premium income. It does not include the cost of operations such as administrative costs and sales and marketing expenditures, which make up the operating margin. See also Operating Margin.

Universal Billing Form 04 (UB-04)—The paper form that institutions must use if they submit a paper claim to Medicare. Its use is also required by commercial payers for paper claims. The UB-04 form replaced the paper UB-92 form from prior years. The more commonly used (and interchangeable) name for this form is CMS-1450.

Universal Provider Identification Number (UPIN)—An identification number once issued by CMS for use in billing Medicare. The UPIN was replaced by the national provider identifier in 2007 and is no longer in use. See also National Provider Identifier.

Upcoding—The practice of a provider billing for a procedure that pays better than the service actually performed. For example, an office visit for which the maximum allowable charge is $45 may be coded as a complex visit that is paid at $75.

UPIN—See Universal Provider Identification Number.

UR—See Utilization Review.

URAC—A not-for-profit organization that performs reviews on external utilization review agencies (free-standing companies, utilization management departments of insurance companies, or utilization management departments of managed care plans). Its primary focus is payers, although it has expanded its accreditation activities by, for example, accrediting health-related websites. States often require certification by URAC or another accreditation organization to operate. URAC once stood for Utilization Review Accreditation Commission, and the organization was also once known as the American Accreditation HealthCare Commission (AAHC); neither of those names is used today.

URO—See Utilization Review Organization.

Usual, Customary, or Reasonable (UCR)—A statistically based method of profiling prevailing fees in an area and paying providers on the basis of that profile. One archaic method is to average all fees and choose the 80th or 90th percentile. Payers typically use another method to determine what is reasonable. Sometimes this term is used synonymously with "fee allowance schedule" when that schedule is set relatively high.

Utilization Management (UM)—The combined activities of a payer or integrated delivery system to reduce the amount of unnecessary utilization and by manage the cost of utilization. It encompasses the three types of utilization review: prospective review, concurrent review, and retrospective review. It also includes other activities such as case management.

Utilization Review (UR)—An older term for utilization management, and somewhat less encompassing of all UM activities. It is still frequently used to refer to precertification of hospital cases alone. See also Utilization Management.

Utilization Review Organization (URO)—A free-standing organization that performs utilization review for self-funded plans, usually on a remote basis, using the telephone and paper correspondence. It may be independent, or it may be part of another company such as an insurance company that sells UR services on a stand-alone basis.

Value-Based Insurance Benefits Design (VBID, VBBD, or VBD)—A benefits design that allows for improved coverage under certain conditions. For example, a member with congestive heart failure would be able to obtain certain drugs without having to pay a copayment or coinsurance. Unlike a benefits waiver program, the value-based benefits design is applied to all members of the group who meet certain criteria and who are covered by the plan, not on a case-by-case basis.

Value-Based Payment (VBP)—Modifications of payments to hospitals by CMS based on several factors such as efficiency, consumer satisfaction, and other metrics. VBP is required under the ACA.

VBID, VBD or VBBD—See Value-Based Insurance Benefits Design.

Waiting Period—The amount of time a new employee must wait before being eligible for coverage under an employer group plan. The ACA limits the waiting period to no more than 90 days.

Waste, Fraud, and Abuse—See Fraud, Waste, and Abuse.

Workgroup for Electronic Data Interchange (WEDI)—A group that provides input on electronic transaction standards under HIPAA.

Worker's Compensation—A form of social insurance provided through property-casualty insurers. It provides for medical benefits and replacement of lost wages that result from injuries or illnesses that arise from the workplace; in turn, the employee cannot sue the employer unless true negligence exists. It is not considered to be health insurance. Worker's compensation has undergone dramatic increases in cost, resulting in carriers adopting managed care approaches. It is often heavily regulated under state laws that are significantly different than those used for group health insurance. See also Time Loss Management.

Wraparound Plan—Insurance or health plan coverage for copayments and deductibles that are not covered under a member's base plan. MediGap is a form of wraparound. Such options exist for commercial plans as well.

Zero Down—The practice of a medical group or provider system distributing the entire capital surplus in a health plan (except for the surplus required for statutory reserves) or the group to the members of the group, rather than retaining any capital or reinvesting it in the group or plan.

Index

Note: Page numbers followed by *e, f, n,* or *t* indicate material in exhibits, figures, footnotes, or tables, respectively.